THE **WHOLE30**®

FOR ATTICUS STONE
You are the whole world.

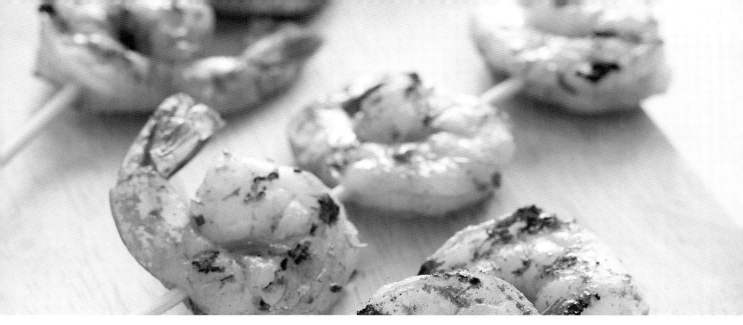

THE WHOLE30®

the 30-day guide
to total health
and food freedom

MELISSA HARTWIG AND DALLAS HARTWIG

with Chef Richard Bradford
Photography by Alexandra Grablewski

HOUGHTON MIFFLIN HARCOURT
Boston New York

Copyright © 2015 by Melissa Hartwig and Dallas Hartwig
Photography copyright © 2015 by Alexandra Grablewski
Whole30® is a registered trademark of Thirty & Co., LLC
The Whole30 logo is a trademark of Thirty & Co., LLC
All rights reserved.
Food styling by Suzanne Lenzer
Prop styling by Nidia Cueva
Design by Vertigo Design NYC
Production by the Stonesong Press

For information about permission to reproduce selections from this book, write to trade.permissions@hmhco.com
or to Permissions, Houghton Mifflin Harcourt Publishing Company, 3 Park Avenue, New York, New York 10016.
www.hmhco.com

Library of Congress Cataloging-in-Publication Data is available
ISBN 978-0-544-60971-6
Printed in China
SCP 30 29 28 27 26
4500745289

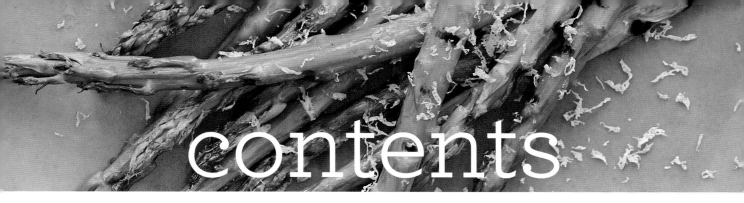

contents

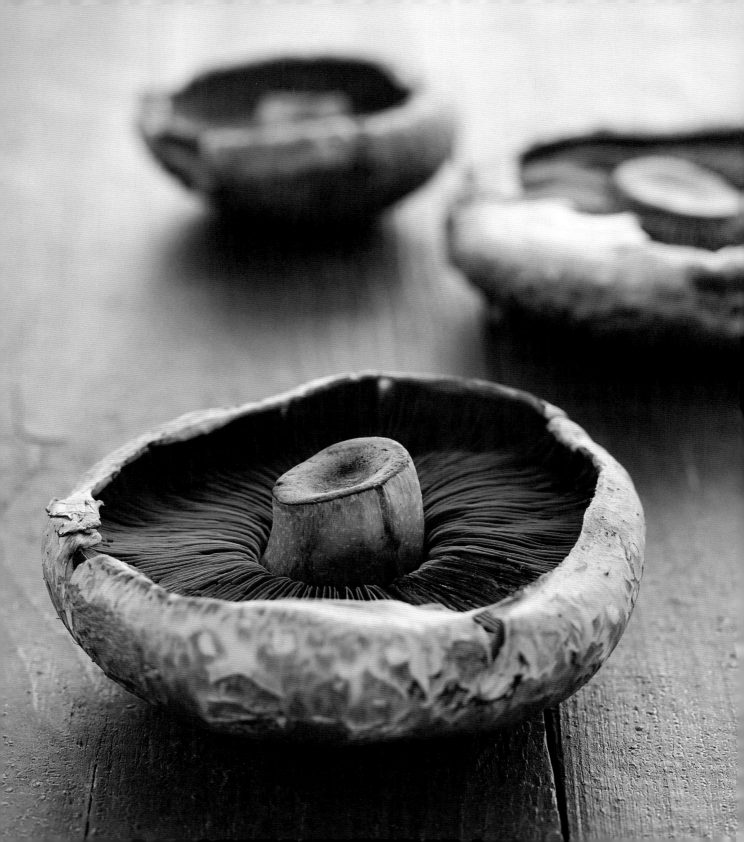

preface

The most often-quoted line in the entire Whole30 program is this one:

"It is not hard. Don't you dare tell us this is hard. Quitting heroin is hard. Fighting cancer is hard. Drinking your coffee black. Is. Not. Hard."

Since we created the Whole30 in April 2009, thousands of people have told us that this line is what finally motivated them to start the program and change their lives. If you're the kind of person who responds well to tough love (for which the Whole30 is famous), this line was written for you. It's a well-meaning kick in the pants to put this challenge into perspective, retire your excuses, and start owning the changes you want to make in your life.

This is not hard. You've done way harder things. You can do this. It's just one month.

We'll always leave that line untouched, because it speaks to where we were when we created the Whole30, and the many people that message has inspired. Now, we want to share something else.

We know this is hard.

It may not be as physically challenging as birthing a baby or as emotionally draining as the death of a loved one, but changing the way you think about food is hard.

Our relationship with food is an emotional one. Food is our comfort, our reward, a trusted friend, a mother's love. You've got food habits, traditions, and associations that go back to childhood. You can't imagine how you would live (happily) without certain foods in your life. And we are asking you to give up those foods for an entire month.

Yes, the idea is threatening. Scary. Downright paralyzing. How will you celebrate, manage your stress, deal with a tough day at the office, bond with your family, enjoy life without cake, chocolate, wine, or bread?

We're not even going to *mention* cheese right now.

If the Whole30 was just another diet, a short-term quick fix, or a 30-day test of willpower, it would be easier. You can do anything for 30 days, and believing you could return to your old habits and foods a few pounds lighter when the month was over would make temporary restriction easier.

But the Whole30 is not a diet. It's not a quick fix. It's not even a weight-loss program. The Whole30 is designed to change your life. It's a monumental transformation in how you think about food, your body, your life, and what you want out of the time you have left on this earth. It's so much bigger than just food. It's a paradigm shift the likes of which you may only experience a few times in your whole life.

Big changes like that are always hard.

So we need you to know that we understand. In fact, that's exactly why we wrote this book. Because we know the Whole30 can be challenging, and we want you to be successful. We want to teach you as much as we can in the next 30 days so that you will succeed in changing your life.

It starts with food.

Improving your sleep, energy levels, mood, attention span, body composition, motivation, self-confidence, self-efficacy, and quality of life starts by changing the food you put on your plate. Yes, the Whole30 eliminates cravings, corrects hormonal imbalances, fixes digestive issues, improves medical conditions, and strengthens the immune system.

But the program will do so much more than you are expecting it will do. We know that, because we've seen it happen with thousands of people. What starts off as a "diet" somehow expands into other areas of your life, areas you didn't even know could be improved simply by eating good food. The next 30 days will initiate a healthy chain reaction throughout your entire life, imparting a sense of control, freedom, stability, and confidence that will inspire you to take on other personal development goals, big and small.

You'll feel better, so you'll want to do more. Which makes you feel even better, and want to do even more. It's the exact opposite of the cycle you've been stuck in—feel bad, eat junk food, feel even worse, eat even more junk food. We carefully designed the Whole30 to jump-start new, healthy habits, and keep you moving forward in a positive way more consistently and sustainably than any quick-fix weight-loss diet ever could.

So we know how powerful this program is, but we also know how hard it can be, which is why we wanted to give you more than just our rules and some recipes. We've created a comprehensive quick-reference guide so that we can be with you every step of the way through the next 30 days. *The Whole30* is the accumulation of more than five years of experience with hundreds of thousands of Whole30 participants, several focus groups, and dozens of community surveys.

> ## IT STARTS WITH FOOD.
>
> Our first book, *It Starts With Food,* shares the behind-the-scenes of our general nutrition recommendations—the science behind our plan, and the background of the Whole30. We highly recommend you read it before tackling the program, especially if you're the kind of person who likes to know why you're doing what you're doing, happily geeks out on the science-y stuff, or needs a little more convincing that we really do have a solid basis for our guidelines.

We know what you'll need to be successful. And we're giving it all to you here, because we want nothing more than to have you experience the miraculous results that so many Whole30 participants have reported to us.

Part 1 of *The Whole30* explains the what, why, and how of the program. We'll detail the Whole30 rules and recommendations, fully prepare you for your 30-day journey, preview a typical program day by day, and walk you through a sample reintroduction schedule.

Part 2: Everything You Need to Know is the most extensive Whole30 FAQ ever compiled.

Seriously.

This is where we pulled out all the stops, combing our website comments, forum, social media posts, and emails to make sure we included all the answers to all the questions ever asked (we hope), and as much advice as we could possibly cull together from our team and experts in our community. We'll talk about what you can and can't eat, drink, and supplement with; how much to eat (not in the way you'd think, though);

how to grocery shop; successfully navigating dining out and travel; managing cravings, stress, and the scale; adapting the program for special populations; troubleshooting your Whole30; and for the first time anywhere in print, our complete guide to Whole30 reintroduction.

There is so much good stuff in Part 2 . . . but there's still more to come.

Part 3: Whole30 Kitchen Basics will help you get your kitchen in order and teach you the cooking skills you'll need for the next 30 days. We knew we needed to include this, because cooking can be one of the most intimidating parts of the Whole30—even scarier than the idea of giving up cheese.

The lesson we hope to teach you here, however, is that you don't have to make complicated meals with fancy ingredients. You just need to know how to prepare and cook the tasty basics, which we'll lay out for you in enough detail to get even the "I can barely boil water" people feeling kitchen-competent. In fact, you could cook your way through the entire Whole30 right here in this section, making what we call "ingredient meals"—delicious, tasty, varied meals that require no recipe, just healthy, fresh ingredients and the proper cooking techniques.

Eventually, however, you're bound to start feeling kitchen-frisky. Which brings us to Part 4.

Part 4: Recipes is the main attraction, so step right up and feast your eyes on all of this gorgeous food you could be eating for the next 30 days. Culinary Institute of America–trained chef Richard Bradford has created more than one hundred recipes in ten different categories, ranging from super-simple to slightly more involved (but still totally accessible). He doesn't use any hard-to-find specialty ingredients, and he doesn't require any exotic kitchen equipment—in fact, we'll give you a list of exactly what you'll need to cook your way through this book starting on page 187.

The best part is that every one of these recipes—even the super-simple ones—are alive with flavor. He's hit the food trifecta here: recipes using simple ingredients that are easy to prepare and incredibly tasty. Don't be fooled by the short list of ingredients or the simple spices; the deliciousness of Part 4 will sneak up on you, you'll see.

Oh . . . and yes, we give you a meal plan. We knew you were going to ask that. It's on page 196. Of course, it may not look like you expect it to look, but we'll explain.

Finally, in the Appendix, we'll give you a comprehensive list of Whole30 resources: where to find more inspiration for sourcing, preparing, and cooking Good Food; where to go if you need Whole30 help; how to connect with us throughout your Whole30 journey; and more.

Now, as you prepare to embark upon your Whole30 journey, we want you to know that we're with you, every step of the way. So before we begin, allow us to rewrite our famous "this is not hard" section, just for you:

It will be hard. You will not be perfect. Don't even try to be perfect. No one is judging, no one is keeping score, and there are no penalties for admitting that this is hard, you are struggling, and you need help. Be patient with yourself, because real change takes time. Be kind to yourself, and celebrate even the smallest of victories, because a series of small victories is all it takes to change your life. Finally, know that it's not 30 days—it's one day. One meal. One bite. Do this one bite at a time if you have to, because it's for the most important and worthwhile cause on earth—you.

Welcome to the Whole30.

Best in health,

MELISSA HARTWIG and
DALLAS HARTWIG

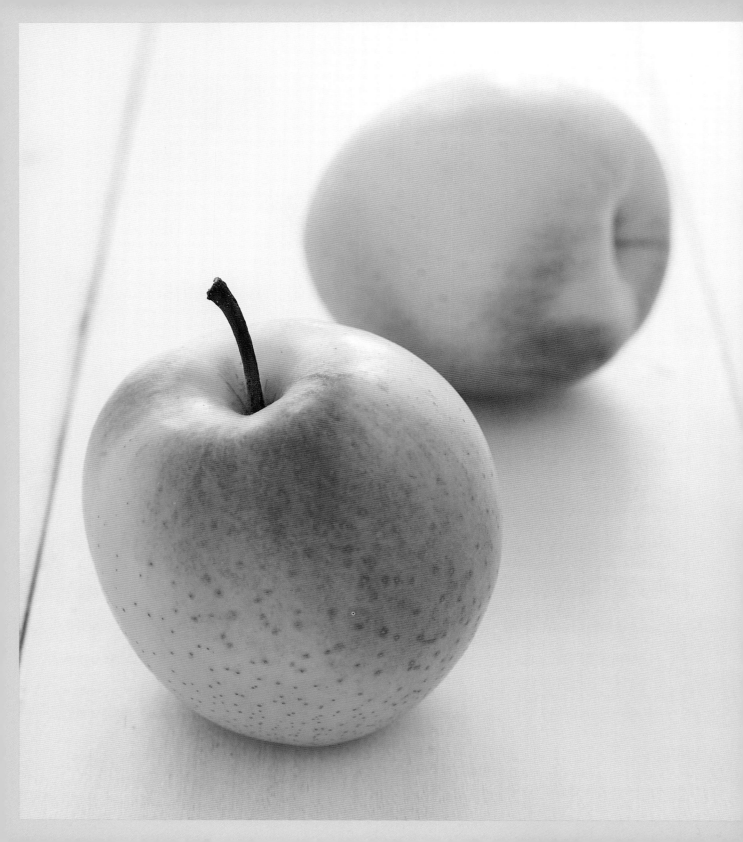

PART 1

welcome to the whole30

"To say that the Whole30 is life-changing would be an understatement. Following the Whole30 has allowed me to take control of my health and that has spilled over to all parts of my life. Of course there are physical changes: definite weight loss, an increase in strength and stamina, and just generally feeling more comfortable in my skin. More important, I've had severe anxiety and panic attacks that came out of nowhere, bordering on agoraphobia. All of that is gone. The mental attitude that I currently have is priceless. I'm naturally, optimistically calm and happy. I still have bad days, but I deal with it so much better. I honestly do not see myself going back to any bad foods that I used to eat. I'm having fun cooking for myself and feel like I've uncovered a new side of myself that has been hiding: a new, happy, optimistic, energetic, and innovative side."

—DOMINIK Z., QUEENS, NY

what is the whole30?

Think of the Whole30 like pushing the "reset" button with your health, your habits, and your relationship with food. Our premise is simple: certain food groups could be having a negative impact on your body composition, health, and quality of life without you even realizing it. Are your energy levels inconsistent or nonexistent? Do you have aches and pains that can't be explained by overuse or injury? Are you having a hard time losing weight no matter how hard you try? Do you have some sort of condition (like skin issues, digestive ailments, seasonal allergies, or chronic fatigue) that medication hasn't helped? These symptoms may be directly related to the foods you eat—even the "healthy" stuff.

So how do you know if (and how) these foods are affecting you? Eliminate them from your diet completely. Cut out all the psychologically unhealthy, hormone-unbalancing, gut-disrupting, inflammatory food groups for a full 30 days. Let your body heal and recover from whatever ailments those foods may be causing. Push the "reset" button with your metabolism, systemic inflammation, and the downstream effects of the food choices you've been making. Learn once and for all how the foods you've been eating are actually affecting your day to day life, and your long-term health.

For 30 days, the program eliminates foods demonstrated by science and our experience to promote unhealthy cravings and habits, disrupt your metabolism, damage your digestive tract, and burden your immune system. After 30 days, you carefully and systematically reintroduce those foods, and pay attention to how they impact your cravings, mood, energy, sleep, digestion, body composition, athletic performance, pain, and the symptoms of your medical

WHAT IS NORMAL?

But wouldn't you know if these foods were making you less healthy? Not necessarily. Say you're allergic to a tree just outside of your house. Every morning, you wake up and your eyes are a little bit itchy, your nose is runny, your head aches just a bit. But day after day, exposed to the same allergy . . . those feelings start to become your "norm." You no longer notice the headache, stuffiness, or itchy eyes, because that's just how you feel every single day. Now, you take a vacation somewhere where there are none of those trees. The first morning you wake up, you're clearheaded, your eyes are bright and your head doesn't ache. You feel fantastic—and when you return home, you are now acutely aware of how terrible those trees make you feel. That's what we're trying to do for you here—remove all common potential dietary triggers, so you can be truly, honestly aware of what your life would be like without them.

condition. With that knowledge, you can then create the perfect diet for you; a nutrition plan that feels balanced and sustainable, grounded in new healthy habits, keeping you looking, feeling, and living your best.

The most important reason to try the Whole30?

This will change your life.

We cannot possibly put enough emphasis on this simple fact—the next 30 days will change your life. It will change the way you think about food, it will change your tastes, it will change your habits and your cravings. It could, quite possibly, change the emotional relationship you have with food, and with your body. It has the potential to change the way you eat for the rest of your life. We know this because we did it, and hundreds of thousands of people have done it since, and it changed our lives (and their lives) in a very permanent fashion.

The physical benefits of the Whole30 are profound. A full 96 percent of participants lose weight and improve their body composition without counting or restricting calories. Also commonly reported: consistently high energy levels, better sleep, improved focus and mental clarity, a return to healthy digestive function, improved athletic performance, and a sunnier disposition. (Yes, many Whole30 graduates say they felt "strangely happy" during and after their program.)

The psychological benefits of the Whole30 may be even more dramatic. Through the program, participants report effectively changing long-standing, unhealthy habits related to food, developing a healthier body image, and dramatically reducing or eliminating cravings, particularly for sugar and carbohydrates. The words so many Whole30 participants use to describe this place?

"Food freedom."

Finally, testimonials from thousands of Whole30 participants document the improvement or "cure" of any number of lifestyle-related diseases and conditions.

high blood pressure • high cholesterol • type 1 diabetes • type 2 diabetes • asthma • allergies • sinus infections • hives • skin conditions • endometriosis • PCOS • infertility • migraines • depression • bipolar disorder • heartburn • GERD • arthritis • joint pain • ADHD • thyroid dysfunction • Lyme disease • fibromyalgia • chronic fatigue • lupus • leaky gut syndrome • Crohn's • IBS • Celiac disease • diverticulitis • ulcerative colitis • multiple sclerosis

BUT I'M NOT SICK—IS THIS FOR ME?

In a word, yes. The Whole30 is for everyone. So many doctors have reached out to us to share their dramatic results using the Whole30 with their patients—improvements in cholesterol, high blood pressure, chronic pain, even the reversal of diabetes—but you don't have to be sick to benefit from the program. If you want more energy, better sleep, sustainable weight loss; if you've tried every diet out there with no long-term success; if you feel helpless and out of control with your food and cravings; the Whole30 is for you.

our good food standards

The success of your Whole30 depends in large part on the 100 percent elimination of the "less healthy" foods (and beverages) we rule out for the duration of the program. We've chosen these foods because they fail some (or all) of the four Good Food Standards we outlined in *It Starts With Food*. We'll talk about specific foods in a minute, but first, let's talk about how the Whole30 targets each of those key areas of health.

TARGET: An (Unhealthy) Relationship with Food

The Whole30 is specifically designed to address any long-standing, unhealthy psychological and emotional relationships with food, helping you break free of cravings and bad habits. We eliminate nutrient-poor, calorie-dense, low-satiety foods that promote overconsumption—the stuff that once you start eating, you just can't stop. These "foods with no brakes" are the cookies, crackers, chips, chocolates, ice creams, and other comfort foods to which you find yourself irresistibly drawn when you're stressed, lonely, anxious, or unhappy.

Over time, overconsumption of these foods rewire reward, pleasure, emotion, and habit pathways in the brain, promoting a vicious cycle of craving, overconsumption, guilt, and remorse. The simple act of giving in to a craving (again) also stresses you out—and emotional and psychological stress have physical consequences that, in part, further exacerbates your desire for sugar.

The Whole30 rules are carefully crafted to quash your cravings (specifically for sugar and empty carbohydrates), identify your food triggers, and teach you to find other sources of comfort and reward, so that you are in control of your food, and not the other way around.

TARGET: A Sluggish Metabolism

The Whole30 rules and meal recommendations also target a sluggish metabolism, helping you restore a healthy hormonal balance, effectively regulate blood sugar, and become "fat adapted" (able to use dietary and body fat as fuel). Over time, the overconsumption of foods with no brakes conditions your body to rely on sugar for energy, leaving you unable to burn the fat stored on your body, and requiring you to eat every few hours to maintain energy, focus, and a pleasant demeanor. It also disrupts your body's ability to manage your blood sugar, the delicate balance of key hormones like insulin and leptin, and how well those hormones' messages get through to your brain. These changes not only promote energy dips, excessive hunger and cravings, and weight gain, but start you down the road to chronic diseases like obesity and diabetes.

The foods you'll eat during your Whole30 will promote stable blood sugar levels, teach your body how to utilize fat as fuel, regulate your hormones, and improve their communications with your brain. As a result, during your Whole30 you'll likely experience an increase in energy, a reduction in hunger between meals, weight loss, and an improvement in biomarkers like blood pressure, "good" cholesterol, and fasting blood sugar.

TARGET: A Disrupted Digestive System

One of the most important targets of the Whole30 program is your gut—specifically, the small intestine, where the vast majority of your food is digested and absorbed. Certain foods promote a "leaky gut," a condition where the small intestine is no longer able to properly absorb the nutrients you eat. This means the healthy foods you chew and swallow aren't actually nourishing your body, and things like partially digested food, bacteria, or other toxins are allowed to "leak" from your intestines into the bloodstream, where they don't belong. This triggers an immune reaction, and promotes chronic systemic inflammation everywhere in the body, not just in the digestive tract.

The Whole30 eliminates the foods shown to cause or promote this leaky gut, allowing your digestive tract to heal and your immune system to calm. This helps to resolve a host of digestive issues (like heartburn, acid reflux, constipation, diarrhea, gas, bloating, and related pain) and reduce or eliminate the wide-ranging systemic effects of chronic inflammation.

TARGET: An Overactive Immune System

Last but certainly not least, the Whole30 is an anti-inflammatory diet, designed to calm an overactive immune system and reduce or eliminate the symptoms of inflammation—aches, pains, and medical issues you may not have ever associated with your food choices. Systemic inflammation starts in your gut, but because the immune activity goes everywhere your bloodstream flows, the symptoms may appear anywhere, in any form—even in the brain.

This kind of inflammation is often referred to as "silent inflammation," but we believe it's not really silent if you know what you're listening for. This is a comprehensive (but not exhaustive) list of conditions and diseases linked to systemic inflammation or having an inflammatory component. If you experience any of these conditions or symptoms, there's a pretty good chance you have some of that "silent" inflammation.

WHAT IS CHRONIC SYSTEMIC INFLAMMATION?

Your immune system's top priority is defense against outside threats, like fighting off a cold or healing tissues when you trip and sprain your ankle. This immune activity is aggressive but short-term—your immune system recognizes the threat, rapidly ramps up to deal with it, and then returns to a "resting" baseline when the job is done. During this resting baseline, your immune system plays a critical role in the repair and maintenance of various body structures. Chronic systemic inflammation is the full-body, long-term up-regulation of immune system activity. Think of chronic systemic inflammation like being a little bit sick all the time; when certain factors (like your food choices) overload the system and keep it working hard all the time, it is less effective at doing its other jobs, like healing that stubborn tendinitis or keeping your arteries clear of plaque. Chronic systemic inflammation is at the heart of an endless number of lifestyle-related diseases and conditions, like allergies, asthma, eczema, autoimmune diseases, high cholesterol, heart disease, stroke, diabetes, and obesity.

Related to Silent Inflammation

acid reflux/heartburn	eczema	multiple sclerosis
acne	edema	myasthenia gravis
allergies	emphysema	myositis
alopecia	endometriosis	nephritis
Alzheimer's disease	essential tremor	obesity
anemia	fibroids	osteopenia
arthritis	fibromyalgia	osteoporosis
asthma	gastroenteritis	Parkinson's disease
atherosclerosis	gingivitis	PCOS
bipolar disorder	gout	periodontal disease
bronchitis	Graves' disease	polychondritis
chronic bursitis	Hashimoto's thyroiditis	psoriasis
cancer	heart disease	Raynaud's phenomenon
carditis	hepatitis	rheumatoid arthritis
celiac disease	high blood pressure	sarcoidosis
chronic pain	high cholesterol	scleroderma
circulation issues	high triglycerides	seizures
cirrhosis	infertility	sinusitis
colitis	inflammatory bowel syndrome	Sjögren's syndrome
Crohn's disease	insulin resistance	spastic colon
dementia	interstitial cystitis	chronic tendonitis
depression	joint pain	trichotillomania
dermatitis	lupus	ulcerative colitis
diabetes (types 1 & 2)	Lyme disease	vasculitis
diverticulitis	migraines	vitiligo

By removing the foods most likely to contribute to both an impaired gut and chronic systemic inflammation, the Whole30 can reduce or eliminate the symptoms related to any number of lifestyle-related diseases and conditions, dramatically improving how you look, how you feel, and your quality of life.

Now it's time we talk about the foods. You know, the ones that mess with your cravings, tank your metabolism, disrupt your gut, and aggravate your immune system. We're just going to come right out and name them.

Added sugar and artificial sweeteners. All alcohol. All grains (even whole grains). Legumes, including peanuts and soy. Nearly all forms of dairy.

Don't freak out.

We know there are a lot of fun foods in this list. Maybe some of your favorite foods. Maybe *all* of your favorite foods. You may be panicking. You may be thinking, "No way can I do this." You may believe you can't live without _____.

You may also be saying things about us that aren't very nice.

It's okay. We can take it.

We assure you, you can do this. And you will. We will walk you through it. We will give you all the information, support, and resources you need. We will teach you how to live without the foods you thought you couldn't live without. We will bring you new favorite foods—foods that are just as delicious, even more satisfying, and won't promote that awful crave-overconsume-guilt-remorse cycle from which you are so desperate to be free.

The Whole30 can bring you food freedom.

Just keep reading with an open mind.

WHAT ABOUT WEIGHT LOSS?

Since the inception of our Whole30 program in April 2009, we've made one thing abundantly clear: This is not a weight-loss program. It's not a diet, it's not a quick fix, and it's certainly not a "17 Day Get Skinnier Than Your Friends" kind of approach. But that doesn't mean we don't recognize or value your weight loss goals. We know most of you want to lose weight, and we want to help you do it—healthfully and sustainably, by encouraging you to focus on your health.

When you make yourself healthier from the inside out, improved body composition, self-esteem, and happiness generally follow, but it doesn't work the other way around. In addition, scale weight is one of the fastest ways to lose motivation, even if you thought you were making great progress in other areas. ("I only lost half a pound today. This program isn't working at all!") It's okay to take on the Whole30 with weight loss in the back of your mind. Just don't allow that focus to take you to an unhealthy place with the program, mentally or physically. See pages 98–99 for more on weight loss and the Whole30.

foods that make you less healthy

"I am in my third round of Whole30. Rather than thinking of sugar, cookies, bread, or chocolate bars, I now think of protein, veggies, and fruits. I am now a master salad mixer, a creative whiz with the blender, and am enjoying food prep in the kitchen. I am amazed at the change and the fact that I have a very different perspective on food. I've lost 13 pounds, dropped a dress size or two, and feel terrific. I know I'm on the right track with the Whole30."
—ETHEL LEE-MILLER, TUCSON, AZ

Here is a big-picture view on why these five food groups fail our Good Food Standards, and why they're out for the duration of your Whole30. (For a much more detailed analysis, read Chapters 8, 10, 11, and 12 in *It Starts With Food*.)

Slay the Sugar Dragon

Added sugars in your diet do not make you healthier . . . but you already knew that. Added sugars, whether from table sugar, honey, agave nectar, or maple syrup, do not contain the vitamins, minerals, and phytochemicals that contribute to your overall health, but they do contain lots of empty calories.

Added sugar promotes overconsumption via pleasure and reward pathways in the brain. This creates an unhealthy psychological relationship with your food and creates hard-to-break habits, leading to further overconsumption and sugar "addiction." Overconsumption leads to hormonal and metabolic dysregulation, which are inflammatory in the body, and promote disorders like insulin resistance, diabetes, and obesity. In addition, sugar disrupts the delicate balance of gut bacteria, which promotes digestive issues and inflammation in the gut.

LESS HEALTHY

To be fair, we're not saying there's nothing good to be found here; grains and beans contain fiber, and dairy has calcium. However, there is no vitamin, mineral, or phytonutrient that you could get from these foods that can't be found (often in a more bioavailable form) in high-quality meats, vegetables, fruits, and natural fats . . . without the potential metabolic, digestive, and inflammatory downsides that come with these "less healthy" food groups. Read on. . . .

Artificial or "non-nutritive" sweeteners (including Splenda/sucralose, Equal/Nutra-Sweet/aspartame, Truvia/stevia, Sweet'N Low/saccharin, xylitol, maltitol, etc.) may also promote ongoing metabolic dysfunction. In fact, studies show people who switch from real sugar to artificial sweeteners don't lose weight or improve their hormonal balance. New research suggests some artificial sweeteners may even disrupt gut bacteria just like real sugar! And from a psychological perspective, artificial sweeteners are not a solution for banishing your sugar cravings; in fact, they only continue the cycle of craving, reward, and overconsumption.

It's the Alcohol

Alcohol (like sugar) does not make you healthier. It is neurotoxic, which is why your brain doesn't work quite right after a few drinks. It is a very concentrated source of calories (nearly twice as calorie-dense as sugar, gram for gram!) but contains no actual "nutrition."

In addition, consumption of alcohol often sets us up to make poor choices*—the after-effects of which can turn one late-night pizza into a whole weekend of carb-a-palooza.

In addition, alcohol makes it harder for your body to properly control blood-sugar levels, and directly promotes changes in your intestinal lining which contributes to "leaky gut," promoting inflammation that starts in the gut, but travels everywhere in the body.

Whether your vice is red wine, tequila, gluten-free beer, or potato vodka, the common denominator—and what makes you less healthy—is the alcohol itself.

*Poor choices with food. We're not even going to touch those other poor choices.

Not Even Whole Grains

This section is referring to grains and grain-like seeds—wheat, oats, barley, corn, rice, millet, buckwheat, quinoa, and the like. (Yes, we said rice and corn!) Both refined and whole grains promote overconsumption, which creates hormonal and metabolic disruption. They also contain inflammatory proteins (like gluten) and fermentable carbohydrates that can promote an imbalance of gut bacteria and provoke inflammation in the body.

The inflammation that starts in your gut, often causing a plethora of digestive issues, also "travels" throughout the body, as the inflammatory components of grains allow various substances to improperly cross your intestinal lining and go everywhere your bloodstream goes. This often manifests itself as things like asthma, allergies, skin conditions, fertility issues, migraines, joint pain, and other symptoms that you might never have associated with the food that you eat.

Grains also contain "anti-nutrients" called phytates or phytic acid that make valuable minerals like the calcium, magnesium, and zinc found in the grains themselves unavailable for use in your body. In part because of these phytates, all grains (even whole grains) are relatively nutrient-poor, especially compared to vegetables and fruit.

Pass on the Peanuts (and Beans, and Soy)

Legumes (beans, peas, lentils, soy, and peanuts) have similar issues as those with grains. First, they are generally nutrient-poor when compared to vegetables and fruit. In addition, they contain anti-nutrients (phytates) that can't be completely neutralized by usual preparation methods of prolonged soaking and rinsing, cooking, sprouting, or fermenting. These anti-nutrients rob the body of valuable minerals, and if cooked improperly, could even cause damage to your intestinal lining and provoke systemic inflammation.

More significantly, legumes also contain fermentable carbohydrates that can disrupt your gut bacteria, and commonly cause gas, bloating, cramps, pain, and other digestive issues when consumed.

Another concern, specific to soybeans and even more so with processed soy products, is the content of compounds that behave like estrogen (that female sex hormone) in the human body. These compounds, classified as phytoestrogens or isoflavones, bind to and stimulate (or in some tissues, block) estrogen receptors. And while the overall research on soy products is inconsistent, in our view there are some alarming issues related to the consumption of soy and soy products. We think you shouldn't mess with your delicate sex hormone balance, and ingesting phytoestrogens in an unknown "dose" via soy products does just that.

Finally, peanuts are especially problematic, as they contain proteins (called lectins) that are resistant to digestion. These lectins can cross into our bloodstream, and promote inflammation anywhere and everywhere in the body. These lectins may be why the incidence of peanut allergies are so prevalent today.

Milk (and Cheese, and Yogurt) Don't Do a Body Good

Dairy (from cow, sheep, and goat's milk) contains factors designed to help little mammals (like calves and human infants) grow fast. But the growth factors found in milk and milk products, along with some immune factors and inflammatory proteins, may not do our adult bodies any good.

The carbohydrate portion of milk (lactose) together with the milk proteins produce a surprisingly high insulin response, which could be inflammatory in our bodies and further promotes disorders like obesity and diabetes. In addition, high levels of insulin along with other dairy growth factors promote unregulated cell growth. (Makes sense if you are a calf trying to triple your body weight in a matter of months, but not so much sense for us human adults.) In fact, unregulated cell growth is the underlying cause of cancer (the uncontrolled reproduction of mutated cells), and is why, in some studies, dairy consumption has been shown to be associated with some types of hormonally driven cancers.

Dairy proteins can also be inflammatory in the body (especially casein, which is concentrated in cheese), and have been associated with an increased risk of autoimmune diseases like rheumatoid arthritis. Finally, immune factors and hormones in the milk proteins can cross-react with our immune system, leading milk drinkers to report a worsening of their seasonal allergies, asthma, acne, and other related conditions.

The Wrap-Up

Now, hear us clearly. We're not saying these foods are "bad." There is no morality when it comes to food—foods aren't bad or good, and you're not bad or good for eating (or avoiding) them. We're not even saying these foods are bad for you. We don't know that yet.

The thing is, neither do you.

Until you eliminate these foods, you won't know how these foods have been impacting how you look, feel, or live. Is dairy making you stuffy or wheezy? Are grains making you bloated or sad? Is your diet in general what's keeping you in chronic pain, making your joints swollen, or harming your thyroid?

Science suggests they could be, but the truth is, you don't know. But you can, in just 30 days. Commit to pushing these foods off your plate completely for the next month. Not one bite, not one sip, not one taste. Give your body a chance to restore its natural balance, heal, and recover. Give your brain a chance to change your tastes, create new habits, and find new rewards. Pay attention. See what changes. Take good notes. Be brutally honest.

At the end of the 30 days, you'll reintroduce these foods one at a time, carefully, systematically, evaluating if or how they push you off your healthy balance. Pay attention. See what changes. Take good notes. Be brutally honest.

Now you know.

In just a few weeks, you've figured out what mainstream media, other diets, nutrition coaches, even your own medical doctors haven't been able to give you—the perfect diet for *you*. The diet that feels sustainable, satisfying, deliciously freeing. The diet that keeps you looking and feeling your best, while still enjoying less healthy foods when, where, and how often you choose. The diet that was specifically created for you, because through our protocol, your awareness, and your determination, *you* created it.

Now that is food freedom.

And now, you're ready for the Whole30.

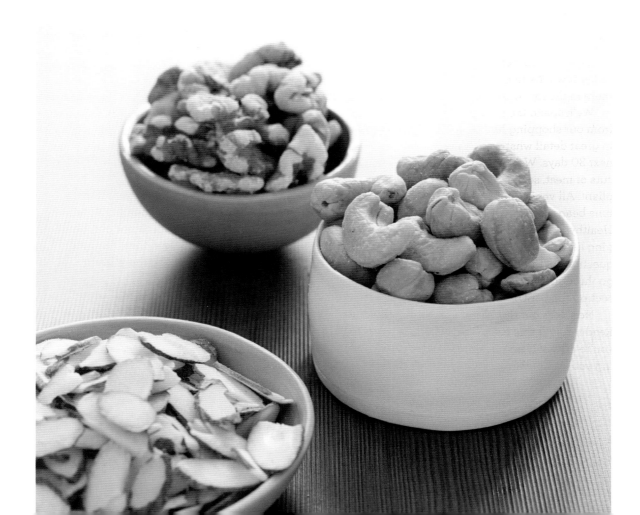

the whole30 program rules

"Here is the truth: six weeks ago, I weighed 346 pounds, walked with a cane because of terrible joint pain, and took 16 units of NovoLog (injectable insulin) three times a day. I started the Whole30 and committed. Today I weigh 294 pounds, my sugars are level with no insulin, and I have tolerable pain with no cane!" —DAVE S., CHANDLER, AZ

The first step in your journey is to familiarize yourself with the Whole30 program rules. These are the guidelines you'll be following for the next 30 days, and the better you know the rules, the easier it will be to make good food choices out there in the real world.

We'll spend the vast majority of this book, from our shopping list to our recipes, explaining in great detail what you will be eating for the next 30 days. We'll even simplify it here: basic cuts of meat, seafood, and eggs are always compliant. All vegetables except for corn, peas, and lima beans are compliant. All fruit is compliant. Healthy fats are outlined in detail on our shopping list (page 192–193). And if you have more questions about specific foods or drinks, we'll go through them one by one in our Can I Have? section (page 60).

Now, let's get the "no" items out of the way. Read through this list in detail a few times, so you're crystal clear on exactly what to avoid during your Whole30.

The Whole30 Program Rules

We ask that you dedicate yourself to following these rules 100 percent for the duration of your program—no slips, cheats, or special occasions.

- **DO NOT CONSUME ADDED SUGAR OF ANY KIND, REAL OR ARTIFICIAL.** No maple syrup, honey, agave nectar, coconut sugar, Splenda, Equal, NutraSweet, xylitol, stevia, etc. Read your labels, because companies sneak sugar into products in ways you might not recognize.

HERE ARE THE MOST BASIC GUIDELINES:

YES: Eat meat, seafood, eggs, vegetables, fruit, and natural fats.

NO: Do not consume sugar, alcohol, grains, legumes, or dairy. Do not consume baked goods or "treats." Do not weigh or measure yourself.

- **DO NOT CONSUME ALCOHOL IN ANY FORM.** No wine, beer, champagne, vodka, rum, whiskey, tequila, etc., whether drunk on its own or used as an ingredient—not even for cooking.

- **DO NOT EAT GRAINS.** This includes wheat, rye, barley, oats, corn, rice, millet, bulgur, sorghum, sprouted grains, and all gluten-free pseudo-cereals like amaranth, buckwheat, or quinoa. This also includes all the ways we add wheat, corn, and rice into our foods in the form of bran, germ, starch, and so on. Again, read your labels.

- **DO NOT EAT LEGUMES.** This includes beans of all kinds (black, red, pinto, navy, white, kidney, lima, fava, etc.), peas, chickpeas, lentils, and peanuts. No peanut butter, either. This also includes all forms of soy—soy sauce, miso, tofu, tempeh, edamame, and all the ways we sneak soy into foods (like soybean oil or soy lecithin). The only exceptions are green beans, snow peas, and sugar snap peas—refer to page 63.

- **DO NOT EAT DAIRY.** This includes cow, goat, or sheep's milk products such as cream, cheese, kefir, yogurt, and sour cream. The only exceptions are clarified butter or ghee—refer to page 183.

- **DO NOT CONSUME CARRAGEENAN, MSG, OR ADDED SULFITES.** If these ingredients appear in any form in the ingredient list of your processed food or beverage, it's out for the Whole30.

- **DO NOT RECREATE BAKED GOODS, "TREATS," OR JUNK FOODS WITH APPROVED INGREDIENTS.** No banana-egg pancakes, almond-flour muffins, Paleo bread, or coconut milk ice cream. Your cravings and habits won't change if you keep eating these foods, even if they are made with Whole30 ingredients. (Refer to page 95 for more information.)

- **DO NOT STEP ON THE SCALE OR TAKE MEASUREMENTS.** This is about so much more than just weight loss, and to focus on your body composition means you'll miss out on the most dramatic and lifelong benefits this plan has to offer. So, no weighing yourself, analyzing body fat, or breaking out the tape measure during your Whole30. (Start on page 29 for details.)

The Fine Print

These foods are exceptions to the rule, and are allowed during your Whole30.

- **CLARIFIED BUTTER OR GHEE.** Clarified butter (page 183) or ghee are the only sources of dairy allowed during your Whole30. Plain old butter is not allowed, as its milk proteins could impact the results of your program.

- **FRUIT JUICE AS A SWEETENER.** Products or recipes including orange, apple, or other fruit juices are permitted on the program, although we encourage you not to go overboard here.

- **GREEN BEANS, SNOW PEAS, AND SUGAR SNAP PEAS.** While these are technically legumes, they are far more "pod" than "bean," and green plant matter is generally good for you.

- **VINEGAR.** Most forms of vinegar, including white, balsamic, apple cider, red wine, white wine, champagne, and rice, are allowed during your Whole30 program. The only exceptions are flavored vinegars with added sugar, or malt vinegar, which is thought to contain gluten.

DEEP BREATH

We know this seems like a lot to remember, but we promise you'll get the hang of it fast. It's easy to avoid big categories of foods, like bread, cereal, pasta, and beans, and if you're buying foods without a label (like ground beef, spinach, or apples), you know you're in the clear. The key to success with pre-packaged foods or processed meats that may or may not be compliant is learning how to read your labels. If you're buying broth, canned tomatoes, turkey burgers, or coconut milk, take a look at the ingredient list. If it contains anything off-plan, it's out for your program. This may require a little detective work, though—companies sneak sugar into products under a variety of names, and chemical-sounding ingredients may be unhealthy or totally harmless. Download our Guide to Sneaky Sugars and Common Additives Cheat-Sheet at www.whole30.com/pdf-downloads to help you translate your labels with ease.

Give Us 30 Days

Your only job during the Whole30 is to focus on making good food choices. You don't need to weigh or measure, you don't need to count calories, you don't need to stress about organic, grass-fed, pastured, or local. Just figure out how to stick to the Whole30 in any setting, around every special circumstance, under any amount of stress, for 30 straight days.

Your only job? Eat. Good. Food.

The only way this will work is if you give it the full 30 days: no cheats, slips, or "special occasions." You need such a small amount of any of these inflammatory foods to break the healing cycle—one bite of pizza, one splash of milk in your coffee, one lick of the spoon mixing the batter within the 30-day period and you've broken your health and healing "reset," and have to start over again on Day 1.*

You must commit to the full program, exactly as written, for the full 30 days. Anything less and we make no claims as to your results, or the chances of your success. Anything less and you are selling yourself—and your potential results—short.

It's only 30 days.

It's for Your Own Good

Here comes the tough love—perhaps the most famous part of the Whole30. This is for those of you who are considering taking on this life-changing month, but aren't sure you can actually pull it off, cheat free, for a full 30 days. This is for the people who have tried to make lifestyle changes, but "slipped" or "fell off the wagon" or "just had to eat _____ because of this _____."

We say this with love.

---

*This isn't us playing the tough guy, attempting to ruin your life, or trying to turn the Whole30 into a hazing. There is science behind this. See page 56 for details.

- **IT IS NOT HARD.** Don't you dare tell us this is hard. Fighting cancer is hard. Birthing a baby is hard. Losing a parent is hard. Drinking your coffee black is. not. hard. You've done harder things than this, and you have no excuse not to complete the program as written. It's only 30 days, and it's for the most important health cause on earth—the only physical body you will ever have in this lifetime.

- **DON'T EVEN CONSIDER THE POSSIBILITY OF A "SLIP."** Unless you physically trip and your face lands in a box of donuts, there is no "slip." You make a choice to eat something unhealthy. It is always a choice, so do not phrase it as if you had an accident. Commit to the program 100 percent for the full 30 days. Don't give yourself an excuse to fail before you've even started.

- **YOU NEVER, EVER, EVER HAVE TO EAT ANYTHING YOU DON'T WANT TO EAT.** You're all big boys and girls. Toughen up. Learn to say no (or make your mom proud and say, "No, thank you"). Learn to stick up for yourself. Just because it's your sister's birthday, or your best friend's wedding, or your company picnic does not mean you have to eat anything. It's always a choice, and we would hope that you stopped succumbing to peer pressure in seventh grade.

- **THIS DOES REQUIRE A BIT OF EFFORT.** Grocery shopping, meal planning, dining out, explaining the program to friends and family, and dealing with stress will all prove challenging at some point during your program. We've given you all the

tools, guidelines, and resources you'll need in this book and our website, but you also have to take responsibility for your own plan. Improved health, fitness, and quality of life doesn't happen automatically just because you're now taking a pass on bread.

- **YOU CAN DO THIS.** You've come too far to back out now. You want to do this. You need to do this. And we know that you can do this. So stop thinking about it, and start doing. Right now, this very minute, commit to the Whole30.

We want you to participate. We want you to take this seriously, and see amazing results in unexpected areas. Even if you don't believe this will actually change your life, if you're willing to give it 30 short days, try it. It is that important. We believe in it that much. It changed our lives, and we want it to change yours too.

Welcome to the Whole30.

getting started with the whole30

"Whole30 has changed my life. In December of 2011, I was topping the scale at 200 pounds. My body and joints ached every day. I was always tired, not sleeping well, fighting acne and eczema. I wanted to change but didn't know how. I bought your book, and jumped right into the Whole30 in January 2012. Needless to say, I was blown away! I ended up doing a Whole90, and lost 30 pounds in three months. I was sleeping like a baby, my eczema cleared up, my acne went away, my period cramps lessened, my energy skyrocketed, and I was so much more positive! Three years and five Whole30s later, I was 60 pounds lighter, and went from barely squeezing into a size 15 to wearing a size 4. I've become so passionate about health that I am now a certified health coach and just finished a 200-hour yoga teacher training."

—HEATHER F., BOSTON, MA

Now that you know what you're signing up for, it's time to actually sign up. Yes, we're asking you to commit to the program now—but that doesn't mean starting right this minute. We're excited that you're excited, but there's a whole lot of preparation to be done before you can successfully kick off your Whole30.

You may need just a day or two to get ready, or you may need a week or two to get your house (and your head) around the changes you're about to introduce. There is no one perfect timeline—you'll have to decide what works best for you.

In this mega-chapter, we'll outline our five-step process to fully prepare you for the Whole30; things you'll have to consider, strategize, and get in order before Day 1.

Speaking of Day 1 . . .

STEP 1: Choose Your Start Date

While we do encourage you to start as soon as you possibly can, there are a few things to consider before you circle that date on your calendar. While it represents just a blip in your whole lifespan, 30 days is still a long time, and we want you to think about what's coming up during and immediately after your Whole30.

If you've got a once-in-a-lifetime vacation, a planned trip to an unfamiliar location, or a wedding (especially your own!) in your immediate future, consider starting the Whole30 after those events. Navigating the Whole30 for the first time under those conditions may prove extremely difficult, and we don't want you stressed out before your program even begins. In addition, you may end up resenting the Whole30 instead of learning from it if you are reintroduction) exactly which foods you want to avoid going forward, because their negative consequences just aren't worth it. What a great time to head into a vacation or special event—with all the self-confidence, energy, and awareness that the Whole30 has to offer. We bet if you set it up this way, you'll find your vacation is healthier and happier, and you won't have to spend the next six weeks struggling to get "back on track" like every other vacation you've ever taken.

In addition, if you've got an important athletic event or an A-level race in the coming month, consider starting the program after your

forced to pass up pasta in Italy or your own wedding cake because you're on Day 15.

We're tough, but not so tough we'd want you to miss out on your own wedding cake.

It's also important not to have your Whole30 end the day before a vacation, holiday, or special event where you know you'll want to eat All the Things. As you'll read in the Reintroduction FAQ on page 132, the Reintroduction portion of the program is just as critical as the 30-day elimination. Ideally, you'll allow a full ten days after your Whole30 is done to go through the schedule as outlined, then enjoy your vacation, honeymoon, or family reunion.

In fact, if you can plan well enough in advance, starting your Whole30 exactly 40 days before your special event is actually perfect timing. You'll be feeling so good from your Whole30 experience, your new habits will feel solidly in place, and you'll know (thanks to your camaraderie, and memories than they are about your finish time or score, aren't they?

Finally, take a look at your calendar during the proposed 30-day period and see what business or personal commitments you have in place. If you've got a family dinner, a business lunch, or a bridal shower in your imminent future, excellent! Consider it an opportunity to take your Whole30 skills out on the town. You'll have to deal with lots of new situations during your program, so write these events into your plan for the month (see page 26), but don't let them push your Whole30 off.

In summary, there will never be a "perfect" time to do the Whole30, so think about what you have coming up, choose a date, and circle it on your calendar in permanent marker. (Really—write it down. Habit research shows that putting your commitment on paper makes you more likely to succeed.)

And with that, it's official—you have your Whole30 start date!

STEP 2: Build Your Support Team

For many of you, the Whole30 will be a radical lifestyle change—and that kind of change is hard when you're going it alone. Finding the right support network will be critical to keeping you motivated, inspired, and accountable during your program. You've already done the first step—choosing a start date, and publicly announcing your commitment. Why not take that opportunity to recruit some in-person support from the people who care about you the most? They don't have to do the Whole30 with you—they just have to support your health efforts for the next 30 days.

Maybe you're nervous about asking friends and family for help. It's really not that hard.

event is over, as your performance may suffer during the first few weeks of the program. (See page 127 for details.)

Now here's a little bit of tough love.

If you're not getting paid for your performance, it's not that important.

Not compared to your health, at least. If you've got a community-wide exercise competition, an obstacle race, or a charity 5K, don't let that hold you up from starting your Whole30. Those events are more about the socialization,

Remember they love you, and only want the best for you.

The first step is sharing a bit about the program. Explain that this is a lifestyle change, not a crash diet or weight-loss plan. Describe it as a 30-day experiment, after which you'll know a lot more about what foods are having a negative impact on your cravings, energy, sleep, and health. Be sure to mention that you aren't cutting calories, carbs, or fat—in fact, you'll be eating as much real, whole, nutrient-dense food as you want—and that there are no pills, meal replacements, or packaged foods to buy. In fact, the entire program and a ton of resources are available for free online!

You should also share why you are choosing to embark upon this journey with those you care about. If you're looking for their support, now is not the time to be vague—things like, "it can really help with energy" aren't going to be very engaging. Make it personal. Share your current struggles, your goals, and all of the ways you believe the program will make you healthier and happier.

If you're speaking to those closest to you, share from the heart, and let them know the challenges you've been facing with your emotional relationship with food, your cravings, your habits, and your health. When it comes to co-workers, don't get into graphic detail; try something like, "Every day at 3 p.m., I feel like I need a nap. I'm hoping the Whole30 will help me keep my energy up without my usual afternoon soda and candy bar."

Finally, don't forget to ask for their support. It's nice that you're telling them more about your life and your aspirations, but how are they supposed to know they have a role to play here unless you tell them? Saying very directly, "Can I count on you to support me for the next 30

HOW NOT TO MAKE FRIENDS AND INFLUENCE PEOPLE

If you want to get people on your side, you have to lead with the things you *will* be eating, not the list of things you're *not* eating. If you start the conversation with "I'm not eating sugar, grains, legumes, or dairy, and no alcohol—turns out those things are really bad for you," you'll probably alienate them immediately. First, they almost certainly have some of those foods in their diet, and they may feel like now that you're on this healthy plan, you'll be judging their food choices. Second, they may look at the list of "can't" items, think, "What the heck do you eat?" and immediately write the Whole30 off as some extreme fad diet. Now, imagine leading with this: "For 30 days, I'll eat lots of whole, fresh, nutritious foods—no calorie counting at all! Breakfast could be a vegetable frittata, fresh fruit, and avocado; lunch is a spinach salad with grilled chicken, apples, pecans, and a raspberry-walnut vinaigrette; and dinner is pulled pork carnitas with roasted sweet potato and a cabbage slaw. Sounds good, right?" Now that's a totally different conversation—one that's likely to earn you a high-five, and maybe even a "Where do I sign up for that?"

days?" lets them know how important these efforts are to you, and how much you'd value their encouragement and help. Even better, ask them how they think they could support you. They may come up with some creative ideas you'd never considered, and asking them to participate in the process will make them feel even more engaged.

Still, despite all your best efforts, there are reasons that family and friends may be less than supportive of your Whole30 plan. They could be a little jaded—be honest, have you announced your "commitment" to every diet on the planet, only to crash and burn a week into it? They could be worried about your health, misunderstanding the principles of the Whole30 or confusing it for a crash or fad diet. They could be feeling slightly defensive, wondering if your new, healthy habits will make them feel guilty for their less-than-ideal behaviors. Or they could be plain old jealous, wanting to make lifestyle changes themselves, but not knowing where or how to start. If you find yourself doing the Whole30 alone, we've created a variety of ways to find the support you need virtually, through our community.

First, you can subscribe to the Whole30 Daily (www.w30.co/w30daily), a newsletter service straight to your inbox, every day of your Whole30. We've created 32 days of information (including a Day 0 and Day 31) written just for you, specific to that particular day of your Whole30. (After watching hundreds of thousands of people run through our program, we know exactly the kind of guidance you need, and when you need it.)

It's our way of checking in with you during every day of your Whole30, filling your inbox with positive messages, helpful instructions, and a vast number of resources. We'll provide you with specially developed guidance (especially in the first week); resources to make shopping, prepping, cooking, avoiding temptation, exercising, sleeping, and managing your stress that much easier during your program; and give you

introspective assignments designed to keep you focused and aware during every stage of your Whole30.

We've also built in some accountability—at the end of every day, you'll have to click the button that says, "I completed another day of the Whole30!" Yep, that means we're waiting to hear how you did on your program every single day, which gives you even more incentive to stay committed and see your program through.

Next, make friends on the Whole30 Forum (www.w30.co/joinw30). The Forum is another way to connect with others doing the program, and learn from the many "veterans" who stick around to offer support to the new folks. With tens of thousands of participants and a fantastic

RECRUIT

If you're hoping to find someone to do the program with you, be strategic in sharing your motivations for completing the program. Chances are, your sedentary best friend won't relate to you saying, "I really want to cut my 5K time by five minutes, and the Whole30 helps with recovery from exercise." But if you can find some common ground, or something you know he's been troubled by, all of a sudden your pitch takes on more relevance. Tell your skin-sensitive buddy, "My skin was breaking out like crazy for a while. The Whole30 will help me figure out which foods make my skin freak out—the before and after pictures I've seen are amazing." Sneaky? Maybe a little . . . but we like to think it's for the greater good.

team of Whole30 expert moderators, our Forum is the friendliest, most collaborative, most supportive community you could imagine.

In particular, the Whole30 Logs allow you to share your day-to-day experience with our community, and stay in touch with others who started their program on the same day you did. Feel free to start your own threads, search for specific questions, and post on others' threads to connect with our fantastic members during (and after) your program.

Finally, connect with other Whole30 participants on social media. Our Facebook, Twitter, and Instagram feeds are a thriving part of our Whole30 community, and a fun way for you to participate and connect. Our Instagram feed and #whole30 hashtag are particularly active—we post new, fun content several times a day, and connect with program participants when they tag us in their posts. If you need support at 2 a.m., want a quick recipe for dinner, or have a grocery shopping moment of crisis, our social media pages are the place to get sympathy, support, and advice fast. (See page 405 for our social media feeds.)

STEP 3: Get Your House Ready

Now that you've chosen a start date and lined up your supporters, it's time to get your house in order. This means, in part, cleaning out the junk food and creating a structured plan to work around family members not participating in the program. This is a critical step in ensuring your Whole30 success, so don't skip it! Remember, planning and preparation is everything when it comes to making a dramatic lifestyle change like the Whole30.

You also need to do this because of a concept called "hyperbolic discounting."

This is an economics term that, if you're generous, could be applied to this "clean out the junk" situation. The idea is that you pay lots of attention to what's happening today, but pay less attention to what's happening in the future, because you think that Future You has way more free time, strength, and capacity. How does this apply here?

Today, you're on fire. You're feeling strong and confident and so excited about your Whole30 journey. You look at the chocolate, cookies, and chips sitting in your pantry and think, "I don't need those. I don't even want those." And you'll smugly just push them a little to the side and leave them there, because it's a pain to figure out what to do with them, and you think Future You will feel just as strong, confident, and excited as Today You.

But you won't.

At some point (many points), Future You will be stressed, craving, cranky, and doubting your own capacity. Future You will see that chocolate bar, package of cookies, and bag of chips and be so incredibly tormented by them. So much so that Future You may actually cave to the stress and temptation and eat one, bringing about the familiar cycle of guilt, shame, and remorse and breaking your Whole30 reset.

Don't discount Future You. Deal with the junk now, *because* you're feeling strong, so you have some breathing room when things get tough.

Future You will be grateful.

WHERE ARE MY KEYS?

Habit research shows that the average craving lasts only 3–5 minutes. If the stuff you're craving is anywhere nearby, that spells trouble. If it's not in the house, however, you've bought yourself some time. By the time you change out of your pajama pants, find your keys, grab your wallet, and head for the door, the craving has passed, and you've stuck to your Whole30 another day. Whew. For more craving-busting tips, see page 38.

Clean house

First, get all the stuff you won't be eating out of the house. Having tempting food-with-no-brakes just sitting around is a recipe for home-alone emotional binging, late-night stress eating, and enough constant temptation to wear out your willpower fast. So let's put some distance between you and those potato chips, shall we?

It's time to clean out the pantry—and we mean clean. it. out. Be rigorous here! The more thorough you are now, the easier time Future You will have distracting him- or herself from cravings. (Don't think you can get away with sticking it in a shoe box way in the back of your closet, either. Do you think Future You won't know it's there?)

So throw out the foods you won't be eating, give them to a neighbor for safekeeping, or (if you feel right about this) donate them to a local food bank.

Flying solo

One of the best parts of being an adult is the ability to make big decisions about your own life. Unfortunately, we don't get to make those decisions for the other adults in our lives, even when we think they're the right ones. You can't force your spouse or partner to eat what you eat, but you can (and should) commit to the Whole30 whole-heartedly if you believe it's the right thing for your health and happiness, even if no one else is on board.

You may also propose bringing kids along for the journey, but if your spouse insists they "deserve" their treats (and even undermines your authority on this one), don't fight it right now. This month is about changing your life and settling into your own new habits—that has to take priority until this lifestyle feels manageable and easy for you.

If you're the only one at home doing the Whole30, chances are your family isn't going to take kindly to you tossing out their favorite snacks and desserts. Dedicate one drawer in your fridge and one out-of-the-way cabinet for your family's off-plan items, so you don't have to reach around the Oreos every time you need a can of coconut milk.

At the same time, be very clear about how their actions could either help or hinder your efforts. Be specific about your expectations around junk or snack food: "Please don't offer me chocolate, even as a joke. That would be hard for me to turn down, and I really want to stay committed to this program for my health." However, don't expect them to totally change

their habits just to accommodate you. Know that if family movie night generally involves popcorn and candy, you're going to need a plan to participate without feeling left out, so have a plan (like making a batch of kale chips and brewing a cup of herbal tea) before they break out the air-popper.

Your family may be worried that you'll "spoil" family traditions like movie night or Sunday pancake breakfast because you're now making different food choices. As always, communication here is key. Talk to your family about their concerns, and get their input on how to preserve the tradition in a way that works for everyone. Institute a family bike ride or board game after dinner instead of an ice-cream fest, and assure your kids that you'll still enjoy breakfast in your pajamas with them on Sunday morning. Don't become a Whole30 hermit! Find ways to enjoy the social interaction of date night, birthday parties, or other family gatherings while staying true to the Whole30. You'll get support simply by socializing, and your family will see this lifestyle isn't so limiting after all.

Finally, if you're the primary grocery shopper and cook in your household, determine ahead of time how much modification you're willing to make to your shopping list and the meals you prepare. Will you still buy their chips, snack cakes, and candy, or will they have to buy those things themselves? Will you make separate breakfasts and lunches, but only one compliant dinner? Will you make only Whole30 meals, and they can add their own dinner roll, side of rice, or soy sauce if they choose?

Communicate your decision ahead of time to your family—don't wait until dinnertime to announce that you're not making the pasta they requested. Involve them in the process, if they're

---

SET THE STAGE

Even if your family won't do the program with you, it's still important that they support you in your journey. Write down your motivation for completing the program specific to your family: "I want more energy to play with you on the weekend" or "I want less joint pain so we can hike as a family." Hang it somewhere you can all see it every day. Share your motivation with your family and explain to them why you are committed to this program. Communicate why it's important to you, but agree not to nag, fuss, or fight about what they choose to eat. Finally, make a list of ways you can all treat yourselves (without food) during these 30 days, and then make the time as a family to do it.

willing. ("Would you rather have sweet potato or roasted butternut squash tonight?") And try to find at least one part of each meal that everyone at the table can enjoy together, like a salad with homemade ranch dressing, a grilled steak, or our Watermelon Salad (page 359), to give them a taste (literally) of your Whole30.

Now that you've got space in your pantry and a family food strategy, it's time to focus on what you'll be eating for the next 30 days.

Plan some meals

Even if you're not the planning type, you really want to have at least the first few days of Whole30 meals planned. First, as we'll explain in our Grocery Shopping section (page 192), it's economical, ensuring you'll buy only what you need and won't have to throw away food you ended up not eating. But more important than that, we want to do everything we can to keep our brain happy during what is sure to be a tumultuous ride, and . . .

The brain loves a plan.

Back in the 1920s, a Russian psychologist discovered that incomplete or interrupted tasks tend to "stick around" in people's brains, distracting us and stressing us out. This preoccupation with things left undone requires so much cognitive effort that it keeps our brains from focusing on other (more important) things. We suspect you've all experienced this—the distraction, unease, and restless sleep that comes from the half-completed paper due next week, the work project you're behind on, or the email you really need to send tomorrow.

Now, let's apply this to the Whole30.

You're ready to start the program. You've got some friends supporting you. Of course, you plan on grocery shopping for some Whole30 food. But you're going to play your meals by ear. After all, how hard can it be? A hunk of meat, fill your plate with vegetables, add some fat. Simple.

Not so simple for your brain, which senses there's some unfinished business here. What, exactly, will you eat? Will Monday's dinner make good leftovers for Tuesday's lunch? You have an early meeting on Wednesday, what can you make for breakfast in under ten minutes? What the heck will you do with the Brussels sprouts you bought, anyway? This uncertainty makes your brain very unhappy, which makes *you* distracted, stressed, and unhappy.

Don't underestimate how different your next 30 days are going to look from how you used to eat, even if you used to eat pretty healthy. There's no more picking up pizza when you're really tired, unwinding with a glass of wine after a long day, or relying on the whole-grain bagel on the breakroom counter to get you through your mid-afternoon meeting.

You cannot eat raw Brussels sprouts in a business meeting. Well, you could, but that would be weird, and not very tasty.

You really need a plan.

Make a plan for what you'll eat for breakfast, lunch, and dinner for the first three to seven days of your Whole30. Write it down, in detail: the complete meal, the page of the recipe or cooking technique, the ingredients you need to buy, whether you'll make extra for leftovers. ("Cook extra chicken breasts on Tuesday, use leftovers in Harvest Chicken Salad for Wednesday lunch.") Look at your calendar and identify challenging circumstances during this time period—early meetings, business lunches, sports matches, travel—and write down how you'll handle them. ("Pack a Primal Pac and an RxBar on Wednesday in case my plane is delayed.")

Now your brain is happy.

Even though you haven't prepared, cooked, or eaten the meals, your brain still has a sense of completion because you have a *plan*. (Bonus: without the thought of "what am I going to eat for breakfast?" swirling around your head at midnight, you'll sleep better, too!) So even if you're a competent cook, a healthy eater, or a die-hard fly-by-the-seat-of-your-pants kind of person . . . trust us on this one. At least for the first few days, make a plan.

If you want to wing it for the rest of your Whole30, go right ahead . . . but if that ever stresses you out, you know exactly what to do to make your brain happy again.

Go shopping

Time to stock up on Whole30 foods! If you're planning to use our seven-day meal plan, we've made this task really easy for you. Just download our ready-to-go shopping list at www.whole30.com/pdf-downloads and fill your cart.

> ### OUR WHOLE30 MEAL PLAN
>
> We've given you a detailed seven-day meal plan on page 196, but this is more for inspiration than an absolute directive. You're all grown-ups, and you are fully capable of deciding for yourself what to eat for breakfast on Thursday. Read through our general plan and adapt it for your own tastes, lifestyle, family, and budget. Or, keep it simple and just do exactly what we tell you for the first week, just to get you started. We (and your brain) won't mind that one bit.

If you're going to create your own meal plan, you'll want to read our best tips for saving time and money at the grocery store before you decide what you'll be eating. (A budget-conscious shopping strategy may actually influence your breakfast, lunch, and dinner choices!) Turn to page 194 and read through this section before creating your meal plan and hitting the grocery store.

STEP 4: Plan for Success

Unless you plan on living like a recluse for the next 30 days, your Whole30 will likely be littered with obstacles. Spur-of-the-moment dinner invitations, meetings that run long, travel delays, a stressful encounter the likes of which you used to manage with wine and ice cream . . . Unfortunately, when people hit some of these unexpected tough situations, they often quit their Whole30 right then and there. Why?

Because they have no plan.

Are you seeing a theme here?

So right now, before your Whole30 actually starts, we're going to sit down and think about the next 30 days. Let's anticipate all of your obstacles, and make a plan for what you'll do when you face them. We like using if/then statements when crafting our plans, so we'll follow this template for helping you map out your best Whole30 success strategies.

Prepare, prepare, prepare some more

First, write down every potential stressful, difficult, or complicated situation you may encounter during your Whole30. These may include business lunches, family dinners, travel plans, a long day at work, birthday parties, holiday celebrations, office gatherings, family stress, job stress, financial

IF/THEN

Studies show you are two to three times more likely to succeed in your goal if you use an if/then plan than if you don't. Here's how it works: Habits have three parts: the cue, the routine, and the reward. If/then statements create a really strong link between the cue (the "if") with the routine (the "then"). That strong link means you're more likely to follow through with the action automatically, with far less effort. And "less effort" translates to "less willpower required," which is always a good thing when highly tempting, rewarding comfort foods are involved.

stress . . . really, anything you think might come along and attempt to derail your Whole30 train.

If there's nothing definitive on your calendar, use history as your guide. If the last three times you visited your mom you came home and binged on chocolate, that's one "if." If the last time you had a late, stressful night at the office, you broke open the wine, that's another. It won't hurt for you to over-plan at this juncture—the more situations you've accounted for, the more relaxed your brain will be, and the more likely you are to stick to your Whole30 when challenges come up.

The next step is to create the "then" part of your plan for each potentially difficult situation: "If this happens, then I'll do this." Again, you'll want to write this down. Here are some examples:

BUSINESS LUNCH: If my co-workers pressure me to have a drink, then I'll say, "I'm doing this food experiment to see if I can make my allergies better—I'll just have a mineral water, please." (Or, use a strategy outlined in our Dining Out chapter on page 89.)

FAMILY DINNER: If Mom invites me out for dinner, then I'll remind her I'm doing the Whole30, and ask if I can cook for her instead.

FAMILY DINNER PART 2: If my mom insists on taking me out, then I'll ask her if we can go to (Whole30-friendly restaurant), because it's my favorite and I haven't been in ages.

FAMILY DINNER PART 3: If dinner at my mom's turns into an inquisition about my "crazy diet," then I'll tell them I'm happy to share all the details after dinner, and change the subject by asking someone a question about their life.

TRAVEL DAY: If I get to the airport and my flight is delayed, then I'll snack on the Primal Pacs, apples, carrot sticks, and the individually sized packet of almond butter I brought in my carry-on.

STUCK IN TRAFFIC: If I get stuck in bad traffic, then I'll put on my favorite podcast and snack on the dried fruit-and-nut bar I keep in my glove compartment for emergencies.

BIRTHDAY PARTY: If my office has a birthday celebration, then I'll make sure I've already eaten when I arrive at the party, politely refuse the cake, but stick around and socialize with all of my co-workers.

HOLIDAY: If I'm invited to a holiday cookout, then I'll ask the host about the menu and bring an appetizer and a compliant side dish so I know there will be something I can eat.

FAMILY TRADITION: If my spouse makes pancakes on Sunday, then I'll also make a hearty frittata so we can still eat together and I won't be tempted.

DAILY RITUAL: If I'm tempted to munch on potato chips during our nightly TV time, then I'll make a cup of herbal tea, or skip TV and read a book or take a bath instead.

WINE RITUALS: (yes, these deserve their own category): If I'm craving a glass of wine after work, then I'll create a new ritual: pour some kombucha into a fancy glass and relax with my spouse/kids for 20 minutes.

STRESSFUL SITUATION: If I find myself stressed/lonely/anxious and tempted to eat my usual comfort foods, then I'll call one of the people on my support list and ask them to talk it through with me, then make a delicious Whole30 dinner so I'm well-fed.

KNOWN "TRIGGER": If I have a fight with my spouse, then I'll call my friend and we'll go out for coffee or a healthy Whole30-compliant meal.

LONG DAY AT THE OFFICE: If I get home from work starving and cranky and I'm tempted to order take-out, then I'll cook a meal from my go-to list.

EMERGENCY DINNERS

Plan three quick and easy "go-to" meals you can make in ten minutes or less, with foods you always have on hand. Some examples are a Kitchen Sink Scrambled Eggs (page 202) using whatever veggies you have on hand and topped with hot sauce; our No-Fuss Salmon Cakes (page 346); a can of tuna mixed with homemade mayo, fresh fruit, and walnuts over salad greens; or a Pre-Made Paleo meal (see page 403) straight out of the freezer. Write your list down and pin it to your fridge, so you'll always have a plan for nights when things just get crazy.

Whew. Do you have a long list? Good! That means you've really thought through all of the challenges you might face in the coming days, and given your brain a good plan so it knows exactly where to steer you if your "if" situation comes up.

Finally, it's always a good thing to have a catchall if/then scenario here, so if you find yourself caught unawares, you still have a way to deal with it that doesn't involve ditching your Whole30. Try this: "If something comes up that I didn't anticipate and I feel tempted to go off-plan, then I'll . . ." Fill in your own blank—call a friend, go for a walk, make yourself a cup of tea, jump on our Forums for support, anything you think will help you overcome the challenge and stick to your Whole30 for yet another day.

Because sometimes, that's how you work this program.

One day, one meal, one bite at a time.

STEP 5: Toss That Scale

This is your last and final step in preparing for the Whole30, and it's the one you may have the hardest time following. However, we take this rule very seriously, and you should, too.

There is no faster way to sabotage your Whole30 than to subject yourself to weekly (or daily) weigh-ins. If you've been a slave to that numerical readout, it's time to set yourself free, at least for the next 30 days. Why are we so dead-set against tracking your "progress" based on body weight?

Oh, there are so many reasons. We'll narrow it down to four.

First, scale weight fluctuates wildly. It's good to measure things to track progress, and if you weighed yourself monthly, that might help you spot a trend in your body weight (gaining, losing, or maintaining). However, over the course of a day (or even a few hours) your weight can go up or down by as much as five or six pounds, and that fluctuation isn't at all representative of body fat gained or lost. You can eat a few higher-carb meals and gain a few pounds of water weight, or wake up dehydrated and "lose" a pound or two.

When it comes to your body weight, the time of day matters, what you're wearing matters, even where you step on your scale matters, assuming you don't have a doctor-grade scale in your home bathroom. Allow us to remind you, that number is coming from a $20 hunk of plastic you bought at the local value store. Weighing yourself daily tells you nothing about your big-picture trend, and only serves to reinforce the next three points.

Second, scale weight says nothing of your health. You want to lose 20 pounds? We can make that happen. Cut your daily calories in half

and spend two hours a day doing low-intensity cardio. That'll make that scale show the "right" number . . . for about a month. Until your willpower runs out (as those behaviors aren't at all sustainable), and your messed-up metabolism fights back. At which point, you gain all the weight back and then some. But hey, for a few weeks, your scale said you were down 20 pounds!

Does that digital readout moving in either direction tell you anything about whether you're in worse or better health? Of course not. (In our scenario, the scale is going down, but your health certainly isn't improving! Conversely, you could be doing some smart strength training, sleeping well, and eating healthy, and be gaining weight in muscle mass—but that weight gain doesn't mean your health is declining!) That scale number alone tells you nothing about what's going on with your relationship with food, hormones, digestive system, or inflammatory status. That number on the scale doesn't reflect improved cravings, better sleep, a happier mood, or a boost in self-esteem. And those are the factors that impact your health far more directly than your body weight.

Third, the scale blinds you to the real results you are achieving every day you are on the Whole30. By focusing so much of your attention on that number on the scale, you effectively miss out on observing the other, more significant, results of your efforts. Your skin is clearing up. Your wedding ring slides on easier. Your mobility is increasing. You breathe easier when you run. Your nose isn't as stuffy. You passed up donuts at work without a second thought. Your kids made a mess and you didn't snap at them. You've discovered a love of cooking. Those results could be motivating you to continue with your new healthy habits—but until you stop obsessing about gaining or losing half a pound, you'll never be able to see the emotional, mental, and physical progress you've actually been making.

Fourth, the scale maintains control of your self-esteem. This is perhaps the most important reason of all to break up with your scale. It's psychologically unhealthy to allow a number—any number—to determine your sense of self-worth, value, or self-confidence. And yet, that's exactly what happens to people who are overly invested in their scale.

This breaks our heart.

It's downright tragic that your daily weigh-in determines whether you have a good day or bad day, and whether or not you feel good about yourself. The scale results can take you from confident to self-loathing in under 5 seconds, but what the scale is telling you *is not real*. You are working hard to change your habits. You are overcoming obstacles on a daily basis. You are taking better care of yourself than you have in years. You are actually doing what people every day wish they could do—change their lives for the better.

You know what this makes us want to say?

Very bad words about your scale.

So please, for the next 30 days, get rid of your scale. Put it in the garage, give it to a friend to "hold," or better yet, take it out back and introduce it to your sledgehammer in a nice little pre-Whole30 ritual.

If you do that, please video it and send it to us. We'd love to see that.

You deserve better, and your daily weigh-in is one more habit we really want you to conquer on the Whole30.

Do measure "before and after"

We'll give you a very long list of ways to measure your Whole30 success starting on page 43, including the many physical benefits of the program. However, though we don't focus on weight loss, most people do lose weight or improve their body composition, and that certainly can be part of what motivates you to keep up with your new healthy habits when your Whole30 is over.

> **SOUND FAMILIAR?**
>
> You hop out of bed and head straight for your scale—buck naked, of course. (Can't let clothing factor into your daily weigh-in.) You hop on, close your eyes, cross your fingers, and then peek. Whoo-hoo! Down one pound! It's going to be a great day! You jump into the shower refreshed and invigorated, ready to tackle your morning. The next day, the routine repeats itself—only today, you open your eyes to find you're up two pounds. Two. Whole. Pounds. Immediately, your heart sinks, and you run through all the "bad" food you ate yesterday. Was it that extra helping of potatoes? The snack you had before dinner? The kombucha? You immediately calculate a "fix" for the situation—today, you'll only have two eggs for breakfast, no snacking no matter what, and maybe you'll do a little extra cardio at the gym. You get dressed for work convinced you look awful (wearing the pants that were your favorite just last week), and dejectedly start your day feeling fat and ugly.

MEASURING SUCCESS

We don't want you to ignore your body for the next 30 days—just the force of attraction between you and the earth. (That's all your scale measures, after all!) You can still observe changes in your body and see them as progress. Keep an eye on how your clothes are fitting—are they hanging easier, fitting looser, or are they easier to button or zip? (Pay close attention to your "usual" belt loop here—you may have to adjust by a notch or two before your program is over.) Is your stomach flatter, indicating less bloating, constipation, or water retention? Are your rings slipping on or off easier, demonstrating a decrease in swelling or inflammation? Examine your skin—is it less dry, flaky, or broken out? Are your nails starting to grow, is your hair shedding less or feeling thicker? All of these physical changes are yet another sign that your Whole30 is moving you in the right direction!

However, we understand it's really hard for you to evaluate your own physical progress just using a mirror. You see yourself every day, and small daily changes are easy to go unnoticed. So while we don't want to see any of this weighing or measuring during your program, we encourage you to set yourself up for comparison for the day your Whole30 is over.

Weigh yourself on Day 0, before your Whole30 starts. You can also take body measurements if you like—try upper arms, chest, waist, hips, and thighs. We also encourage you to take a before picture, even if it feels embarrassing. You never have to show anyone, but we really want you to have it for posterity.

Trust us on this one.

Find a plain backdrop, stand in as little clothing as you're comfortable in (no shirt and shorts for men, and a jog bra and shorts or bathing suit for women), and have someone take a full-body shot from the front, back, and side. Then, repeat the process in the same manner (ideally wearing the same clothing) on Day 31.

You may be so proud of your accomplishment that you want to share them with us! If so, turn to page 405 and we'll tell you how.

And with that, now it's almost time to kick off your Whole30 program, using the plan you've created and the many resources we've got available for you here. But first . . .

Want a sneak preview of what's likely to happen during your Whole30? We've created a Whole30 Timeline as a tongue-in-cheek (but eerily accurate) way to help new participants anticipate what to expect. As with any process that involves personal experience, your results may vary, but here's what your program might look like.

the whole30 timeline

"I was diagnosed with Mast Cell Disease (Systemic Mastocytosis) several years ago. With this condition, you can experience severe allergic types of reactions, and I have struggled with hives, joint pain, and gastro-intestinal issues for years. Within seven days of my first Whole30, I popped out of bed without joint pain. Within ten days, I had lost the GI distress and bloating that's been a 'normal' part of my existence. The Whole30 has definitely changed my life! My energy is way up, my constant food demons are gone (no more cravings for the stuff that makes me sick) and I just plain old feel great!" —ANNEMARIE G., NEWBURYPORT, MA

You've read up on the program, chosen your start date, and signed up for the Whole30 Daily. You've even recruited friends or family to do the program with you, or at the very least, shared your commitment with them.

It's official: you are doing the Whole30!

But before you actually begin, we should talk about what you can expect to happen over the next 30 days: the ups and the downs.

Wait—the downs?

Yes, downs. Because despite how amazing most people feel at the end of their Whole30 journey, the path you'll be walking for the next month will be rough in spots, and we want to be up front about that. We want you to trust us, and know that we care so much about you and your Whole30 experience that we're willing to shine a bright light on some of the more difficult parts of the program.

In a nutshell, the next month will likely play out like a Telemundo soap opera. As one Whole30 participant put it on Twitter, "Week 1 on the #Whole30 recap: I'm starving, I'm tired, I don't like you, I feel GREAT, I'm hungry again, I feel GREAT, this is stupid."

We found this tweet surprisingly quite accurate.

You'll be exhilarated! You'll be exhausted. You'll be happy! You'll be Señor Crankypants. You'll be feeling fit, healthy, and gorgeous today, and tomorrow believe this isn't working at all. You'll find yourself thinking at the same time that the Whole30 is the best thing that's ever happened to you, and you cannot wait for it to be over.

All of these things will happen, because when you take on something as big as changing your life, it's kind of a big deal. We know our Whole30 "tough love" says this is not hard, and that's true in some ways; after all, you've made it through way harder things than passing up a stale muffin at your weekly staff meeting. But we also acknowledge that this *is* hard. Examining your emotional relationship with food is hard. Breaking habits that started in childhood is hard. Learning to love, comfort, and bond with others (and yourself) without using junk food as an offering is hard.

And that's just the mental stuff.

Physically, you've been throwing your body off balance for the last five (ten? twenty?) years by overconsuming foods that promote cravings, disrupt your hormones, damage your gut, and overwork your immune system. Through your food choices, you've been unknowingly waging a war with your body. Starting the Whole30 is like calling a ceasefire, which means things will eventually get better . . . but first comes a massive clean up effort, which can be just as disruptive and feel just as chaotic as the war itself.

It's not all sunshine and rainbows, and things may get worse before they get better.

But during the process, you will also gain confidence. You will feel proud of yourself. You will be happier, you will feel more energetic, you will "show up" more in life. Your energy will increase, you'll be sleeping more soundly, and your cravings will diminish, if not vanish.

There is lots of sunshine and likely more than a few rainbows in your future.

Hundreds of thousands of people have already completed a Whole30 (and most have returned for more). Through their experience and our scientific research, we've created this Whole30 Timeline—a detailed outline of common experiences to prepare you for some of the physical and emotional challenges you may face, and give you something to look forward to if the days get hard.

The Whole30 Timeline

DAY 1: No big deal/what have I done

It's 3 p.m. on Day 1. You effortlessly breezed past the break room donuts, feeling smug and satisfied after your breakfast frittata. Coffee

with coconut milk actually isn't that bad, and you've packed a big protein salad for lunch. You resisted the pull of a mid-afternoon treat and munched on some jerky and an apple instead. You have a slow cooker full of chili infusing your kitchen with a heavenly smell, and right now, you just can't see why anyone thinks this Whole30 stuff is hard.

This delusion is somewhat akin to the first episode of any reality show where the contestants are herded together and forced to live in one house. At the end of the first episode, everyone just knows they are going to be best friends for life.

Those of us on the other side of the screen know better.

We're thrilled that you're feeling empowered by making one good choice after another all day long. Take note of that Rock Star feeling, stash it away, and bring it back out about an hour later.

You'll likely need it.

Today you may spend the hours bouncing between feeling really energized and completely overwhelmed. You could be wondering how you'll make it 30 days without your favorite foods, or maybe the general "differentness" of the coming days just freaks you out. The idea of changing your life is super exciting, but it's also a little scary.

Our good friend Melissa Joulwan coined a term for this: "frexcited."

This is totally normal.

Share your excitement when you're excited. Allow yourself to feel nervous, too, but remember you have a great plan, lots of support, and some fantastic resources to see you through the next 30 days—so you really have no reason to be nervous.

Well, maybe one.

Because after years (or decades) of less-than-healthy food habits, the next few days may be seriously deficient in sunshine or rainbows.

DAYS 2 TO 3: The hangover

The alarm rings on Day 2 and you pop out of bed expecting to feel great, just like you did yesterday. Instead, you feel headache-y, a little sore, foggy . . . kind of like a hangover. You're pretty sure you didn't down a fifth of tequila in your sleep, so what happened?

Let's revisit what you were consuming before you started the Whole30.

Pizzas, cookies, beer or wine, fast food, potato chips, candy, muffins, bagels, bread (so much bread). This is when the ghost of your high-sugar, high-carb, nutrient-poor past comes back to kick you in the butt—and apparently, the head.

Here's a little math equation for Days 2 to 3. The amount of suck you experience in this phase is directly proportional to the amount of junk you consumed before you began the program. Especially if you consumed it consistently. (This phase is also approximately 34 percent harder for the habitual soda drinkers, as you are eliminating not just the massive hit of sweetness, but the extra caffeine, too.)

Nearly all Whole30ers report headaches, fatigue, brain fog, and general malaise during this part of the program. Your body is having a hard time adjusting to the new foods you're eating, and going without the sugary food-like products you used to eat. (See page 5 for a more detailed explanation.) This process lasts a day for some lucky folks, but for others it can last several. Relax, drink a lot of water, take it easy in the gym, and keep making good food choices.

Now would also be a good time to recruit the sympathy and support of friends and family, because . . .

DAYS 4 TO 5: Kill all the things

Day 4 dawns and you tentatively step out of bed, expecting to feel like you took a headshot from Thor's hammer. Instead, your brain is surprisingly clear. Your limbs feel functional. This could be a good day. You walk into the kitchen and, upon being greeted by the smiling face of your significant other, you are suddenly overcome with the desire to punch them in the face for being so darn cheerful this early in the morning.

EAT ALL THE THINGS

You may also notice a desire to Eat All the Things in this stage, too. That's pretty common, as your body demands the sugar it's been running on, and your brain is craving the sweet, salty, fatty rewards you used to feed it. Focus on making each of your three meals a day a little bigger, include a mini-meal if needed to see you through, and use our Craving vs. Hunger test on page 129 to help you distinguish between actual hunger and your brain throwing a tantrum.

Congratulations! You've made it to Day 4.

Over the next two days, prepare yourself for the overwhelming urge to Kill All the Things. Your kids will forever be working your last nerve, the way co-workers talk, chew, and breathe will annoy you, and chipper cashiers and baristas will cower in your crankiness.

Your brain won't be happy when you withhold your previously generous rewards of super-sweet, salty, and fatty junk foods—and an unhappy brain is a stressed and anxious brain. Not to mention your hormones are desperately trying to keep up with your new food choices, your gut is trying to heal, you've had a headache for the last three days, and you really miss your diet soda.

This too shall pass.

Beg your spouse, children, parents, and co-workers for patience and forgiveness as nicely as you can, preferably before you tell them to stop breathing so loud. Take a deep breath, eat some sweet potato, and remind yourself of why you took on the Whole30 in the first place. We promise you will feel better soon.

DAYS 6 TO 7: I just want a nap

It's Day 6, and you made it through the last phase without smiting anyone. Hoorah! The thing is, today you don't feel like you could smite anyone if your life depended on it. It's 10 a.m. and all you can think about is crawling under your desk for a catnap. As the day drags on, your desk is morphing from hard wooden surface to snuggly warm pillow right before your eyes. You hit the gym in a daze and wonder if you fell asleep in child's pose, would anyone notice?

You hold off crawling into bed until the reasonable hour of 8 p.m., only to drag yourself up eleven hours later feeling no more rested than you did the day before.

We know exactly what you're thinking.

For the love of Oprah, I thought this Whole30 thing was supposed to make me feel better. Isn't eating like this supposed to *increase* my energy levels?

Yes, in the long run. See, you've been reliant on sugar for energy for a really long time. Because of all the muffins, mocha lattes, and junk foods you've been eating, you trained your body to need sugar every few hours to function. Now, your body can also run very well on fat as fuel, but your mitochondria (the cellular "powerhouses") need time to learn how to use body and dietary fat to power you. Which means you're stuck in this limbo where you aren't eating the energy you know how to run on, and you're not good at using the energy you've got on hand. (See page 124 for more information.)

Studies show the process of "fat adaption" (the ability to use fat as fuel) actually starts in just a few days, but takes a few weeks to fully ramp up. The good news is that people generally experience this switch by the second week of the program, so if you can hold out just a bit longer, you'll reap the major benefits of fat adaption—namely, consistently high energy morning, noon, and night.

Besides, you could probably use a day off from the gym anyway.

DAYS 8 TO 9: NOOO! my pants are TIGHTER!

You've made it through the Hangover, managed not to Kill All the Things, and are feeling far more peppy.

Then, you put on your jeans.

They're just jeans—not your skinniest jeans, just normal, comfortable jeans. In fact, they're the jeans you wore just three days ago. (You were too tired to wash them. It's okay, we understand.) Three days ago, they fit. But this morning you had to take a big deep breath to get that button where it ought to be.

Seriously, Whole30? Seriously?

Luckily, this phase doesn't happen to everyone—but if it's happening to you, here's why: The same processes that ran over you like a truck a few days ago are still working their magic in your body. Your body composition is not actually changing for the worse, we assure you. But the enzymes that digest your food and the millions of bacteria that live in your gut are adjusting to your new intake of meat and vegetables, and the lack of easy-access sugars. This is something they do naturally, and these adjustments will go a long way to improve your gut function long-term. However, these adjustments can be a bit uncomfortable. Bloating, constipation, diarrhea, or all three may appear (or reappear) as your gut starts to heal, rebalance, and process this new food effectively.

The good news is that most people find this phase passes relatively quickly, and their pants are easy to button again within just a few days.

WHAT-MAPS?

Your increased intake of fruits and vegetables may be the culprit here. First, while these plants are nutrient-dense, they also contain something called FODMAPs—a collection of fermentable carbohydrates and sugar alcohols found in various foods, including vegetables and fruits. FODMAPs are poorly absorbed, thereby "feeding" gut bacteria and causing a host of symptoms, including gas, bloating, digestive distress, and systemic inflammation. Plus, while fiber is healthy, the sudden increase in insoluble fiber from things like leafy greens, broccoli, and cauliflower may be irritating your digestive tract. Refer to our Troubleshooting guide on page 124 if you want a little digestive help during this phase.

DAYS 10 TO 11: The hardest days

Fact: based on observing hundreds of thousands of people run through the program, we know you are most likely to quit your Whole30 program on day 10 or 11. By this point, the newness of the program has worn off. You've already experienced most of the unpleasant physical milestones, but you've yet to see any of the "magic" the program promises. You're still struggling to establish a new routine (you are so. tired. of. eggs.), and while you've been trying really hard to have a good attitude, today you are incredibly aware of all the foods you're "choosing not to eat right now." Everywhere you look, you see the things you can't have: the melted cheese on your co-worker's burger, the creaminess of your neighbor's coffee, the cold beer in your friend's tailgate cooler.

Arghh! This is hard! Will the results really be as good as "they" all say it is?

You are cranky. You are impatient. You are a grown-up person who can eat cheese if you decide you want to eat cheese. And the Whole30 is just some stupid challenge anyway.

This is where you really start to experience the psychological power of your food choices and habits. You've put in a lot of effort to get to where you are right now. Your brain demands some kind of reward (but you deserve it!) and food has always been your go-to prize. But instead of a treat, you're standing face-to-face with the realization that you have twenty more days of perceived deprivation ahead of you.

First, if you know these days are coming, they won't come hurtling out of nowhere and knock you off your game. Prepare for them and you'll have a much easier time. Yes, you do deserve a reward for working so hard and staying on point—but it's time you redefine your idea of reward. Think long and hard about the foods you're grieving and ask yourself what need you're expecting them to fulfill. Are you feeling anxious and looking for reassurance? Are you feeling sad, and looking for something to cheer you up? Are you worried you won't successfully finish the program, and it's easier to self-sabotage than fail?

Remind yourself that food cannot fill that void for you. When has a cupcake ever made you feel truly accomplished, comforted, calm, or beautiful? So find another way to fill that need. Schedule a date with a friend, treat yourself to a new kitchen gadget (look for inspiration on pages 140–145), or get a massage. Rely on support from friends, family, or our online Forum

or social media community to see you through. (A quick post that says, "Help!" always has our attention.)

The good news? Just get through these two days and things will be much better.

DAYS 12 TO 15: I dream of . . . junk food?

Hurrah! The slump is over! Most people report that most of the negative symptoms we've been describing are gone by the end of the second week. Your pants fit again! Your energy levels are back to normal! You're back to feeling confident in your commitment!

But something weird is happening.

You're dreaming. Not crazy nightmare or strange surrealist dreams. Incredibly normal and realistic dreams—about donuts. Or Twinkies. Or fast-food hamburgers. Often, people dream of things they'd never actually eat or drink in real life! This experience is incredibly common on the Whole30, and some say rivals the kinds of weird cravings and dreams you get during pregnancy. (One Whole30er reported craving pickles and Doritos together during this phase! We're pretty sure he wasn't pregnant.)

These dreams usually go one of two ways. You either enjoy the heck out of it and wake up laughing, or you believe you're doing something wrong in your dream, and you wake up feeling guilty.

Please. There is no guilt about what you do when you dream. The Whole30 rules are pretty comprehensive, but they can't touch what happens in your subconscious. Which is really good news, because some of you seriously pig out while you're REM-ing.

The trouble is, sometimes these dreams and cravings carry over into real life. The diet soda ad on the billboard is calling your name, and your co-workers' heads transform into giant Girl Scout cookies as you gaze on in disbelief.

All joking aside, this phase can be really intense for some people. This is the part of the program where our brains are desperate to drive us back to the comfort of the foods we used to reward ourselves with. Our food relationships are deeply rooted and strongly reinforced throughout the course of our lives, and trying to change them is a difficult, emotional process.

CRAVING BUSTERS

Based on studies of people resisting temptation, the average craving lasts around three minutes, and the most effective way to get through it is to distract yourself. Go for a short walk (even if it's just around the office), pay a bill or two, drink a glass of water, take a sniff of some peppermint essential oils, text a friend, or read a few pages of a good book. Now is not the time to indulge in a sweet Whole30 treat like a dried-fruit-and-nut bar—that's just changing the ingredients in your reward, and it won't help you break that giving-in-to-a-craving habit.

DAYS 16 TO 27: Tiger blood!

You've hit the downhill slope of your Whole30 and life is beautiful—which means different things for different people. For some (generally people who came to the program eating well, exercising regularly, and feeling pretty good to begin with), Tiger Blood means you woke up feeling like someone flipped a switch and turned on the awesome. Your energy is through the roof, cravings are under control, clothes are fitting better, workouts are stronger—you feel unstoppable!

For others, this Tiger Blood stage feels more like a real sense of self-efficacy. It doesn't mean things are perfect or even easy, but you're proving to yourself that you can do this, things are getting better, and you're seeing small improvements almost daily. Your energy is steadier, you have a firmer handle on the cravings, and you're experimenting with new, delicious foods. You may notice that your ability to focus is keener, your body composition is changing, your moods are more stable, you're stepping up your exercise, or you're just plain happier these days.

Of course, this may not happen like magic at the halfway point. There are a huge number of factors that influence which benefits you see and when. If you're one of those folks who has hit the halfway mark and isn't seeing or feeling the dramatic changes others have reported, know this:

You're not doing it wrong.

If you began the Whole30 with a medical condition, a long history of unhealthy food habits, or a chronically stressful lifestyle, your magic may take longer to appear, and probably won't be a "light switch" moment. So don't stress about whether you're feeling honest-to-goodness "Tiger Blood"—be patient, and be on the lookout for small, gradual improvements to keep you motivated. Slow and steady still wins this race.

DAY 21 (INTERLUDE): I am so over this.

You've solidly settled into week three of the program, but despite the benefits you're seeing, you went to bed last night dreading the thought of breakfast. You weren't much more excited about it this morning, either. Come to think of it, you're so un-thrilled with any of your meal options right now that if Iron Chef Bobby Flay were to waltz into your kitchen and ask you what you wanted to eat, you'd probably just say, "Ugh."

You're loving the way your body is responding to the program, but you're just not sure if you can make it through nine more days. The culprit? A major case of food boredom. For some folks, it gets so overwhelming that they lose their appetite altogether for a day or two.

You know that being bored and hungry is just a recipe for disaster.

The solution: don't let the food fatigue overtake you! Rekindle your appetite and your enthusiasm for the program by making something new from the @whole30recipes Instagram feed, schedule a potluck with your Whole30 friends, or treat yourself to a new cookbook (see page 402). We guarantee you haven't tried all the combinations of food available to you on the Whole30, so make a little effort and you'll get over this hump all the faster.

DAYS 22 TO 25: The scale (and mirror) are calling . . .

In your third week, you may notice yourself pausing in front of the mirror a little more frequently, taking an embarrassing number of half-naked selfies, and staring longingly at the spot on your bathroom floor where your scale used to live. You've been focusing on all of your non-scale victories for the last three weeks, but now you're just dying to know . . . has anything really changed? (And by *anything*, you mean *your body*.)

Fact: this is the period of time when you are most likely to break our "no scale" rule, or find yourself analyzing, scrutinizing, and judging whether individual body parts have shrunk, firmed up, or look any different at all. This can be *very* distracting. In fact, this is quite likely to pull you right out of the positive, self-confident space you've been occupying for the last week or so, and send you spiraling right back down into self-doubt, negative self-talk, and discouragement. (This is even more likely to happen if you've been white-knuckling your way through our "no scale" rule all along, continually fantasizing about stepping on the scale.)

Know this time period is coming, and resist the "craving" to weigh or over-analyze. Go back to your original Whole30 non-scale goals, and note the progress you've made. Create a list of everything you want to accomplish before your program is over, and focus on making it happen. Make a conscious effort to bypass the mirror unless you really need it (yes, you do have kale stuck in your teeth), and compliment your friends and family for something *other* than their appearance. We guarantee if you change your focus, your urge to weigh or measure will pass fast, and you'll slip right back into your happy, confident, proud Whole30 routine.

DAY 28: 28 is as good as 30 . . . right?

It's Day 28. DAY 28! You're almost there! You've pushed through all the rough spots, fought off the food boredom, and you really love where you are right now. This Whole30 thing is like second nature by now, and you're primed to make it through Day 28 without breaking a sweat—until you get to work.

Today is your department's monthly birthday celebration, and at the break a co-worker teases, "You've been so good for 28 days! You can have just one cupcake with us to celebrate." You brush the comment off (you're used to them at this point), but it really gets you thinking. You *have* been so good. And it's been *so long*. You're practically done already.

Aren't 28 days just as good as 30?

Um, no. Twenty-eight days is not as good as 30.

You made a commitment to give yourself 30 full days of Good Food and improved habits. You made a commitment to finish the Whole30, and reintroduce foods in a systematic, deliberate fashion. You made a commitment to changing your life, and the specific commitment you made was to last 30 full days.

Take these promises seriously. If you cop out now, you're telling yourself that the commitments you make to yourself are open to compromise. You're telling yourself that you are not important enough to honor your promise to you. But that is simply not true.

You are important.

You are worth the promise.

So take a deep breath, say "No, thank you," and celebrate with a self-five for seeing your commitment through. (We promise it's much more satisfying than a store-bought cupcake.)

DAYS 29 AND 30: Holyoprahitsalmost overwhatamigoingtoeatnow?

It's Day 29, and you are winning the Whole30. The thoughts you had yesterday of throwing in the towel were gone as fast as they arrived. You effortlessly cruise through the day and crawl into bed thinking happily, "Tomorrow is Day 30!"

Wait. TOMORROW IS DAY 30.

This small thought grows into full-blown, cold-sweat panic. Tomorrow is your last day on the Whole30! What are you going to do after that? You've worked so hard, fought through all the anger, the naps, the cravings to get to the awesome you're feeling now. All the while, the rules have been your backbone, your lifeline, your excuse for being "that person" in social situations.

Now what are heck are you supposed to do on Day 31?

First, breathe, then relax.

It is totally normal to feel a twinge of panic as your Whole30 comes to a close. For the past 30 days, you've lived, breathed, and literally eaten the rules. You look and feel better than you have in years. It's natural to hesitate at the thought of making any changes, especially if you're afraid reintroducing things will knock the Tiger Blood right out of you. But keep in mind that the Whole30 was intended to be a short-term reset and learning experience, not a permanent plan. We know it's scary, but you have to learn how to take the habits you've created here out into the real world—what we call "riding your own bike."

We've given you two different options for your Reintroduction protocol (see page 42 for details), and both of them are really detailed, spelling out exactly what you do during this part of the program. Plus, if you're not quite ready to dive back into some of the foods you used to eat, know that we do offer a gradual approach to this process— you certainly don't have to bring back bread, cereal, and pasta right away if you don't want to.

Whew.

DAY 31: Deep breathing, and maybe some wine.

Congratulations—you've finished the Whole30. It's time to give one of our reintroduction protocols (starting on page 42) the same attention you gave the last 30 days, and be honest with yourself about your mental, physical, and emotional reactions to the foods and drinks you're bringing back.

Tonight, that process might just start with a glass of wine. And that would be perfectly okay.

Cheers to you, Whole30 graduate!

whole30: reintroduction

"I was having severe stomach pains, which my family doctor diagnosed as IBS. The stomach pain was always there and it didn't matter what I ate. The pain continued through two specialists, a nutritionist, and an acupuncturist. I felt like I was crazy. The pain was at its worst and had been like that for a year, I wanted to go to the emergency room but I could not get out of bed. I was on three different stomach medicines, a sleeping and an anxiety medication. I gave the Whole30 a try because I had nothing to lose—and with my first Whole30, I didn't have pain, and now I'm not on any medications! I also lost 15 pounds and 2 dress sizes. The Whole30 has changed my life."

— STEPHANIE J., COATESVILLE, PA

It's Day 31—high five! You've officially completed our Whole30 program. You still have a little more work to do with our reintroduction protocol, but before you move on, let's take a minute to evaluate your progress before you jump on the scale.

Wait, what?

We can hear you already: "I've been dying to get on the scale for 30 days, and now you want me to wait even longer?"

Yes, we do.

That scale still has the potential to steal your Tiger Blood. Maybe you wanted to lose fifteen pounds and you only lost ten, or you went down two belt holes, but the scale didn't change.

You're going to jump on that scale the morning of Day 31 and think, "The Whole30 didn't work!" But you'd be wrong, and we want to help you see the real benefits you've achieved.

Here is a very, very long list of the Whole30 benefits you may have experienced. (And we're sure you'll find a few that aren't detailed here!) We call these "non-scale victories"—in fact, that phrase even has its own hashtag on social media, because we believe it's so critical to evaluating your Whole30 results. So take a moment before you get on that scale to check off everything you've noticed in the last 30 days. Be generous here—you worked hard, and you deserve to be proud of what you've accomplished!

Whole30 Non-Scale Victories!

Physical (outside)

- Fewer blemishes
- Glowing skin
- No more under-eye circles
- Improvement in rashes or patches
- Less dimpled skin
- Longer, stronger nails
- Stronger, thicker hair
- Brighter eyes
- Fresher breath
- Whiter teeth
- Flatter stomach
- Leaner appearance
- Clothes fitting better
- Rings fitting better
- Less bloating
- More defined muscle tone
- Less joint swelling
- Looking younger
- Feeling more confident in your appearance

Physical (inside)

- Healthier gums
- Less stiff joints
- Less painful joints
- Fewer PMS symptoms
- A more regular monthly cycle
- Increased libido
- Less stomach pain
- Less diarrhea
- Less constipation
- Less gas
- Less bloating
- Improved "regularity"

- Fewer episodes of illness
- Fewer seasonal allergies
- Reduction in food allergies
- Fewer migraines
- Fewer asthma attacks
- Less acid reflux
- Less heartburn
- Less chronic pain
- Less chronic fatigue
- Less tendonitis/bursitis
- Less shoulder/back/knee pain
- Improved blood pressure
- Improved cholesterol numbers
- Improved circulation
- Improved blood sugar regulation
- Improved symptoms of your medical condition
- Reduced or eliminated medications
- Recovering faster from injury or illness

Mood, emotion, and psychology

- You're happier
- You're more outgoing
- You're more patient
- You're more optimistic
- You laugh more
- You're less anxious
- You're less stressed
- You handle stress better
- Your kids say you're more fun
- Fewer mood swings
- Improved behavior (kids)

- Fewer tantrums (kids)
- Improved depression symptoms
- Improvement in your mental health condition
- Fewer sugar cravings
- Fewer carb cravings
- Improved body image
- Improved self-esteem
- Improved self-confidence
- Less reliance on the scale
- Feeling in control of your food

Brain function

- Improved attention span
- Improved performance at your job or school
- Improved memory
- Faster reaction times
- Fewer ADD/ADHD symptoms
- Clearer thinking
- Higher productivity

Sleep

- You're sleeping more
- You fall asleep more easily
- You sleep more soundly
- You no longer need a sleep aid
- You no longer need to hit the "snooze" button
- You awaken feeling refreshed
- Less snoring
- Less night sweats
- Less sleep apnea
- Fewer restless leg syndrome symptoms
- Fewer night cramps

Energy

- Energy levels are higher
- Energy levels are more even
- More energy in the morning
- No more mid-day energy slump
- More energy to play with your kids
- More energy to exercise
- More energy to socialize
- More energy at work or school
- You no longer need to eat every two hours
- You no longer get cranky if you don't eat
- You feel energetic between meals
- You need less sugar or caffeine to prop up energy levels

Sport, exercise, and play

- You started moving or exercising
- You became more consistent with exercise
- You can exercise longer, harder, or faster
- You feel more athletic
- You can lift heavier things
- You hit new "personal bests" in the gym or at your sport
- You recover more effectively from exercise or sport
- You have the confidence to try a new activity
- You play more with your kids or dog
- You're more coordinated
- Your balance is better
- You're outside more

Food and behaviors

- Healthier relationship with food
- Reduction in disordered eating habits
- Practicing mindful eating
- Learned how to read a label
- Know which foods make you more healthy or less healthy
- Eat to satiety
- Listening to your body
- Abandoned yo-yo dieting or crash dieting
- No longer afraid of dietary fat
- Learned how to cook
- Don't use food for comfort
- Don't use food as reward
- Don't use food as punishment
- Don't use food as stress management
- No longer a slave to sugar and carbs
- Know the difference between hunger and cravings
- Fewer cravings
- Healthy coping strategies to deal with cravings
- More variety, color, vitamins, and minerals in your diet
- Food no longer has unwanted "side effects"
- No more food guilt or shame
- No more bingeing
- When you do indulge, it's deliberate
- When you do indulge, you savor it

Lifestyle and social

- New healthy habits to pass down to your kids
- More knowledgeable about nutrition
- You shop locally and eat seasonally
- New cooking skills
- New recipes
- Meal prep is organized and efficient
- You've made new like-minded friends who support your lifestyle
- You maximize your food budget
- Spend less time and money at the doctor's office
- You've created other health goals
- Healthy eating habits have brought your family closer
- You've joined a new community
- Your kids have the best school lunches
- People ask you what you're doing differently
- People come to you for health, food, or lifestyle advice
- You are Whole30

Whew. Now look back at all your checkmarks, and don't deny yourself a moment (or longer!) to be proud of what you've accomplished and give yourself the much-deserved credit for all of your hard work. Remember, the Whole30 is just the first step in changing your life—and the benefits continue to roll in the longer you embrace the new, healthy habits you've learned.

SHOULD YOU CONTINUE?

If you're still feeling underwhelmed when you look at your list of results, you may need a little more time on the program to experience the maximum benefit. Thirty days is a great start, but you can't always correct medical conditions, long-standing habits, or years of consistent weight gain in just one month. Many people report benefitting greatly from adding another 15, 30, even 60 days to their program—and you've come so far now, what's another few weeks? If you've experienced some benefits from the program but still hope to see even more improvement, consider extending your Whole30. This is especially true if you are managing diseases (like arthritis, Lyme disease, or diabetes), lifestyle conditions (like allergies or eczema), and serious cravings for sugar or junk foods. If you think you'd benefit from some additional time on the Whole30, keep on keeping on, and come back to this section when you're ready for reintroduction.

Okay, *now* you can step on the scale, take measurements, and take your "after" photo for comparison. (We bet you'll be 72 percent happier with your scale and measurement results after completing our non-scale victory exercise.)

Whole30 Reintroduction

Now it's time for phase two of the Whole30: reintroduction. The reintroduction process is critical to your learning experience, so please don't skip over this part.

Seriously.

This is your one opportunity to slowly, carefully, systematically reintroduce some of the off-plan foods you've been missing into the "clean" environment you've created with the Whole30. Now is your chance to really evaluate how these foods make you feel in the context of a better relationship with food, improved metabolism, healthier digestive tract, and more balanced immune system. Let's illustrate the importance of this process with a story.

It's Day 31, and you decide to celebrate your Whole30 completion by indulging in pancakes, a sandwich with potato chips, a beer (or two), a slice of pizza, a bowl of ice cream . . . oh, and that half a donut you found on the break room counter. Hey, you worked hard—you deserve it!

And on Day 32, when you feel like you've been hit by a truck—when your Sugar Dragon is raging, your energy is non-existent, your stomach feels like you swallowed a bowling ball, and you're crankier than you've been in a month, you won't know why. Was it the pizza or the bread that made your skin break out? Did the pancakes set off your carb cravings, or was it the ice cream? Is your stomach reacting to the donut, the beer, or (most likely) the entirety of the junk food party you threw in your digestive tract?

Thirty days of so much hard work completely wasted, because you've learned *nothing* about how these less healthy foods impact you.

Don't do that. Please.

You've come this far—take the extra time to really reap the benefits of our carefully crafted reintroduction schedules. Be patient, and take the lessons you'll learn in the coming days with you for the rest of your life. Rush this process, and you'll be selling yourself short. Way short.

Okay, now that we got that out of the way, we've created two reintroduction schedules for you to choose from—the Fast Track, and the Slow Roll. What's the difference?

The Fast Track reintroduction schedule is just that—our complete reintroduction protocol in just ten days. This is for people who know exactly what they've been missing and want to figure out as soon as possible how these foods impact them, so they can start implementing what they learned out in the real world. If you're satisfied with your Whole30 results and feel ready to bring some of these other foods back into your life, this is the plan for you.

Our Slow Roll schedule is far more gradual, lasting as long as you choose, based not on our timeline, but your own. It's for people who feel so amazing post-Whole30 that they're not ready to reintroduce less healthy foods just for the sake of reintroducing them—in fact, they're happy to keep eating mostly Whole30 until something really amazing comes along, even if that's a month from now. This scenario especially applies to those who experienced a significant improvement in a medical condition during their Whole30, and suspect their symptoms will come back with a vengeance once they start eating off-plan again.

With both of these plans, the premise is simple: treat it like a scientific trial, where the Whole30 is your "control group," and each individual food or food group is the "experimental group." You'll reintroduce foods back into your diet one at a time, while keeping the rest of your diet in line with the Whole30 rules. This means you'll have to plan carefully, and not combine major food groups during your reintroduction period. (Don't worry—we'll give you a detailed schedule and sample reintroduction days for each plan.)

Note, we aren't adding a set timeline to reintroduce added sugar in either plan. There's really no need, as you'll be eating some added sugar when you reintroduce these off-plan foods, and it's nearly impossible to separate the effects of the sugar or high carbohydrate content from the impact of the other less healthy elements in these foods. Just pay attention to the impact of sugar plus other food groups—for example, if you react far more negatively to eating a donut than you do

DON'T MISS IT?

For both plans, if you don't miss a particular food or drink that you know makes you less healthy, don't bother to reintroduce it. Not missing tofu, black beans, cottage cheese, or pasta? With evidence pointing toward these foods making you less healthy and no vital nutrients you aren't already getting from the healthy foods you are eating, there's no reason whatsoever to add them back into your diet. Only reintroduce those foods that you suspect you'll really want to include back into your diet once in a while, and leave the rest happily behind.

to eating pizza crust, you can be sure the combination of gluten containing grains plus sugar is an especially nasty one for you. (If you really want to pursue the idea of reintroducing sugar on its own, see page 133 for our best advice.)

We'll outline our reintroduction plans one at a time, giving specific timelines and sample reintroduction days for each. Read through both options carefully before deciding which one to follow, as you will likely learn valuable information from the description of each approach.

The Whole30 Fast Track Reintroduction

The benefit of our Fast Track schedule is that you get your reintroduction over relatively quickly, and are then free to take what you've learned out into the real world. You may find great freedom and joy in being able to quickly reincorporate some of these foods back into your regular diet in a way that still keeps you moving in the direction of "more healthy." Plus, because the schedule is very structured, you'll have a clear method of reevaluating these foods without the effects of one food group conflicting with another. Finally, because you have the benefit of knowing exactly when you'll be reintroducing these foods, you can structure things such that any negative side effects won't completely ruin your life.

The biggest downside is that you may have a pretty miserable two weeks. Reintroducing so many off-plan foods in such a short period of time (especially when your system has been so happy without them) means your energy, sleep, mood, cravings, skin, digestion, and medical symptoms may all blow up at once.

Remember how just a few days ago you were looking forward to bringing back your beloved pizza, beer, and ice cream?

EAT ALL THE THINGS

Actually, we'd actually be surprised if you were still planning on an epic junk-food rampage come Day 31. In a 2014 study of more than 1,300 Whole30 participants, 76 percent said while they were planning on eating all kinds of treats on Day 31, by the time their Whole30 was over they didn't even want those foods anymore!

All we're saying is . . . brace yourself.

The good news? Once you're done, you'll be able to move forward implementing a healthy, balanced nutrition plan that will last the rest of your life.

Below is a sample Fast Track Reintroduction Schedule. (Keep in mind the foods we select in these sample days don't have to be your choices.)

DAY 1 (optional): Evaluate gluten-free alcohol, while keeping the rest of your diet Whole30-compliant. For those of you missing your red wine, 100 percent agave tequila, or gluten-free beer, take this opportunity to reintroduce. Have a drink or two (don't go overboard!) at some point today, paying attention to how you feel during and after your experience. Then, go back to the Whole30 for the next two days, and see how things go. Pay attention, evaluate, and decide how, how often, and how much to incorporate alcohol into your lifestyle—if at all.

DAY 1 (OR 4): Evaluate legumes, while keeping the rest of your diet Whole30-compliant. Try a thick slather of peanut butter on your green apple with breakfast, a bowl of miso soup and soy sauce on your sashimi at lunch, and a side of black beans with dinner, while paying attention to how you feel. Then, go back to the Whole30 for the next two days, and see how things go. Pay attention, evaluate, and decide how, how often, and how much to incorporate legumes into your regular diet—if at all.

DAY 4 (OR 7): Evaluate non-gluten grains*, while keeping the rest of your diet Whole30-compliant. Eat a bowl of oatmeal, a serving of white rice, some corn tortilla chips, and a sandwich made from gluten-free bread, while paying attention to how you feel. Then, return to the Whole30 for the next two days, and see how things go. Pay attention, evaluate, and decide how, how often, and how much to incorporate non-gluten grains into your regular diet—if at all.

DAY 7 (OR 10): Evaluate dairy, while keeping the rest of your diet Whole30-compliant. Have plain yogurt in the morning, add milk or cream to your coffee, top your salad with cheese in the afternoon, and use ordinary butter and sour cream on your baked potato with dinner, while paying attention to how you feel. Then, return to the Whole30 for the next two days, and see how things go. Pay attention, evaluate, and decide how, how often, and how much to incorporate dairy into your regular diet—if at all.

DAY 10 (OR 13): Evaluate gluten-containing grains**, while keeping the rest of your diet Whole30-compliant. Over the course of your day, have a bowl of whole-wheat cereal or a muffin, two slices of whole grain bread, some wheat crackers, and a beer, while paying

> ## A WORD OF CAUTION
> It's Fast Track, not Shortcut. You really don't want to trim this schedule down any more than it already is, or these less healthy side effects could start to pile up, making you feel even worse and making it harder to determine which food caused which negative symptom. Stick to two days of Whole30 eating between each reintroduction group at a minimum—refer to our Reintroduction FAQ on page 132 for more information.

attention to how you feel. Then, return to the Whole30 for the next two days, and see how things go. Pay attention, evaluate, and decide how, how often, and how much to incorporate gluten grains into your regular diet—if at all.

Congratulations! Your reintroduction is technically over, and you can now implement what you've learned in the rest of your life. Of course, only you can decide what's worth it for you. If wine gave you a migraine, milk gave you major gas, or bread made your eczema worse, it's up to *you* to figure out whether those side effects are worth it. Maybe you love wine so much that you'll happily trade a glass for a headache. Well then cheers to you! You're now in charge of when, how much, and how often to reincorporate these foods back into your own life—and where you draw that line is entirely up to you.

Still, aren't you glad you know?

*Corn, brown or white rice, certified gluten-free oats, quinoa, etc.
**Any product made from wheat, rye, or barley—bread, cereal, pasta, crackers, beer, etc.

Thanks to your Whole30 awareness, you know it's a bad idea to have a glass of wine during a work lunch, a big glass of milk on a first date, or bread before your photo shoot. You know exactly how good Whole30 foods make you feel, and exactly how these off-plan foods will affect you. That's the benefit of reintroduction—the awareness it brings, and the freedom you'll now have to create a healthy, balanced, sustainable diet that will keep you moving in the direction of "more healthy" for the rest of your life.

Not bad for just over a month's worth of work.

The Whole30 Slow Roll Reintroduction

The Slow Roll schedule doesn't follow any particular timeline. The whole point is for you to continue eating mostly Whole30 until something so special or delicious comes along that you decide you're ready to indulge, and evaluate the effects.

The benefit is that you get to continue your everyday life feeling unstoppable, powered by the Whole30 diet that works so well for you. You'll also maintain your current quality of life, living symptom-free (or with reduced symptoms) as long as you stick to the plan. Plus, when you're only reintroducing foods you find absolutely irresistible, you'll savor them more, and be less tempted by not-so-special "just because it's there and you can" options. Finally, because you're only reintroducing a small amount of off-plan food at once (one special occasion dessert, a glass of your favorite wine, your mom's homemade bread), the side effects may not be as severe or last as long as a Fast Track reintroduction day.

The downside is that instead of setting aside a dedicated three days to reintroduce and evaluate specific foods, you'll be testing them "in the wild," not knowing how they'll affect you. This means you may spend your anniversary weekend dealing with stomach cramps, bloating, and irregularity—not very romantic.

ONE SLOW ROLL CONSIDERATION

There is one way to keep your daily diet feeling more sustainable without jeopardizing your Tiger Blood. To give yourself a little breathing room on this stretched-out reintroduction schedule, consider relaxing on the Whole30 "no added sugar" rule come Day 31. This doesn't mean you're eating frosting washed down with energy drinks, but if you want sugar-cured bacon with your eggs, ketchup on your burger, or the vinaigrette dressing that comes with your restaurant salad, go right ahead. Note that we're not actually changing your diet much here—you were already eating meat, condiments, and salads with dressing on the Whole30. We're just broadening your choices a bit, in a way that won't send you running for the nearest donut shop. Of course, if there are some foods you suspect (or know) will be "triggers" for your Sugar Dragon, stay away! Sweetened nut butters or coconut butters, dark chocolate, or coffee creamers may send you hurtling down the path of cravings and overconsumption.

Plus, when there's a "worth it" conflict, you'll have to either pass up a food or beverage you really want, or lose some of the awareness you could have gained from a stricter schedule. For example, say you attend a family dinner, and you really want both your mom's homemade cornbread and your grandma's apple pie. You've got a dilemma—eat both, and you won't be sure whether any negative effects came from the corn, the gluten, the sugar, or a combination of all three. Pass up one and you're going to be sad about what you missed.

If the benefits of a Slow Roll reintroduction outweigh the potential downsides for you, here's a sample diary we created to illustrate how this works. Understand, however, this is only an example—your schedule will depend on you stumbling across something that's worth it for you.

DAY 31: My Whole30 is done! I'm celebrating with some 90 percent chocolate, but not bringing anything else back just yet. This Tiger Blood feels too good!

DAY 35: My mom baked an apple pie for dessert, but that's not my favorite, and I didn't really want it, so I passed. And it was easy!

DAY 42: Tonight's my birthday, and I really want a glass of wine at dinner, but I may also want dessert. When I get to the restaurant, I'll decide if I really want either.

DAY 43: Wine gives me a headache, but boy it was delicious. Back to my Whole30-ish (basically Whole30 + ketchup and a teaspoon of honey in my tea).

DAY 47: Movie night at home, and I'm dying for a bowl of hot, buttered popcorn. I'm going for it! I've still got clarified butter left over, so we'll see how corn goes.

DAY 48: Not bad! No noticeable effects, except eating a little popcorn made me want to eat a LOT of popcorn. Back to Whole30 for a few days.

DAY 50: We're in Mexico, and I'm dying for a fresh churro! Bring on the gluten. (Not really, but I really want a churro.)

DAY 51: Bad, bad, bad. My body does not like churros. At all. Gluten is not my friend, and I'll be thinking long and hard about whether I eat it again.

You get the point—you continue with your Whole30-ish diet until something amazing comes along. You decide to reintroduce. You pay attention, return to the Whole30 for at least two days (if not longer), and repeat.

It's a Marathon, Not a Sprint

One of the things we really like about the Slow Roll reintroduction is that it emphasizes a very important point: reintroduction is actually a lifelong process. Now that you have a baseline for looking and feeling your best (the Whole30), every time you eat a potentially less-healthy food, you should both savor it immensely and pay close attention to how it impacts you.

The more experience you have with the Whole30 program, the more your awareness will grow, and the more you'll be able to identify the subtle nuances of how food affects you. By your second or third Whole30 and reintroduction, you'll find you're paying attention to things you never would have noticed—the fact that eating gluten makes you sad, or how too much sugar puts you in a bad mood for two days straight.

Finally, if you're really paying attention, you'll also notice your definition of "worth it" changes as time goes on. What's worth it for you should be critically evaluated on a regular basis by paying close attention to your experience when eating certain foods. Was the idea of the food better than actually eating it? Did you used to love the food, but today it's just "meh"? Could you happily do without something today that yesterday you thought you couldn't live without? Don't be afraid of flip-flopping here—you're the one who calls the shots, and your favorite "treat" today may be tomorrow's "this just isn't doing it for me."

Proceed with (Craving) Caution

One last important point, and something that trips up many a Whole30er during their reintroduction. If at any point you start to feel out of control with your food choices (like what you've reintroduced woke up your Sugar Dragon), get back on the Whole30 for as long as it takes to stabilize. Don't wait, don't delay, and don't try to talk yourself out of it. Otherwise, you'll find yourself covered in powdered sugar sipping a large mocha latte while ordering pizza for lunch and wondering why your pants are so tight again.

You know exactly what we're talking about.

This is most common with the reintroduction of sugary foods or gluten grains—eating muffins, chocolate, "dessert," or bread again can make some people rabid with desire for processed carbs and sugar. So be on the lookout for cravings rearing their ugly heads, and halt that process before it takes over your brain by returning to a strict Whole30.

Does this advice sound a little extreme? Like, really, will I feel out of control after just a day of off-plan food? Yeah, you might. And we take sugar and carb addiction very seriously around here so please, listen to us, and don't feel like a failure if you have to jump back on the Whole30 for a few days to calm things down. You're actually *succeeding*, because you're not afraid to do the best thing for you, your long-term health, and your relationship with food. Winning!

The good news? Chances are it will only take a few days before you're back in comfortable territory, feeling great and back in control—and will know to be even more careful when reintroducing those "trigger foods."

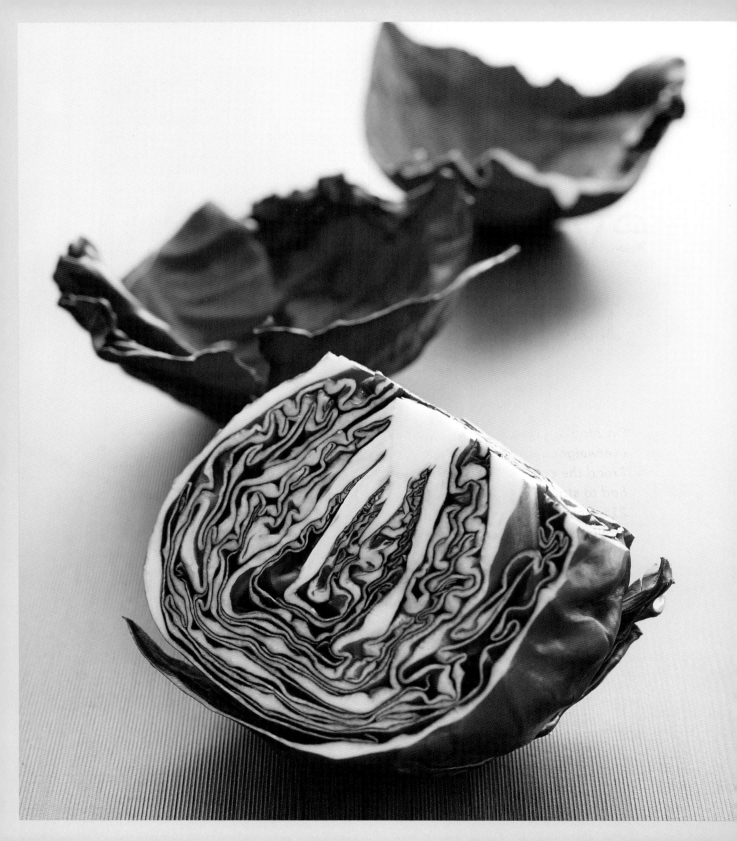

everything you need to know

"On May 4, 2014, I happened across It Starts With Food. *I was 25 pounds overweight, and scheduled to leave for my first-ever trip to Italy the next day. I read the entire book that night, and canceled the trip. Lost all the money. I had to start. I began my Whole30 on May 5th. I've gone from 245 pounds to 215, from a 44 waist to a 38. But the best of all, I have absolutely no sugar cravings. I'm 65, and my biggest regret is not discovering this 60 years ago. Every day, I am in awe of the fact that, for the first time in my life... I AM NOT ON A DIET. Thank you so, so much.*" — JEFF M., THE VILLAGES, FL

you've got questions, we've got answers

By now, you are an expert on the Whole30 rules, have a cadre of friends and family supporting you in your journey (whether in person or online), and have run through our five easy steps designed to get your house, your head, and your Whole30 plan in order. But you still have questions.

We know. We expected this. In fact, we *love* questions. Even questions you think are stupid or silly. Know why?

Questions mean you are really trying to do this right.

We answer every single question we receive from Whole30 participants on social media or via the Forum. Even questions we've already answered 1,343 times. Because when you ask a question, it tells us that your Whole30 is important to you. It tells us that you are thinking critically about the next 30 days, deepening your understanding of the rules and embracing the spirit and intention of the program. Your questions mean you are engaged and enthusiastic and most important, committed. And we *love* that.

So in the next 15 sections, we've documented more than five years' worth of Whole30 questions and answers: the technicalities, like "Can I have hummus?" and "Can I take communion?"; the lifestyle-related challenges, like "How do I manage a restaurant?" and "What do I take on a long plane ride?"; and the emotional worries, like "Why can't I weigh myself?" and "What if I accidentally eat something off-plan?"

We've answered all of those and more, sometimes in question-and-answer format, sometimes in narrative form. We've put all of our Whole30 education, experience, proficiency, and common sense all in one place.

It's called "everything you need to know" for a reason, and that's the "love" part.

But now for a little "tough."

We're more "teach you how to fish" than "give you a fish" people. That means we'd rather help you figure out where to find the answers than spoon-feed them all to you. Of course, we've given you a massive head start in these sections—but even so, you may still find yourself asking a question we haven't covered here.

Can I have bee pollen? (Yes.)

Will the Whole30 grow my hair back? (Probably not.)

Can I use milk in my coffee if it's my own breast milk? (This is an actual thing that actually happened, and yes, you may, but your husband may not.)

So if you find yourself stuck with a question that isn't in this book, here's what you do:

Search our whole30.com online Forum.

It's free, it's quick to search, and we practically guarantee your question has been asked and answered there already. If not, feel free to start a new thread and ask away—our seasoned Whole30 veterans and Forum moderators will give you their best advice straightaway.

Not a Forum person? Google! That will bring up results from our Forum, things we may have already said on social media, or blog posts on the subject by other Whole30ers.

Still can't find what you're looking for? Your last option is to ask us directly on social media. Pick a medium—Facebook, Twitter, or Instagram, refer to page 405 for exactly how to find us. You'll get an authoritative answer from someone on the Whole30 team within a day or so, although our community members may weigh in even sooner than that. (New Whole30 friends! Yay!)

So there you go—so many answers, so many options, all right at your capable, confident fingertips. We're not sure what else we could do, short of coming to your house and cooking your food for you. Which someone recently asked us to do on Twitter.

Denise, we wish we could have. Really.

You overachievers can read through this entire section start to finish now, helping you get even better prepared before your program starts. For those of you already feeling a little overwhelmed, it's okay. Just know these answers, tips, and tricks are here when you need them, so get going on your Whole30 and come back to this section if a specific question or need comes up. Or, do a combination of both—skim through

FACEBOOK GROUPS

There are lots of Whole30-related Facebook groups out there, and we love seeing members of our community band together to support each other on their journey. But use caution, especially if you're new to the program. These groups aren't run or monitored by the Whole30 team, which means the information you're getting may not be accurate. By all means, join (or create) a group for the friendship, support, and sharing of good recipes. But if you have a question about the rules, the foods, or the science behind the program, make sure you visit the official Whole30 Facebook page or our online Forum to get the answer straight from us.

this section now, then come back to it if you need a little reminder or extra motivation during your Whole30.

Ready?

You sure are.

the general whole30 FAQ

"I just finished my first Whole30 and wanted to say thanks. I have always been fit and have eaten well, but my 50-year-old body really needed a tune-up. I also had high cholesterol (252) that gave concern to my doctor. Enter the Whole30. I lost 4 pounds, mostly around the waist area, which is nice; my waist is now a 31. I also got a blood workup and my results were excellent. My cholesterol is down to 207, triglycerides are normal, LDL-C is normal, and HDL-C is now in the healthy range. On top of all that, I am really enjoying cooking for myself and my family." —BILL B., ELMHURST, IL

Does one bite of pizza or one glass of beer really make a difference?

YES, IT DOES. That's not us being the tough guys, that's science. The point of any elimination diet is to completely remove 100 percent of the potentially problematic foods from your life for a full 30 days straight. Without the complete removal, your body won't experience what life is really like without these triggers. You may think one bite or sip here or there won't really make a difference, but if you're sensitive to these foods,* you require only a tiny amount to break the Whole30 "reset"—to disrupt the gut, fire up the immune system, and potentially trigger the symptoms of your condition.

Now, you might say, "But if I was sensitive, I'd know it." Uh, no. You would not. Nobody knows they're sensitive until something happens to make them *realize* they're sensitive. We know people with celiac disease who walked around eating bread for decades before they realized there was a problem. The point of the Whole30 is to identify sensitivities. So until

you've done the full Whole30 by the books (which means 100 percent compliance for at least 30 days), you may *not* know.

I ate something off-plan. Do I have to start over?

THE SHORT ANSWER IS YES, first and foremost because of the science. You introduce something inflammatory into your newly "clean" environment and you have to start all over again. In addition, those are the rules. The Whole30 program is black and white: no slips, no cheats, no special occasions. The program requires 30 days straight of complete compliance, otherwise it's back to Day 1 for you. There, wasn't that easy? But don't start over because *we* want you to— start over because you promised yourself you'd see this through. Because you made a commitment to yourself. You decided to push the "reset" button on your health, your habits, and your relationship with food, and change your life through the Whole30. So see that commitment through, because you deserve it.

*This is especially true of grains (especially gluten), dairy products, soy, peanuts, and alcohol.

I accidentally ate something off-plan. Do I really have to start over?

SAY YOU FIND YOURSELF at Mom's house for dinner on Day 22 triple-confirming the meal has no grains or legumes. Then halfway through the main course Mom says, "The secret ingredient in this meatloaf—soy sauce!" (Double whammy—soy sauce usually contains both soy and wheat.) In this context, you've done everything you can do. You asked the right questions, got the right answers, and proceeded exactly on plan with the Whole30, as far as you knew.

We'd still tell you to start over. The rules are the rules, and you'll only achieve maximum benefit if you give yourself a full 30 days on the protocol. However, if the stress of starting from scratch or the amount of resentment you'd feel toward your mother would do more harm than good, we could understand if you chalked it up to a learning experience and just finished out your program. Ultimately, you're all grown-ups, and it's always up to you as to whether or not to start over.

Is the Whole30 low-carb?

THE WHOLE30 IS NOT A LOW-CARB DIET BY DESIGN. We don't count calories or carbohydrates, restrict carbohydrates, or give you any sort of guidance as to how many grams of carbohydrates you should be eating. (It's also not a no-carb diet: people think of "carbs" as breads, cereals, and pastas, but vegetables and fruit contain carbohydrates, too!) By virtue of the nutrient-dense foods you'll be choosing, your diet will likely include less carbohydrate than you used to eat, but that's probably a good thing. Unless you're incredibly active, do high-intensity activity or exercise a few times a week, or are in hard training for endurance sports, you don't need piles of carbohydrates for energy. However, if you find yourself in one of these categories, you will have to purposefully include carb-dense vegetables and fruits into your daily diet, to ensure you have enough to fuel your activity level. Make it a point to eat potatoes, winter squashes like butternut and acorn, bananas or plantains, and other fruits every day, so your energy stores are sufficient to see you through your workout or long training run.

Is the Whole30 like the Atkins Diet?

NOT REALLY. Atkins is a deliberately low-carb, high-fat diet with the primary purpose of helping participants lose weight. Tracking your caloric and carbohydrate intake is a mandatory part of staying in compliance with the given carb-gram ranges for each phase. Participants are encouraged to eat real food, but are also offered a prepackaged line of meals, shakes, and bars to supplement their meals. Cheese, milk, artificial sweeteners, and diet sodas are also allowed on the program.

By comparison, the Whole30 is not low- or high-anything—our Meal Template (page 194) is actually quite moderate in terms of recommended amounts of protein, carbohydrates, and fat. More significant, the purpose of the Whole30 is to reset your health, your habits, and your relationship with food. It's not designed for weight loss, although participants do lose weight as a result of improving their health. Finally, the Whole30 has no required weighing or measuring (in fact, that's frowned upon), a much stronger focus on food quality, and specifically targets cravings and food addictions.

Is the Whole30 like Paleo?

IN A GENERAL SENSE, YES. The Whole30 was originally based on a Paleo framework, and generally omits foods that aren't part of a typical Paleo diet, like grains and legumes. However, we don't focus on evolution or history (what our Paleolithic ancestors may or may not have eaten). Our program is primarily concerned with how food in today's modern world impacts our health and habits. We exclude some foods that some would consider technically "Paleo" (like honey or baked goods made with almond flour), and allow some foods that aren't usually part of a Paleo plan (like potatoes and green beans). However, there is an awful lot of overlap; many people come to the Whole30 from a Paleo diet, or find a more general Paleo template works well for them when their Whole30 is over.

Why 30 days?

HABIT RESEARCH SHOWS the average number of days to make a new habit stick is 66—but the harder and more complicated the change, the longer it will take you to really solidify the new behavior. Understanding habit research, we had a few choices to make when designing the program. We could have made it a Whole66 (or longer), but the idea of changing your diet in this fashion for more than two months would have scared a lot of people away. We could have made it short (like a Whole14), but we knew that wasn't likely to bring you the stunning benefits of the program. So we chose a middle ground. Thirty days is long enough to create new habits and bring you stunning results, but not so long that you are afraid to take it on.

Can I do the program for less than 30 days?

UNDER SPECIAL CIRCUMSTANCES, YES. We think inserting a "Whole7" or a "Whole10" into your life at key times is a great way to get an effective reset and get you back on track. The caveat? You have to have done a full Whole30 and be practicing your new, healthy habits more

often than not in your everyday life to benefit. The more you do the Whole30 and the closer you live to these standards on a day-to-day basis, the faster you'll be able to get through any negative consequences and jump into the Tiger Blood stage. (Remember "Tiger Blood" from our Whole30 Timeline?) Attempt a Whole7 on your first go-round or after six months of carb-a-palooza and you'll end up with all of the unpleasant side effects, and none of the benefits!

For the experienced Whole30 participant, we recommend throwing in a Whole7 or Whole10 in the week before or after a vacation, just before a holiday, or during a time of stress, when eating healthy will help you better handle the challenge. The rules are exactly the same, and don't limit yourself to seven or ten days—keep going until you feel like you're back on healthy ground and in control of your food habits.

Should I consider extending my Whole30 to 45 or 60 days?

WE TALK ABOUT THIS IN THE REINTRODUCTION SECTION (page 45), but if you've got a chronic medical condition, an autoimmune disease, or a long history of unhealthy food habits or addictions, you may want to plan on being on the program longer than 30 days. While the basic program is long enough to steer you in the right direction and bring you some of the results you're hoping to see, you can't expect to fully reverse years (or decades!) of medical symptoms or food-related habits in just a month. Autoimmune conditions are especially stubborn, often requiring six months or more of dietary and lifestyle intervention to bring significant healing and resolution of symptoms. If you feel like you can commit to a Whole45, 60, or 90 right out of the gate, go for it! You can also take a wait-and-see approach, and decide whether or not to keep going come Day 31.

Can you do the Whole30 forever?

IF YOU REALLY WANTED TO, you could absolutely do the Whole30 for the rest of your life. Unlike other "diet" programs, the Whole30 has no temporary induction period, doesn't restrict calories, and provides you with an abundance of the vitamins, minerals, phytonutrients, and fiber essential for excellent long-term health, which means if you stayed on the program forever, you'd actually be optimally healthy. However, we don't think you should make it a Whole365. From a practical perspective, following the Whole30 rules every single day could get pretty stressful. Plus, doing the Whole30 for the rest of your life would completely eliminate the opportunity to indulge in some truly extraordinary, really special off-plan foods. (You wouldn't *have* to eat fresh pasta in Italy or toast with champagne at your best friend's wedding, but we'd want you to feel like you could if you wanted to.) Remember, at some point, you have to take the things you've learned on the program out into the real world, and make your own decisions about what you think is "worth it" or not. If you never practice—if you always use the rules of the Whole30 to make those decisions for you—you will never truly attain food freedom.

Should I do the Whole30 over the holiday season (Thanksgiving, Christmas, Hanukkah, etc.)?

WE DON'T RECOMMEND IT. First, the Whole30 is primarily about awareness. The only way to learn how certain foods are actually affecting your health is by paying close attention during the 30-day elimination and the subsequent reintroduction period. But during the holidays, nobody has time to pay attention to anything—you simply can't give the program the energy and attention it deserves. In addition, the holidays are already pretty stressful with events, gifts, and travel—not to mention the treats and temptations! You could be setting yourself up for a fall if you try to take on a program as rigorous as the Whole30 on top of an already stressful season. Finally, the holiday season is meant to celebrate family traditions, honoring your culture and heritage, and that celebration almost always includes special handmade foods. That kind of food should be honored, savored, and shared in the company of those you love, and you'll miss out on that once-a-year experience if you are doing a Whole30.

That's not to say you should dive face-first into every candy bowl you stumble across—feel free to throw in a Whole30 before the season to set yourself up for holiday success, and intersperse days of Whole30-style eating in between parties, gatherings, and events. (And make sure you join us at whole30.com every year on January 1st for our official New Year Whole30 kick-off!)

Where is the science behind your recommendations?

THE SCIENTIFIC BACKGROUND of our general nutrition recommendations and the Whole30 program is outlined in detail in *It Starts With Food*. In addition, we have included more than 400 peer-reviewed studies supporting our recommendations in that book's references.

food

"I was never a cook. I only craved sweets, and eating healthy to me was chicken and a vegetable—boring! The Whole30 has really inspired me in a whole new direction. It is so much fun using your guidelines and recipes and experimenting to see what flavors we like, and the Whole30 encouraged us to try more than just lettuce, green beans, and broccoli. My goal this year was to become 'a cook' and thanks to you, I am well on my way."

—AMANDA M., TOKYO, JAPAN

ADDITIVES: read your labels

Most processed foods contain additives to maintain color, preserve shelf life, stabilize, or emulsify. It's not always easy to determine which are healthy and which aren't, but we've simplified it for you during your Whole30 by excluding only MSG, sulfites, and carrageenan during the program. (See these individual entries to learn why we singled them out.) All other additives, including citric acid, ferrous gluconate, and guar gum, are acceptable—although we encourage you to try to find products with no additives whatsoever.

⭐ TIP: *If you're not sure what an additive is or does, Google it! Wikipedia is a pretty good source of basic information, and it may put your mind at ease to find that the scary-sounding "ascorbic acid" in your dried cranberries is really just a fancy word for vitamin C.*

ALMOND FLOUR/COCONUT FLOUR: yes

Yes, you can have almond flour, coconut flour, tapioca flour, and other non-grain flours, but it's context-dependent. You can use them in place

of breadcrumbs in your meatballs, to dredge a piece of chicken, or to thicken a sauce or stew. You may not use them for "Paleo" baking—to make pancakes, bread, tortillas, biscuits, muffins, cupcakes, cookies, pizza crust, waffles, or anything of that nature. Remember, these foods are expressly off-limits during your Whole30. (See "Treats, Food Fixations, and the Scale" on page 95.)

ARROWROOT POWDER: yes

Arrowroot powder is a fine choice as a thickener, and can be especially helpful in sauces and gravies. Like almond flour, though, it's not appropriate for use in baked goods.

BACON: read your labels

It's really, really hard to find bacon without any added sugar, but if you can, you're in the clear. (Remember, if there is any form of sugar in the ingredients list the product is out for the Whole30, even if the label says, "Sugar = 0 grams.") The best option is choosing one of our Whole30 Approved bacons (page 404), but you can also check with your local natural foods store, or ask a local farmer or butcher shop.

> TIP: *For the healthiest bacon, look for "pastured" and "organic" on the label—or better yet, ask your local farmer if his pigs are raised in a natural environment and fed a natural diet.*

BEAN SPROUTS: yes
The plant part of the bean (the sprout) is fine to eat. The problematic compounds are found in the bean (the seed) itself.

BRAGG'S AMINO ACIDS: no
Bragg's Amino Acids are made from soy, and all forms of soy are out for your Whole30. A great Whole30-compliant substitute, however, is Coconut Secret's coconut aminos. It tastes just like soy sauce, without the soy or gluten! (Available online, or in many health food stores.)

BUCKWHEAT: no
Buckwheat is a pseudo-cereal—not botanically a grain, but containing compounds that may cause similar problems. All grains and pseudo-cereals are out for your Whole30.

CACAO (100 PERCENT): yes
Cacao (or 100 percent cocoa) is great when used as a savory spice in recipes, like the Mocha Steak Rub found in *It Starts With Food*. Feel free to add it to your coffee or tea, or brew it on its own as a coffee substitute. However, per the rules of the program, we don't allow the mixing of cocoa and dates or other fruits to make chocolate-y dessert confections or sweetened "hot chocolate" drinks.

CANNED VEGETABLES AND FRUIT: yes
While canned produce may not pack the same micronutritional punch as their fresh or frozen counterparts, we're not going to discriminate. If canned veggies help you up your intake, we'll take it. Just watch out for added ingredients like sugar or sulfites, and avoid any fruits packed in syrup.

CAROB: yes
While carob is technically a legume, carob powder is generally made from the pod of the plant and not the seed. Since all of the potentially problematic parts are contained in the seed, carob powder is fine on your Whole30, but the same no-making-chocolate-y-desserts concept applies.

CARRAGEENAN: no
Carrageenan is a concentrated, processed seaweed extract used to thicken processed foods, and is found in everything from deli meat to yogurt to chocolate. Carrageenan is inflammatory if it gets through the gut lining into the body, which could happen if you have increased gut permeability. (Carrageenan is actually used in laboratory studies to *create* inflammation in animals.) Furthermore, low-quality carrageenan may be degraded to components that can cross even a healthy gut barrier. For these reasons, we specifically exclude carrageenan on the Whole30.

> TIP: *Deli meats (like turkey or roast beef) may be hard to find without added sugar or carrageenan, but there are compliant brands in both health food markets and grocery stores. Be patient, read all your labels, and ask at the deli—sometimes, the prepackaged meats contain carrageenan, but the fresh-sliced meats at the deli counter don't.*

CHIA: yes

These "seeds" aren't the same botanical family of seeds that we eliminate with grains and legumes, so that makes them fine to eat during your Whole30.

⭐ TIP: *Chia seeds aren't likely to cause you any serious trouble, but they're not the omega-3 superfood they're made out to be, either. Chia should be treated like any other nut or seed and consumed in limited quantities.*

CHIPS: no

While we recognize that potatoes are a real food, we also know that eating them in the form of fries and chips has turned them from "produce" into an adulterated commercial "product." It's easy to find sweet potato, beet, or vegetable chips that meet the Whole30 ingredient standards. It is *not* easy, however, to consume those chips in a way that's true to the spirit of the Whole30. It's hard to find a suitable place for them in our meal template (no, half a bag of "Sweets and Beets" is not an appropriate way to fill your plate with vegetables), and even harder to stop yourself from eating them when the designated serving comes to an end. For most of us, chips are a bona fide food-with-no-brakes, and fall into that deep, dark area of less-healthy foods with technically compliant ingredients. For that reason we do not allow frying starchy veggies and turning them into chips during your Whole30. (However, if you want to roast some kale until it's crispy, or thinly slice jicama into a scoop for your guacamole, be our guest.)

CITRIC ACID: yes

This is a common preservative and flavoring agent in canned or jarred foods, like tomatoes or olives. The addition of citric acid to your food won't affect your Whole30 results in any way.

COMMUNION: yes

Let's be clear: God > Whole30, and whether you decide to take communion during your program is entirely up to you. While most communion wafers do contain gluten, and that gluten may impact the "reset" process and your Whole30 results, we would never ask you to compromise your faith for our rules.

⭐ TIP: *Some progressive churches do offer gluten-free wafers these days, which would have less impact on your Whole30 gut-healing efforts. You might take this opportunity to speak with your church group or leaders to see if there are others in the community who would prefer a gluten-free offering.*

CONVENTIONALLY RAISED MEAT, EGGS, AND ANIMAL FATS: yes

We want you to eat the best quality food you can afford, especially when it comes to animal products. In *It Starts With Food*, we discuss how the best meat, seafood, eggs, and animal fats come from animals raised in their natural environments (ideally organically) and fed their natural diets. This means looking for "grass-fed," "organic," "pastured," or "wild-caught" on your labels. However, this is just a best-case recommendation, not a requirement of the Whole30 program. Conventionally raised (factory-farmed) animal products are also acceptable on the program.

DARK CHOCOLATE: no

Anything less than 100 percent cocoa (cacao) is off-limits during your Whole30. Even 90 percent dark chocolate is still sweetened—and therefore candy.

DATES: yes

All fruits, including dates, are allowed on your Whole30. However, please don't try to turn dates into a form of added sweetener (like boiling them down into a syruplike paste)—while technically within the rules, that kind of thing goes against the spirit and intention of the program.

> ⭐ TIP: *These little sugar bombs pack a huge punch—they're as close to candy as you can get on the Whole30. We strongly recommend against using them as a "treat" to feed your Sugar Dragon.*

FLAX SEEDS: yes

These "seeds" aren't the same botanical family of seeds that we eliminate with grains and legumes, so that makes them fine to eat during your Whole30.

> ⭐ TIP: *Flax isn't likely to cause you any serious trouble, but it's not the omega-3 superfood it's made out to be, either. Flax should be treated like any other nut or seed and consumed in limited quantities.*

FRENCH FRIES: no

It's kind of like the argument against chips—anything deep-fried in vegetable oil is by default not that healthy, and fries are one of those foods-with-no-brakes we warned you about. For most of us, fries of any kind fall into that deep, dark area of less-healthy foods with technically compliant ingredients. For that reason we do not allow deep-fried potatoes, whether commercial or homemade, for the duration of Whole30. (Potatoes of any variety in boiled, baked, steamed, pan-fried, grilled, microwaved, or roasted form are good to go, however.)

GREEN BEANS: yes

The problem with legumes comes when you consume the seed. As with snow peas or sugar snap peas, green beans are mostly plant matter (the pod), with only tiny, immature seeds. As such, we're not too worried about their potential downsides—if green beans are the worst thing in your Whole30 diet, you're doing okay.

GUAR GUM: yes

This is a common vegetable gum thickener, often found in canned coconut milk, and should not pose any significant negative health consequences during your Whole30. (This also applies to other thickening, stabilizing, and emulsifying "gums," like locust bean gum, xanthan gum, or gellan gum.)

> ⭐ TIP: *Very few people report a sensitivity to guar gum, but if you notice any digestive issues after consuming coconut milk, first try reducing the quantity you consume in any one sitting. If that doesn't help, switch to a brand without guar gum, like Native Forest.*

GUM: no

All chewing gums contain some form of added sweeteners (including xylitol) that aren't acceptable under Whole30 guidelines.

> ⭐ TIP: *Chewing for hours and hours at a time sends a message to your body that you're eating. If you spend a lot of time chewing but not actually eating, your body is going to get quite confused in its responses, including secreting stomach acid and saliva in the absence of incoming food. Consider brushing your teeth more frequently or eating small amounts of mint leaves or fennel seeds as a fresh-breath alternative.*

HEMP SEEDS: yes

These "seeds" aren't the same botanical family of seeds that we eliminate with grains and legumes, so that makes them fine to eat during your Whole30.

HOT SAUCE: read your labels

Hot sauce is a great way to add spice and flavor to your Whole30 dishes, just read your labels carefully, or choose a Whole30 Approved brand like Tessemae's or Horsetooth Hot Sauce, both available online. (See page 403 for details.)

⭐ TIP: *Many national hot sauce brands include only Whole30 Approved ingredients, including Frank's Red Hot (Original, Chili and Lime, and Extra Hot), Tabasco (Original, Buffalo Style, and Garlic Pepper), Cholula, Texas Pete Hot Sauce, Valentina Mexican Hot Sauce, Tapatio, Louisiana Hot Sauce, and Crystal Hot Sauce.*

HUMMUS: no

Traditional hummus is made from garbanzo beans, which are a legume. Consider eggplant-based baba ghanoush instead.

KETCHUP: make your own

All commercial ketchups contain added sugar in some form, with the exception of Tessemae's (the only Whole30 Approved ketchup). Otherwise, you can substitute salsa, or make your own with our recipe on page 323. Note, don't expect these to taste super-sweet like your old ketchup. Whole30 ketchup tends to have more of a vinegar tang than a syrupy sweetness.

LARABARS (and other fruit/nut bars): read labels and use with caution

There are many brands and varieties of fruit and nut bars that are acceptable during your Whole30, but you have to read your labels. Make sure there is no added sugar in any form, or other off-plan ingredients like peanuts or gluten-free grains.

⭐ TIP: *We highly recommend using these bars as emergency snacks, on-the-go or travel food, or as fuel during endurance athletics. They're as close to candy as you can get on the Whole30 (using dates as a binder), so don't use them to satisfy sugar cravings. Your brain doesn't know the difference between a Snickers bar and a Larabar!*

MAYONNAISE: make your own

You'll be hard-pressed to find a commercial mayonnaise that doesn't contain off-plan ingredients—especially added sugar. Even the "olive oil" mayo is mostly soybean oil. The good news is that making your own compliant mayo is easy! (See our Basic Mayonnaise recipe on page 179.)

MSG: no

Monosodium glutamate (MSG) is a common flavor enhancer in many processed foods. This chemically structured ingredient is shown to have neurotoxic effects and is also linked to obesity. Because we think it's such noxious stuff, it's specifically off-limits for your Whole30, so if you see it on the label (like with some canned tunas), find a healthier alternative. The good news is that most of the foods that contain MSG are already off your plate on the program, but you can download our Common Additive Cheat-Sheet at www.whole30.com/pdf-downloads to learn other sneaky names for MSG.

MUSTARD: read your labels

Mustard is a fine choice, just read your labels carefully. Yellow mustards are generally compliant, but most other varieties often contain sulfites, which are out for the program.

⭐ TIP: *Many national mustard brands include only Whole30 Approved ingredients, including Annie's Naturals Organic Dijon and Horseradish Mustards, French's Yellow, Nathan's Deli-Style Mustard, and Gulden's Spicy Brown. Be extra careful with Dijon flavors, as most contain white wine.*

NATURAL FLAVORS: yes

The ingredient category "Natural Flavors" can stump even the most diligent label reader. It's impossible to say what's included in these flavors or where they come from, but they're not explicitly ruled out on the Whole30.

NIGHTSHADES: yes

Nightshades are a group of plants that contain compounds that may be inflammatory in certain populations (like those with an autoimmune disease, or those with chronic inflammation or joint pain). While nightshades may prove inflammatory in special populations, they're a healthy, nutrient-dense choice for most. Feel free to enjoy all forms of nightshades during your Whole30, unless you are specifically eliminating them due to a known sensitivity.

⭐ TIP: *Nightshades include: ashwagandha, bell peppers (aka sweet peppers), bush tomato, cape gooseberries, cocona, eggplant, garden huckleberries, goji berries (aka wolfberry), hot peppers (such as chili peppers, jalapeños, and habaneros), kutjera, naranjillas, pepinos, pimentos, potatoes (red, white, Yukon gold, baby, purple, etc.; but not sweet potatoes or yams), tamarillos, tomatillos, tomatoes, and spices like cayenne, chili pepper flakes, chili powder, curry, paprika, and red pepper.*

NUTRITIONAL YEAST: yes

Nutritional yeast can add a delicious texture and nutty flavor to casseroles, vegetable side dishes, and salads. Just consider your source carefully and make sure the option you choose is gluten-free.

"PALEO" BREAD: no

What we actually wanted to say here was, "Hell, no." Buying (or baking) Paleo bread during your Whole30 is an exercise in missing the point. We're asking you to change your food habits here, not just your ingredients. Bread is the very definition of nutrient-poor food-with-no-brakes, and is as off-limits as it gets, even if it is made from coconut flour. In addition, all bread pushes more nutritious foods off your plate. Just say no, and sandwich your meat in lettuce leaves, Portobello mushroom caps, or grilled eggplant instead.

⭐ TIP: *This goes for tortillas, wraps, biscuits, English muffins, flatbread, pita bread, and any other breadlike products that you may see recreated with Whole30-compliant ingredients on a Pinterest board. We'd say sorry but we wouldn't mean it—your bread-lovin' brain will thank us when your 30 days are over.*

"PALEO" CEREALS: no

Paleo cereal recreations are generally made with a base of nuts and seeds, and are almost always sweetened to mimic your favorite childhood cereal. While nuts and seeds are a fine inclusion in your Whole30, we recommend them in limited quantities because the kind of fat they contain isn't the healthiest. In addition, eating a big bowl of "cereal" doesn't leave much room for more nutrient-dense foods (like eggs, salmon, spinach, and berries) on your breakfast plate. Finally, replicating cereal—which many of us used to consume by the box—isn't the habit-changing behavior we want to encourage on the program. You can do better.

"PALEO" ICE CREAM: no

It doesn't matter whether it's made from coconut milk or frozen bananas—the only purpose of this confection is to replicate the taste, texture, and reward sensation of ice cream. (Don't tell us you'd get the same satisfaction from eating a frozen banana because *we call your bluff*.) Plus the addition of cocoa, nut butters, nuts, or other fruits to your creamy concoction takes this recipe straight into "sugar treat" territory, which is expressly forbidden during your Whole30. (See "Treats, Food Fixations, and the Scale" on page 95.)

PANCAKES: no

No, you can't have pancakes. Yes, even if they're just bananas and eggs. First, they are explicitly ruled out in the Whole30 program guidelines. This should be enough of a reason, but in case you're still wondering why (they're just bananas and eggs!) . . .

Pancakes in any form do not facilitate success with the Whole30 program. Reaching your health goals depends on committing to the rules, spirit, and intention of the program. The Whole30 is designed first and foremost to change your relationship with food. And the psychological impact of eating pancakes as part of your healthy eating, life-changing plan cannot be ignored.

Eating eggs, a banana, and some olive oil is not the same as combining those ingredients into a pancake. There are studies that show that how your brain perceives the food influences satiation. This is often cited with liquid food (smoothies or shakes), but experientially we see this with whole foods as well, depending on how they are combined. Pancakes bring up a totally different psychological response than frying some eggs and eating a banana. And it's that psychological (and emotional) response that we are trying to target with the program.

You may not have an affinity for pancakes, but we find that most people who complete our program do best without any of these comfort/trigger foods. So, because we need to create one program that applies to as many people as possible, we rule these Paleo recreations out. In our experience, this sets everyone up for the best Whole30 success possible. And, of course, what you choose to do after your 30 days are up is entirely up to you. (Also see "Treats, Food Fixations, and the Scale" on page 95.)

PICKLES: read your labels

Many big-name brands of pickles contain off-plan ingredients (like sugar) or chemical-sounding additives (like polysorbate 80). Just read your labels, and perhaps visit a local health food store if you have a craving for pickles.

⭐ TIP: *Many national pickle brands are Whole30-compliant, including Cascadian Farms Kosher Dill, Bubbies Kosher Dill, Trader Joe's Kosher Dill, and Whole Foods 365 Organic Baby Dills. Also, Rick's Picks (a national brand sold at many health food stores) pickles some really interesting vegetables. Try the Whole30-compliant Mean Beans, Classic Sours, or Smokra.*

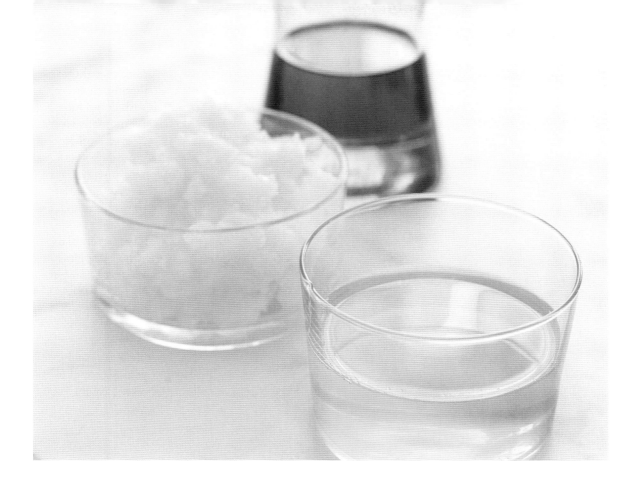

QUINOA: no

Quinoa is a pseudo-cereal—not botanically a grain, but containing compounds that may cause similar problems. All grains and pseudo-cereals are out for your Whole30.

SALAD DRESSINGS: make your own

Nearly all commercial salad dressings contain off-plan ingredients like soybean oil or added sugar. Tessemae's makes the only Whole30 Approved dressing and marinade line, but it's just as easy to make your own. (See page 302 for our dressing recipes.)

SALT: yes

When you cut out processed and packaged foods, you remove the vast majority of sodium from your diet. Adding salt to your Whole30 plate won't push you above healthy sodium limits, and if you avoid salt altogether, you run the risk of an electrolyte imbalance (not to mention serious food boredom). We encourage a mix of iodized table salt and sea salt.

TIP: *Did you know that all iodized table salt contains sugar? Sugar (often in the form of dextrose) is chemically essential to keep the potassium iodide from oxidizing and being lost. That's why salt is an exception to the Whole30 "no added sugar" rules. Without this exception, you'd never be able to eat outside of your own home, because iodized table salt is added to all restaurant and prepackaged foods.*

SAUSAGE: read your labels

Like bacon, it can be hard to find sausage without any added sugar or other off-plan ingredients, but if you can, you're in the clear. (Remember, if there is any form of sugar in the ingredient list the product is out for the Whole30, even if the label says, "Sugar = 0 grams.") Check with your local natural foods store, ask a local farmer or butcher shop, or make your own sausage, using our recipe on page 162.

⭐ TIP: *For the healthiest sausage, look for "pastured" and "organic" on the label—or better yet, ask your local farmer if his pigs are raised in a natural environment and fed a natural diet.*

SESAME OIL: yes

Sesame oil is approved for the program, but the healthiest way to use it is in small quantities as part of a dressing or sauce, or splashed on food just before you pull it off the stove. Cooking such a fragile oil (especially with high heat) can lead to oxidation, which then promotes inflammation in the body when consumed.

SNOW PEAS AND SUGAR SNAP PEAS: yes

The problem with legumes comes when you consume the seed. As with green beans, snow peas and sugar snap peas are mostly plant matter (the pod), with only tiny, immature seeds. As such, we're not too worried about their potential downsides.

SPICES: read your labels

Spices, herbs, and spice mixtures are a great way to add flavor and excitement to your food, but when it comes to spices and spice mixtures, read your labels and avoid those with off-plan ingredients.

⭐ TIP: *Whole30 Approved Spice Hound has over 100 spices and spice mixtures compliant with the program. (See page 403 for where to buy Spice Hound products.)*

STEVIA LEAF: no

While it's not highly processed like its liquid or powdery cousins, the only purpose of stevia leaf is to sweeten something that was not already sweet. This is something we want you to avoid during your Whole30. Instead, learn to appreciate the natural flavors of your foods, and don't rely on sweet tastes to prop up sugar cravings.

⭐ TIP: *Remember, just because a food is "natural" doesn't automatically make it healthy. You'll see sales pitches for things like stevia, coconut nectar, and agave syrup as a healthier alternative to white sugar, but the reward and habit centers in your brain don't know the difference between those and high-fructose corn syrup or table sugar. That's why we say "sugar is sugar"—because from a psychological perspective, it's all the same.*

SULFITES: not as additives (but naturally occurring are fine)

Sulfites occur naturally in many foods and beverages, and are a by-product of fermentation. Found in most wines and balsamic and red wine vinegars, they are also added to processed foods to increase shelf life, preserve color, and inhibit microbial growth. Sulfites can cause significant dermatological, pulmonary, gastrointestinal, and cardiovascular symptoms in sensitive people, which is why we explicitly exclude them during the Whole30. Read your labels: if any form of sulfite is listed in the ingredients (including potassium metabisulfite, a common additive in coconut milk), it's off-limits.

TAHINI: yes

Tahini is a paste made from sesame seeds. Sesame seeds are compliant with the Whole30 program, so tahini paste is too, if all the other ingredients in the paste are compliant.

TAPIOCA: yes

Tapioca is the starch extracted from the root of the cassava plant. It may come in the form of flour, flakes, or pearls. It's perfectly acceptable on the Whole30 as a thickener, and may be used by those needing lots of calories or carbohydrates. Use caution, however—some "tapioca flour" is actually a mix of tapioca and wheat. As always, read your labels.

> ⭐ TIP: *Tapioca is pure starch—practically no nutrition and all carbohydrate. This may come in handy for very active carb-driven athletes, but most of us don't need that concentration of calories or energy on a daily basis. If you're coming from a place of metabolic dysfunction or inflammation, tapioca-based dishes aren't the right choice for your Whole30.*

VANILLA EXTRACT: no

We'll be honest—we think this ruling is kind of silly (nobody uses vanilla extract for the buzz), but we must be consistent with the guidelines to avoid confusion. All vanilla extracts contain alcohol or sugar alcohol, which are off-limits for your Whole30. (If you see vanilla extract listed as an ingredient, you can count that product out for your Whole30, too.)

> ⭐ TIP: *You can use 100 percent vanilla bean powder in place of vanilla extract, or just scrape the inside of a vanilla bean pod. We use it in a 1:1 ratio in recipes; 1 tsp. vanilla extract = 1 tsp. vanilla bean or vanilla bean powder.*

VEGETABLE OILS: some, reluctantly (because sometimes, you have to dine out)

While we don't think vegetable oils are ever a healthy choice, we don't expressly rule them all out on the Whole30. If we did, you'd never be able to eat outside of your own kitchen, because all restaurants use them in some form in their cooking. We wanted to create the healthiest program we could, but we also need it to be possible for those who travel for business or pleasure, or simply want to dine out during the month.

Corn, rice bran, soybean, and peanut oils are out for your program because we rule out all forms of grains (corn and rice) and legumes (soy and peanuts) on the Whole30. However, canola (also known as rapeseed), safflower, sunflower, and grapeseed oils are all allowed—just not encouraged.

> ⭐ TIP: *Eliminate the consumption of vegetable oils at home, even if you're not on the Whole30, and make sure the rest of your diet is focused on the most nutritious choices possible, especially if you dine out frequently. For our best tips and tricks on dining out on the Whole30, see page 89.*

drink

"I started the Whole30 at 218 pounds, a 37-inch waist, and no energy. I also started with over eight years of acid reflux medication under my belt. I could not skip one dose of my medication without experiencing severe heartburn. After just 30 days, I now weigh 199 pounds, my waist is at 34 inches, I have not taken a single dose of my medication for the entire program." — JEREMY M., EAGLE RIVER, AK

ALMOND MILK: read your labels, or make your own

Though it does exist, compliant commercially produced almond milk is hard to find. Ingredients like added sugar (in any form) or carrageenan will render most store-bought almond milks off-limits for your Whole30. The alternative is to make your own—but remember, no added sweetener!

⭐ TIP: *Nuts and seeds aren't your best fat choice in general, and drinking your food is always less healthy than eating it. So even if you make your own, we'd rather you just eat the almonds! Still, if you're interested in making your own almond milk, check out our friend Stephanie Gaudreau's recipe at StupidEasyPaleo.com.*

CACAO DRINKS: yes

Beverages like Choffy or Crio Brü are made from 100 percent cacao beans that are ground and roasted just like coffee. It contains a small amount of caffeine (about 25 percent of that found in a normal cup of coffee), and may provide a delicious alternative to those looking to cut their caffeine consumption. Don't expect them to taste like hot chocolate, however—pure cacao is more bitter and rich tasting than the sweet stuff that comes from a packet. (And remember, the same Whole30 rules apply in terms of adding sugar or creamers.) See page 404 for where to find Whole30 Approved brands of these cacao-based beverages.

COCONUT WATER: read your labels

Most coconut waters are technically compliant, containing only natural sugars from the coconut. However, some brands add additional sugar to their ingredients, so read your labels. Remember, anything with sugar in the ingredient list is out for your Whole30.

⭐ TIP: *Coconut water is essentially a "light" fruit juice. If you're involved in endurance athletics, work in an environment that leaves you prone to dehydration, or just want a refreshing treat, coconut water can be a fine choice for rehydration. (Although adding a pinch of salt to coconut water makes it a much better hydration drink if dehydration is a legitimate concern.) Just don't let coconut water take the place of plain old water in your daily routine.*

CLUB SODA: yes

Club soda is just carbonated water (and maybe some salt)—perfectly fine for your Whole30.

COFFEE: yes

Yes, you can drink coffee. You're welcome. You can drink it black, add compliant coconut milk or almond milk, or add cinnamon or ground vanilla beans to the brew. But remember, Whole30 guidelines exclude milk, cream, non-compliant milk substitutes, and any form of added sugar or sweeteners. And (tough love ahead), if you "just don't like" black coffee, you are either not buying good coffee or you actually don't like coffee—you just like the sweet, creamy stuff you typically *add* to coffee.

> ⭐ TIP: *We'd generally recommend no more than one to two cups a day, always before noon so the caffeine doesn't interfere with sleep. Not that you asked for our opinion.*

FLAVORED COFFEE: read your labels

Some flavored coffees use natural ingredients like cinnamon and vanilla beans to lend some excitement to their beans, and those are fine on the Whole30. However, avoid coffees flavored with extracts (usually alcohol based), artificial flavors, added sweeteners, or chemicals. Ingredient lists aren't always printed on your bag of beans, so you may have to contact your favorite coffee company for more details on their process.

FRUIT JUICE: yes, but please don't drink it

Fruit juice is an approved added ingredient in dishes or beverages on the Whole30. (Technically, you could think of it as a sweetener, but we had to draw the line with "added sugar" somewhere.)

> ⭐ TIP: *While drinking a glass of fruit juice may be technically compliant, we really can't recommend it, even if you juice it yourself. Juicing strips many of the nutrients out of the fruit (many of which are found in the pulp and skin), but still leaves all of the sugar. You'd never eat eight oranges in a row, but you'd think nothing of gulping down an 8-oz glass of orange juice! From a satiety, sugar, and overall health perspective, we'd much rather you just eat the fruit.*

KOMBUCHA: probably—just read your labels

Kombucha may have probiotic benefits (especially if you make it yourself), and we think it's a fine addition to your Whole30 beverage menu. Just read your labels carefully—sugar listed in the ingredients generally means that it was added after fermentation, and that's a no-go. (Fruits or fruit juice as added ingredients are fine, however.)

> ⭐ TIP: *Interested in making your own kombucha and other fermented goods? Sarah Ramsden of Whole9 Canada has an entire online class dedicated to fermentation! Check it out at www.9life.co/whole9ff.*

MINERAL WATER: yes

Mineral water is just carbonated water plus some minerals (like calcium and sodium), present in the natural source of the water. All brands of plain mineral water are fine for your Whole30.

"PALEO" CREAMERS: no

We know there's a recipe out there where eggs, coconut milk, a significant quantity of dates, and some voodoo magic are combined with prayers to create a thick, creamy concoction designed to take the place of your cream and sugar (or Coffeemate) and once again transform your boring black coffee into a sweet, dreamy treat. But much like pancakes made with almond flour, relying on this technically compliant recreation is not part of a healthy relationship with food (or coffee). Instead, we'd encourage you to take a look at why you need this at all. Do you really like coffee, or are you just drinking it for the sugar hit?

PROTEIN SHAKES: almost always no

Almost all protein powders contain off-limit ingredients like whey, casein, soy, pea protein, rice bran, or added sweeteners. Besides, you can do way better. Anything you can get from protein powder (except maybe chemical extractives, added sugar, and strange-sounding isolates) you can get from whole foods during your Whole30 in a much more nutrient-dense, satisfying form.

In addition, formulated and processed meal-replacement shakes like Shakeology or Visalus are always off-limits. These products don't even come close to our definition of real, whole food—and they all include off-plan ingredients like pea protein, rice bran, and stevia.

However, protein powder from approved ingredients like 100 percent egg whites or crickets (yes, there is such a thing as cricket protein!) are allowed on the Whole30, provided they contain no added sweeteners.

⭐ TIP: *We want you to spend a month learning to appreciate real food, how it tastes, the satisfaction you get from preparing your own meals, and how Whole30 foods work to fuel your body before, during, and after exercise. You can have your shaker cup back in 30 days; for now, focus on getting protein from whole-food sources after your workout. Hard-boiled eggs, compliant deli meat, chicken, or canned tuna are easy, portable protein sources to take with you to the gym.*

SELTZER WATER: yes

This is just a fancy way of saying "club soda"—which is just carbonated water.

SMOOTHIES: we'd rather you didn't

This is a very popular question, with a very unpopular answer. Smoothies (generally made using lots of fruit) are technically compliant on your Whole30, but we strongly recommend against them. Food that you drink sends a different satiety signal to your brain than food that you chew. So when you drink your meal, your brain isn't getting the feedback it needs to tell your body that you've eaten—and you get hungry again fast, even though you just ingested plenty of calories (mostly in the form of sugar). Plus, as they are generally fruit-heavy, a breakfast smoothie sets you up for cravings, hunger, and volatile energy levels throughout the day. In summary, eat your food and skip the smoothie, especially for breakfast.

SPARKLING WATER: read your labels

Sparkling water can be a great way to jazz up your Whole30 drink routine. Look for products that only contain water and natural fruit/herb flavors, and avoid any with added sweeteners. Also, do not confuse mineral water or sparkling water with tonic water—the latter is always sweetened.

TEA: read your labels

Green, black, white, or herbal teas (hot or iced) are a great addition to your Whole30 repertoire, but you have to read your labels. Some teas add non-compliant ingredients like stevia, rice bran, or soy to their ingredients.

TIP: *Remember, many teas contain caffeine, so follow our general guidelines and stick to only decaffeinated or herbal varieties later in the day.*

TONIC WATER: no

Tonic water is a carbonated beverage that always contains sugar, ruling it out for your Whole30.

VEGETABLE JUICE: yes

We aren't big fans of drinking your food, but we approve of using vegetable juice as a way to get extra nutrients into your day. However, juice should never take the place of eating real vegetables! Chewing and swallowing your Good Food is always your top Whole30 priority. You'll probably want to juice it yourself (or use a blender of sorts), as most prepackaged "vegetable juices" are actually mostly fruit, or contain off-plan ingredients.

TIP: *Make sure your concoctions are almost all vegetable (with perhaps just a little fruit for flavor). However, note that even some vegetable-only drinks (like those heavy on beets and carrots) may pack more of a sugar punch than you're willing to add to your day. Read your labels, and do the sugar math!*

WATER KEFIR: read your labels

Following the same logic as kombucha, we're okay with water kefir. If you're making it yourself, do what you can to ensure that the sugar is used by the bacteria (generally by allowing appropriate fermentation time). If you're buying, avoid those brands with added sugar in the ingredient list.

Looking to serve something fancier than plain old water at your next gathering? See our festive drink recipes on page 390.

supplements and miscellaneous

"My cholesterol went down by 70 points . . . Not to mention my mild depression/anxiety is gone, moods definitely improved, itchy ear cleared up, strange tenderness in upper left calf that I've had for more than 15 years is gone, exercise-induced asthma is gone, and I have no allergies this season!" —MARY B., PORTLAND, OR

What supplements should I take during my Whole30?

First, you don't have to take anything at all—supplements aren't a required component of the Whole30 program. Based on our experience and the scientific literature, we believe many people would benefit from taking high-quality fish oil, vitamin D$_3$, magnesium, and maybe some digestive help, like enzymes or probiotics. However, none of these supplements are necessary for you to complete your Whole30 successfully. (Refer to page 404 for brands we like, and Chapter 22 of *It Starts With Food* for a more detailed explanation of these supplements' benefits.)

In addition, the Whole30 is primarily about determining food's effects on how you look, feel, and live. If you start adding a bunch of new supplements on top of your new eating plan, it may be hard to differentiate between the effects of the diet and the effects of the supplement. Be conservative when adding new supplements to your Whole30 routine—more isn't better in this situation. You can always use the first few days after your Whole30 reintroduction to experiment with adding a new supplement or two to your routine.

⭐ TIP: *Magnesium has many benefits, including relieving leg and other muscle cramps and buffering the effects of chronic stress. But you don't need a pill to get extra magnesium into your system—an Epsom salt bath is also effective. Make sure your bath water is warm but not too hot, use 1 to 2 cups of salts (don't be stingy!) and soak for 20 to 30 minutes for maximum benefit.*

Do I need a multivitamin?

It might not be a bad idea. We know, you're eating real, whole, natural foods. And yes, all of this good food is loaded with vitamins, minerals, and phytonutrients. So why would you need a multivitamin? Because our soil isn't as rich in minerals as it used to be—which means the fruits and vegetables we eat may not be as nutrient-dense as the ones our grandparents ate. We're not always able to eat pastured, grass-fed, organic animal products, and factory-farmed meat and seafood aren't as nutritious. And sometimes we dine out, consuming vegetable oils that eat up our antioxidant stores. So even though we're doing the best we can with real food, our health may still benefit from the micronutrient boost found in a good, balanced multivitamin. Just make sure yours doesn't contain any off-plan ingredients. (Refer to page 404 for brands we like.)

Do I need a calcium supplement?

The long answer to this question is in Chapter 11 of *It Starts With Food*, but here's the short answer. Building strong, healthy bones is about way more than just calcium, and (despite what the commercials imply) you don't need dairy for strong bones. If you eat a variety of whole, real foods with micronutrients like vitamins K_2 and C, magnesium, and phosphorous, get adequate vitamin D_3 from the sun or supplementation, build bone density by lifting weights, and manage your stress, you don't need a calcium supplement to keep your bones strong. And studies show that calcium supplementation alone doesn't work to prevent fractures from bone loss—taking calcium supplements gives you a short-term boost in bone density, but over time, your hormones will work against the extra calcium, and may even leave your bones more brittle than before. In summary, skip the calcium supplement and just focus on living a healthy lifestyle—your bones will thank you.

> TIP: *Homemade bone broths (see page 176 for our recipes); vegetables (like kale, spinach, collard greens, mustard greens, turnip greens, and bok choy); sea vegetables like nori; meat and seafood (like sardines, anchovies, shrimp, oysters, and canned salmon with bones); and nuts and seeds (like almonds, hazelnuts, and walnuts) are all excellent sources of the vitamins and minerals necessary to build strong, healthy bones.*

What about "green" (vegetable) supplements?

While the idea of a vegetable supplement sounds healthy, these usually contain off-plan fillers like brown rice bran or oat bran. In addition, there isn't any concerted scientific evidence that these supplements actually benefit your health in the dramatic ways they promise. For fear of sounding like a broken record, eating real food (in this case, vegetables) is always your healthiest bet—so skip the bottled "greens."

Can I take over-the-counter medications?

If you're suffering from a nasty cold, sore throat, or other seasonal illness, you may find that the over-the-counter medications you used to take are far from Whole30-compliant. While we encourage you to treat your illness with more natural methods (see our tip below), if you decide that your good night's sleep or easy breathing are more important than following Whole30 rules, you are always free to make the decision that you believe is best for your health. (At the very least, visit GlutenFreeDrugs.com and choose OTC medications that have been verified as gluten-free.)

> TIP: *Natural ways to treat a cold include vitamin C, zinc, and Echinacea; herbal teas with lemon (we like Traditional Medicinals Throat Coat Gypsy Cold Care); homemade bone broth, and plenty of rest and hydration. However, your comfort (and doctor's orders) always trump Whole30 rules, so if you really need the cough medicine, you have our blessing. Feel better!*

Can I take my prescription medication?

Your health care provider's orders always trump Whole30 rules, even if your prescription contains off-plan ingredients like wheat or cornstarch binders, or added sugar. However, we encourage you to discuss the Whole30 with your doctor, and ask if there are more natural, healthy ways to manage your medical condition than simply relying on prescription drugs. (This would be a great opportunity to share your healthy eating efforts with your doctor!) If your health care provider has prescribed a supplement regimen, read your labels to see if the supplements include off-plan ingredients. If they do, ask your doctor to recommend a comparable (compliant) brand. If none is available, please continue to follow your doctor's orders.

What if my supplement has non-compliant ingredients?

If you are on a supplement regimen of your own design, please read your labels! Non-compliant ingredients include added sugar (in any form), grains (wheat in any form, corn starch, rice bran, oat bran, or any other grain by-products), dairy (whey, casein, or other dairy by-products), or soy (even in "lecithin" form). In addition, some manufacturers refuse to clarify their "proprietary blend," leaving you in the dark as to what their supplement actually contains. This automatically rules the supplement out for your Whole30. You can either stop using the supplement during your Whole30, or look for the same kind of supplement with compliant ingredients. (See page 404 for some of our supplement recommendations.)

⭐ TIP: *Even if a prospective supplement is Whole30-compliant, it's hard to know whether it will really add benefit or just drain your wallet. Use our Supplement Evaluation Checklist to help you determine whether the pill or powder in question is worth it for you.*

- **Is the product designed to replace real, high-quality, fresh food in your diet?** Meal replacement shakes, vegetables-in-a-pill, or breakfast bars all promise to do just as much good as real food in your everyday diet, but there isn't a powder, pill, or shake in the world that can replace the vitamins, minerals, phytochemicals, and fiber found in natural, healthy, fresh foods.

- **Are the product's claims too good to be true?** The supplement industry is wholly unregulated—which means manufacturers can make all sorts of claims about their product's ingredients and benefits. Beware of inflated, unsupported claims that sound too good to be true and have little to no peer-reviewed long-term research to back them up.

- **Does the label focus on aesthetic changes?** Most of these slimming/leaning/trimming pills, powders, and shakes contain ingredients that could be harmful to your health, like stimulants and diuretics. And let's face it—if you lose a few pounds by taking a pill without effectively changing your eating habits, how likely are you to actually stay at that weight?

- Is there a hard and heavy sales pitch behind your consideration? If your motivation to buy is based on an aggressive, big-business marketing campaign, fear-mongering ("If you don't take this pill, you won't succeed!"), or generalized group-think ("All the event competitors use our shakes"), then think twice.

- Is it cost-prohibitive to eating better quality food? Even if the supplement meets all of the above criteria, if the daily cost means you'll have to cut your real-food budget just to afford it, it's simply not worth it.

If you've run the supplement-in-question through our entire checklist and it still makes the cut, then it's time for you to exercise your own judgment. At worst, your vitamin, mineral, or supplement is going to put you out a few dollars and still not provide the purported benefits—a waste of money, but no negative effects on your overall health and fitness. At best, the supplement will provide a boost to the already high-quality food you are eating, and help you fill in those small missing pieces in your daily diet and lifestyle.

Can I smoke cigarettes or e-cigs, or chew tobacco?

No—tobacco or nicotine of any sort are not allowed on the program. If you still smoke, you might be thinking, "There is no way I can quit smoking and make these dietary changes all at the same time." And you might be right. If you feel like all of these changes are too overwhelming, then we'd encourage you to focus on getting rid of your tobacco habit first, and then come back to the Whole30. On the other hand, if you've been looking for a program to help you quit, the Whole30 may just be your ticket. Many former smokers have told us they used the Whole30 in part as a smoking-cessation program, and that eliminating sugar and other psychologically unhealthy foods at the same time made the process that much easier. Either way, we encourage you to seek help for your nicotine addiction, prioritize ditching the smokes, and take on the Whole30 as soon as you are ready.

Can I smoke or consume marijuana?

Of course marijuana is a plant, and it may even be legal in your state, but that doesn't make it a healthy choice. Smoking still has negative health effects, but more immediately, smoking pot tends to promote cravings for less-healthy foods—and inhibits your inhibitory mechanisms. We want to set you up for success with your food choices during the next 30 days, which means unless it's prescribed by your health care provider, no marijuana in any form—especially not baked into Paleo brownies.

your whole30 plate

"Before my first Whole30, I knew how to cook with instructions from a package. Even then, I was actually proud of when those dishes came out correctly. Meat was so foreign to me. I hated to cook it because I was always afraid of undercooking it, or it being bad. Now, my fridge is constantly full with home-cooked meals. I know how to work around what I have, how to food prep, and how to feed my family good food instead of packaged food. I will keep learning, thanks to what my Whole30 taught me."

—KIMBERLY H., FORT WORTH, TX

Should all of my meals follow your meal template?

This isn't an official Whole30 rule, but it's a good general guideline to keep your program on track. The template includes a balance of protein, fat, and carbohydrate in amounts that will keep you full from one meal to the next, give you enough energy to sustain your activity levels, and provide a healthy variety of micronutrients. Of course, not every meal is going to look exactly like the plate on page 194—sometimes you eat a stew, a casserole, or a frittata where your meat, vegetables, and fat are all mixed up together. Don't stress—just estimate your portion, eat slowly and chew thoroughly, wait ten minutes and evaluate whether you're still hungry. If you are, go for seconds! It's really hard to overeat real food, and everything on your Whole30 plate is doing your body good.

Do your recipes follow the meal template?

No, because not all of our recipes include a protein and a side of vegetables or fruit. (Our One Pot Meals on page 332 are the exception.) However, with every dish that doesn't follow our template, we've given you "Make it a Meal" recommendations to help you build your own Whole30 plate. For example, if you're making our Braised Beef Brisket (page 214), we tell you to add sweet potato, butternut squash, or carrots to the dish to make it a complete meal. Or, we'll give you recipe pairing suggestions, like suggesting our Halibut with Citrus-Ginger Glaze (page 240) goes well with Green Cabbage Slaw (page 282) and Coconut Cauliflower Rice (page 366).

If you're cooking from our Fundamentals section (page 146), you'll have to build your own plate there, too. Start with our template, including the appropriate protein amount for your context and goals, fill the rest of your plate with vegetables, add some fruit (if you choose), and build in some healthy fats, either in the form of cooking fat, added fat, or both. For example, make our Perfect Seared Chicken Breast (page 157), grill some green beans, peppers, onions, and mushrooms using the technique found on page 361, then make a garden salad with one of our Vinaigrette Variations (page 326) as your added fat.

Shouldn't I be counting calories?

No! Isn't that good news? One goal of our program is to get you back in touch with your body's natural regulatory mechanisms—in this case, trusting your feelings of hunger, and intuitively knowing when to stop eating. That means after a few weeks of eating foods *with* brakes (providing both nutrition and satiety), you'll be eating when you're hungry, and stopping when you're full. By the end of your Whole30, these signals will actually work, perhaps for the first time in years! And we've specifically designed the amounts and proportions recommended in our meal template so you won't need to count calories or plug your food into a calculator—not even if you're trying to lose weight.

> ⭐ TIP: *Please, trust us on this one. One of the biggest mistakes you could make is listening to some calculator you found on the internet over the cues your own body is sending you. Skip the weighing, measuring, and tracking for the next 30 days—it will help you foster a healthier relationship with food, and turn mealtime into a relaxing, enjoyable experience instead of an arbitrary math session.*

Can I have snacks?

Again, this isn't a Whole30 rule, so if you choose to snack, just make sure they are Whole30-compliant. However, we do not generally recommend snacking for some important reasons. Snacking between meals turns your daily dietary habits into grazing, which can disrupt the normal functioning of your hormones and may promote inadvertent overconsumption. It may take you a while to figure out the right size meals for you, however, so if you find you ate too little in any given meal and need additional nourishment, then we'd rather you have a snack to tide you over than spend the rest of the afternoon cranky, tired, and hungry. Ideally, your snacks are just smaller meals—don't snack on veggies or fruit alone, as they're not very satiating all by themselves.

If you find your meals are never big enough to tide you over, then it's time to start making each one a little bigger. Start by adding a little more protein and a little more fat. (You're already filling your plate with vegetables, so you're good on that front.) You can go slow here—just keep adding to your plate until you find an amount that will successfully get you from one meal to the next comfortably.

> ⭐ TIP: *If you're on the go and can't plan a mini-meal, just follow this rule of thumb: include at least two of the three macronutrients every time you eat. So maybe that's protein and fat (like hard-boiled eggs and a handful of macadamia nuts), or protein and carbs (like deli turkey slices and an apple), or fat and carbs (like carrot sticks dipped in guacamole). Following this rule will ensure your snack actually tides you over until your next meal, and that you get enough overall calories in your day.*

I'm pregnant or nursing—now can I have snacks?

Yes, but we'd still rather you eat more small meals than graze constantly like a gazelle. In the early stages of pregnancy, you may be too nauseous to eat a big meal. In later stages, your stomach may not be able to physically hold enough nutrition in just three meals to keep you healthy. (And when you're nursing, your schedule may be hectic enough that you find yourself eating every three hours, timed around your baby.) In these special circumstances, eat more frequent, smaller meals to ensure you're getting enough calories and nutrition. Try to leave at least 2 to 3 hours between meals, if possible—it's better hormonally to eat five smaller meals than pick at food all day long. (See page 109 for more tips on customizing the Whole30 when pregnant or nursing.)

What about my growing kids— can they survive on just three meals a day?

Kids are another exception—they're growing so fast (and their stomachs are so small) that they'll likely need more frequent, smaller meals or snacks in between meals. Our rule of thumb for growing babies and younger toddlers is, if they're hungry, let them eat! Once they're out of toddler stage, however, transitioning them to three meals a day, preferably with their family, is ideal. Feel free to add a snack between each meal to tide them over and ensure they're getting enough calories and nutrition; just follow our previously mentioned snacking guidelines. (See page 117 for more tips on customizing the Whole30 for kids.)

I work a really long day—can I have more than three meals?

Absolutely. If you're up really early and get to bed pretty late, you may find you need four (or even five) meals to keep you fueled throughout the day. Just try to keep them around 3 to 4 hours apart, if you can—any closer than that and your hormones may not have time to do their proper jobs in between.

I'm really active or regularly exercise—should I have more than three meals?

You can and should, especially if you're participating in a high-intensity exercise program,

bodybuilding program, or endurance activity like running or biking. Eating a bonus post-workout meal (as outlined in our meal template on page 194) is the best way to ensure your body gets extra nutrition and calories to help you sustain your activity levels. Timing this meal right after your workout (ideally within a half-hour) also helps you start the recovery process faster and more effectively. Have a meal-sized serving of an easily digestible protein like egg whites, chicken breast, or salmon; and some carbohydrates in the form of starchy vegetables like potatoes, butternut squash, or acorn squash. (Don't worry about adding fat—that's less important for this post-workout meal.) Then, eat your next normal meal 60–90 minutes later.

⭐ TIP: *We also like the idea of a pre-workout snack, to send a signal to your body that activity is coming. Eat a small serving of protein and a little bit of fat anywhere from 15 to 60 minutes before your workout, but skip the carbs here. Try a hard-boiled egg and a handful of macadamia nuts, or a few pieces of jerky and some avocado. If you exercise first thing in the morning, something is better than nothing, so do the best you can. Not sold on the idea of eating before exercise? Try it for a week! You may be surprised at how much stronger or better your workouts feel with a little something in your stomach.*

I don't like eating breakfast. Can I skip it?

You're an adult, which means you can technically do anything you want. However, since you asked us, we'd strongly recommend against skipping breakfast. If you're not hungry first thing in the morning, it's a good indicator that your hormones are off. One of the best ways to get those hormones back in line is to eat something in the morning, when it's biologically appropriate. If you start eating too late in the day, your entire hormonal rhythm can be thrown off—so come nighttime, you'll tend to crave more food. Usually not the good kind, either. Which means that you'll be prowling through your pantry or freezer after dinner looking for a snack, leading to more hormonal disruption. In summary, eat breakfast within an hour of waking to keep your metabolism on track.

⭐ TIP: *If you're really not hungry first thing in the morning, here's our rule of thumb: no coffee before breakfast. We know, you hate that idea, but coffee is an appetite suppressant, which will make it even harder for you to eat. So fire up the frying pan before the percolator—it's for your own good.*

I'm hungry all the time.

This is common, especially in the first two weeks of the program. You're probably used to running on sugar for energy, but you're not eating sugar all the time anymore, so your body is craving energy. That translates to hunger, even if you don't actually need the calories. The good news is that your body has an alternate fuel source (fat) that you'll be really good at using in the next week or two. So remember, this too shall pass. In the meantime, if you're hungry, go ahead and eat an extra meal or a snack—just make sure it follows our guidelines. Trying to prop up your energy levels with handfuls of dried fruit or a fruit smoothie is only setting your cause back.

I'm never hungry.

This is also common, especially in the first two weeks of the program. The food you're eating on your Whole30 is much more satiating than the foods-with-no-brakes you used to eat, and your body isn't used to being this well fed. This may make you feel less than hungry when lunch or dinner rolls around. However, three meals a day is really the bare minimum you need to stay healthy, both calorie and micronutrient-wise, so stick with it. Generally by the second or third week, your hunger will self-regulate, and you'll find yourself ready for breakfast, lunch, and dinner.

How much fruit is too much?

That depends on a few factors. What season is it? It's really normal to eat lots more fruit in the summer, when it's fresh and available, and you're generally more active (hiking, biking, and spending more time exploring the outdoors). Why are you eating it? If you're reaching for a banana or grapes to prop up your sugar cravings, we'd ask you to rethink that strategy. You don't want to end up with the same cravings after your program, and continuing to feed your brain the sweetest stuff allowed every time it pitches a tantrum isn't really changing your habits. How active are you? If you're an athlete, weekend warrior, or generally active person, you may need to purposefully incorporate fruit into your day to provide more carbohydrates.

In summary, how much fruit you eat is up to you. We generally recommend starting with two servings of fruit a day, eaten with meals (not by itself), but don't stress if you end up with four or five servings on a hot summer day, or no fruit at all over a cold winter weekend.

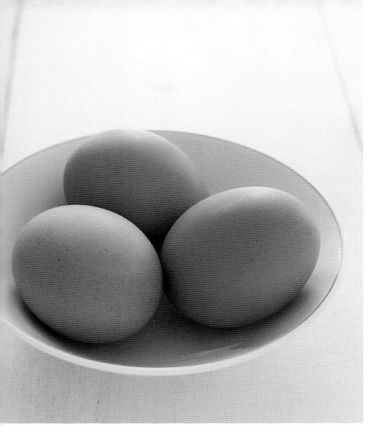

eating a healthy, anti-inflammatory diet like the Whole30. Of course, you should vary your protein sources—if you eat eggs every day for breakfast, you're missing out on the different micronutrients found in salmon, steak, or other protein sources. But don't worry about eating two, three, or even five eggs at a time.

⭐ TIP: *Pastured, organic eggs are a great bang for your protein buck—even at $6 a carton, that's still just $1.50 per (average) meal. Look for words like "pasture-raised" on the carton (which is very different from "free-range" or "cage-free"), or better yet, ask your local farmer what the chickens are fed and how they live.*

That's a lot of meat.

That's not really a question, is it? You may be thinking "so much meat" because we're asking you to include an animal protein source with every meal. Please note, however, that the serving sizes are actually quite moderate (as low as one palm-sized serving three times a day, which is right in line with the U.S. Recommended Daily Allowance), and it's balanced with lots and lots of plant matter. Plus, not every meal needs to include red meat, bacon, or sausage—mix in fish and shellfish, poultry, pork, and eggs to get a good variety of amino acids and micronutrients.

That's a lot of fat.

We know it may look like you're eating tons of fat with each meal, but that's only because we've been conditioned to see all fat as bad. If you're trying to train your body to effectively utilize fat as fuel, you've got to give it some of that fuel, don't you? Plus, fat is a huge player in satiety,

⭐ TIP: *Be extra cautious with dried fruit. It's basically nature's candy—especially dates—so save it for outdoor activities like a long hike or bike ride, or on-the-go emergency food. In addition, read your labels when it comes to things like cranberries or cherries—make sure they're unsweetened (or sweetened with apple juice, not sugar).*

How many eggs are too many?

You'd be hard-pressed to eat too many eggs in one sitting—Dallas will eat a five-egg omelet some mornings. As we explained in Chapter 13 of *It Starts With Food*, you don't have to be afraid of the fat or cholesterol in eggs if you are and makes your food taste 73 percent better. (That's science.) So don't be afraid of a half an avocado or a few tablespoons of cooking oil with each meal. In fact, you may find you need to add even more fat than the meal template calls for, if you're large or active.

⭐ TIP: *We've got safe, healthy, sustainable weight loss built right into our model, because we know that is a major goal for the majority of you—so do not cut your fat intake below the low end of our recommended range. Trying to outsmart the system in an effort to lose weight faster may very well backfire. Your delicate hormone balance will be thrown off if you're chronically underfeeding yourself— plus you'll be hungry all the time, and your energy levels will take a dive, and you'll be cranky because you're tired and hungry. So stick to the lower end of our spectrum if you want, but resist the urge to cut your fat intake even more, because as crazy as it sounds, eating less could be counterproductive to your weight-loss efforts.*

Should I add less fat if my protein source is fatty?

Nope. Some meals, your meat will be fatty (like salmon or a rib eye), other meals it will be lean (like chicken or pork chops). As you are varying your protein throughout the week, it all evens out in the end. Just stick to the template and add the recommended amounts of fat at each meal, regardless of your protein source.

Does cooking fat count as added fat?

It does, but that's generally not enough to satisfy your "added fat" requirement. (You're generally using only a tablespoon or two of fat per meal, and some of that gets left in the pan.) If cooking fat is the only fat in the recipe, and/or if you choose to drain the naturally occurring fat from your meal (like with ground beef), make sure you add some fat back in some other form. Also, feel free to combine fats in any one meal; just choose from the lower end of the spectrum if you're eating more than one. For example, if you want to top your Perfect Burger (page 153) with both Buffalo Sauce (page 304) and Guacamole (page 308), just use a smaller serving of each.

⭐ TIP: *Don't stress about this! Use your body's hunger and fullness signals to guide you, and remember that because you're eating a wide variety of foods and meals, a little more fat in this meal will naturally balance itself out with a little less fat in a meal you'll eat later in the week.*

When I make these recipes, I end up with too much or not enough food for two people.

The serving sizes here are just general guidelines—it's impossible to choose one serving size that will suit everybody's needs. If you find you need more protein in each meal, go ahead and up the amounts in each recipe—unless you need to double the meat, you shouldn't need to adjust the amounts of accompanying dressings, sauces, or spices. If you find you have too many leftovers, scale back appropriately. (And always feel free to add more vegetables to any of our dishes!)

grocery shopping

"As a professional athlete, what I use to fuel my body is of paramount importance. To get the best results, I have to know exactly what I eat for each meal, but before the Whole30, that wasn't easy. I'm sensitive to gluten and dairy, but I never knew where those ingredients were hidden. The Whole30 has been invaluable—it made me a label-reading guru! I look for single, whole ingredients or foods with very few ingredients. I know how to avoid sneaky sugars, gluten, and dairy, and translate labels with science-y or healthy-sounding ingredients that aren't good for me. Since I've done a few Whole30s, I've learned to easily shop for and prepare the most flavorful, healthy foods I've ever had in my life!" —ERICA TINGEY, UCI PROFESSIONAL CYCLIST AND TWO-TIME NATIONAL CHAMPION

One of the most common challenges for people new to the Whole30 is grocery shopping. You can no longer dash through the store picking up the usual—on the Whole30, every product with a label requires a critical review, and you may have to stock your kitchen with some foods you're not used to buying.

Also, this may be more expensive than the way you're used to shopping. We just wanted to address that up front, and put it into perspective. Eating real food does cost more than eating heavily processed fast-food or convenience foods, and stocking your Whole30 kitchen may require some up-front purchases of more costly items things like cooking oils or spices. But isn't eating whole, nutrient-dense, health-promoting foods that make you look, feel, and live your best worth a few extra dollars? Most people find they want to prioritize healthy food once they start feeling better, and are willing to spend a little less in other areas of their lives (like the cable bill, high-priced coffees, or upgrading your smartphone) to make room for grass-fed meats and organic vegetables.

Many people even find they're *saving* money on the Whole30 by cooking at home and not spending money on impulse junk foods, alcohol, and dining out. Regardless, we understand that your budget and time aren't unlimited, so let's talk about making the most of your Whole30 grocery shopping experience.

First, You Must Plan

The most important thing you can do to save time, money, and frustration during your first Whole30 can be summed up in two words: Meal. Plan.

We've already talked about this, right? (Refresh your memory starting on page 25.) By planning your Whole30 meals a few days ahead of time and making a detailed shopping list for each meal, you'll be shopping only for the ingredients you need, and will be less tempted to add "extras" to your cart—these extras can really add up! You'll also be far less likely to waste food, as everything you buy is needed in one recipe or another.

It's also incredible stress-relieving to have a meal plan. Knowing your dinner is already simmering in the slow cooker means far less worry during your work day, and far less temptation to call for pizza when you get home hungry and cranky.

THE PLANNING PLAN

Habit and change research shows that the best plans are detailed, yet not so long-reaching that they become overwhelming. Planning too far in advance (like a whole month of meals) is a lot of work, and what if you don't feel like steak two weeks from Tuesday? Planning for the next three to seven days is perfect; you're not expending effort thinking about what you'll eat every single day, but it's not so long that you feel married to the plan. It also helps your brain achieve some "small wins" quickly—successfully navigating your first few days of Whole30 meals is just the kind of milestone that gives you the self-confidence to keep going. Decide how many days you'll plan based on how often you can go to the grocery store, and how flexible you want to be with your food choices and your budget.

After you've decided which meals to make, you can turn that into a detailed shopping list. To make creating your own shopping list easier, download our free template from www.whole30.com/pdf-downloads, check off the items you need, and write the type (pork shoulder vs. pork ribs), quantity, or amount next to the ingredient.

Now that you have your meal plan and a shopping list, it's time to hit the grocery store. But wait—you should have a plan for this, too!

First, give yourself plenty of time to grocery shop, especially if it's a pre-Whole30 "stock your kitchen" kind of outing. Don't go into the store thinking you'll be out in your usual 20 minutes—reading labels and finding new ingredients takes time. If you have kids, leave them at home if you can. Dedicating an hour alone to shop at your leisure will reduce any stress you might be feeling, and give you the chance to practice some of these guidelines before you shop again with kids in tow.

If your partner or spouse wants to shop and learn with you, even better—unless you're afraid they'll behave like a toddler, in which case you should probably leave them home, too.

Shop Smart

Now you're in the store, shopping list in hand . . . So where do you start?

To make the most of your grocery store budget, shop strategically. There's a reason protein comes first on our shopping list—focus on meat, seafood, and eggs first, buying grass-fed or pastured if you can. If your budget is really tight, you may want to meal plan around what you see on sale in your grocery store flyer, or choose recipes that use more economical cuts of meat (like our Braised Beef Brisket on page 214, Cod with Mushroom and Red Pepper Relish on page 242, or Roasted Pork Shoulder with Butternut Squash, Kale, and Tomatoes on page 344) instead of buying expensive tenderloins or halibut.

Don't overlook frozen burgers, salmon, or shrimp—they're an economical way to buy high-quality meat. Just make sure to read your labels carefully, as many prepackaged burgers or patties include off-plan ingredients. Finally, even at $6 a dozen for pastured and organic, eggs are still your cheapest protein source.

Next, move to the produce section, buying organic vegetables, fruit, and fresh herbs only if you can afford it. Spend your organic dollars on those fruits or vegetables you can't peel (like lettuce or berries), and buy things with a peel or removable skin (like avocado or onions) conventionally. Fresh herbs really add punch to a meal; find them in the produce section, too. (Cilantro and parsley are usually kept by the green onions, while basil, dill, thyme, and others are usually sold in small plastic packages.)

Canned vegetables are also an economical option; you can find canned sweet potato, butternut squash, and pumpkin (not pumpkin pie filling!) at most grocery store chains. Be sure your canned fruit is packed in water or fruit juice, however, not a sugary syrup.

Finally, go frozen! Frozen vegetables are an economical and easy way to get your greens (and reds, and yellows) in. Just make sure your vegetable mix isn't full of corn, lima beans, or other off-plan "vegetables," and don't come swimming in a sugary sauce. Frozen fruit (like berries) are also a great way to get a taste of summertime in February without the high prices of off-season fruit.

The aisles are your next stop, for healthy fats and pantry items. Plan to stock up on healthy fats over time, as these can be the most expensive items on your bill, after protein. First, buy a few different kinds of cooking fats, as you'll use these every day. Prioritize extra-virgin olive oil, unrefined coconut oil, and butter (clarifying it yourself is cheaper than buying ghee), as you'll use these most frequently with these recipes. They're pricey, but you'll only have to stock up once every month or two, so consider them an investment.

Next, add the fats you'll need for your meals, like avocado (back in the produce section), full-fat coconut milk, or coconut flakes, and grab some canned olives as back-up. Finally, shop for nuts and seeds as part of your meal plan, or as an easy on-the-go fat source. Buy just the amount you need from the bulk bins—it's less expensive than buying a whole bag—and if you buy mixed nuts, make sure your mix doesn't contain peanuts!

Finally, stock your pantry with what you'll need for your meal plan, and if you can swing it, pick up a few basics. (Use our shopping list on page 192 as your guide.) This includes checking off at least a few often-used spices (like salt, pepper, ground mustard, cumin, chili powder, garlic powder, and onion powder), and adding to your collection over time as you can afford it.

As for how often you should shop, that's really up to you. There are a few benefits to shopping more frequently (a few times a week, versus once a week). First, because all the ingredients you're buying are perishable, grocery shopping more frequently means all that fresh food is far less likely to spoil before you can use it—another money-saving bonus. Plus, being able to shop a few times a week means you can meal plan just a few days at a time, allowing you more room to include newly discounted foods in

HERB HELP

You can't beat the flavor punch of fresh herbs, but if you're trying to stretch your grocery store dollars, you can substitute dried herbs in any of our recipes. The general ratio is 1:3 (one teaspoon of dried herbs for every tablespoon of fresh). It's not super important to get this ratio exactly right—herbs are very forgiving, and you might discover you like a lot more cilantro or dill than our recipes call for. It's also really easy to grow your own basil, thyme, or rosemary at home! All you need are a few pots, a sunny counter space or table, and a watering can.

your plan, or better accommodate for your family's tastes or requests.

However, you may not have time in your schedule to meal plan, prep, and shop a few times a week. Shopping once a week certainly makes things easy from a time perspective, and can help you better track your grocery budget. If that's the case, you'll want to extend your meal plan out to seven days, and take the time to make a detailed shopping list for every dish. Start with a clean refrigerator (eat up last week's leftovers!), because you'll need the space for your big haul. Finally, let your family know that what's on the plan is exactly what you're eating—but you'll take special requests in time for next week's shopping trip.

dining out

"I followed this plan for the 30 days and a little while afterward. I was an insulin-dependent type 2 diabetic and now I am off of all my medications (under the supervision of my doctor). I did not think that this could happen, but it did. I would like to encourage people to try it for the 30 days suggested. It has truly changed my life."
—JOANN H., CITY/STATE WITHHELD

Your Whole30 will likely involve at least one attempt to navigate a restaurant menu. For those who travel often for work, or "wine and dine" as part of your profession, you may find yourself in a restaurant or airport food court more days than not. When you're new to this way of eating, dining out can be challenging and stressful. Our goal is to make your Whole30 business lunch, family dinner, or cross-country travel easier (and more delicious).

But first, let's get one thing out of the way.

Accept right here and now that at times, you're probably going to feel like "That Person." You know, the one who asks questions about everything, makes about a thousand substitutions, and then still has to send something back?

Yeah. That might be you.

Accept it, embrace it, and then take our advice and do it without ticking off your waiter, the chef, or your dining partners. Follow our strategies and you get what you want, your waiter feels happy to have helped you, and your dining partners don't even notice you didn't eat the bread. Everybody wins.

Here is our timeline for a happy, healthy Whole30 restaurant adventure.

Ahead of Time

First, when dining with a group, take charge and suggest a restaurant that meets your specifications at every opportunity. "Where do you want to go?" "I don't know, where do you want to go?" This is where you step in and say, "Let's go here! The food is great, you'll love it." You'll look like a champ for being decisive, and you get to better control your dining environment.

Do a little research about the restaurant before you go. The more time you have, the more you'll be able to find out. Browse through their menu online, taking note of any table-side

---

GOOGLE!

Smaller, local restaurants are generally more accommodating to substitutions or customization than larger chains. If you don't know the area, search for terms like "organic breakfast," "farm-to-table," or "grass-fed burger" on a review service like Yelp, or search for the same terms on the Web.

specials (like warm bread or chips and salsa), seeking out their allergen statements or gluten-free menu, and noting any special policies—no substitutions could be a problem for you in this situation. Plan your order now, so you won't be tempted by other less healthy dishes when you arrive.

If you have time, call the restaurant. Ask about their cooking fats, and find out how willing they are to accommodate your specific dietary needs. Let the host(ess) or manager know that you're coming, that you'll have some specific food requests, and thank them in advance for accommodating you.

When Ordering

Now, a little pep talk: instead of feeling self-conscious about the requests you're about to make, take ownership! There is a way to be clear in your requests without being bossy, condescending, or difficult. In addition, if you make a big deal out of your "crazy diet," your tablemates will, too. If you order confidently and matter-of-factly, as if it's no big thing, chances are others will follow your lead and not even mention it.

Let your servers know that you have some dietary restrictions, and you'll be asking some questions about the menu. If you know you have legitimate allergies or sensitivities, specify them clearly. Let them know that you really appreciate their help. (We'll talk about how you can show your appreciation later.) If you're patient and respectful with the restaurant staff, they'll show you the same courtesy.

Ask about hidden ingredients (like cheese or croutons on a salad) or preparation methods for everything you're thinking about ordering. Be firm but nice about your requests. Say things like, "Would it be possible to have that steamed instead of fried?" or "May I please have a side of olive oil and lemon instead of the dressing?"

Ask for vegetables to be steamed, grilled, baked, or sautéed with olive oil, instead of fried in vegetable oil. Make sure all baked potatoes come plain, and not smothered in non-clarified butter, cheese, or sour cream. Omelets or scrambled eggs are often infused with milk or pancake batter (!) to make them fluffier, so request shelled eggs, or order them poached. Request individual bottles of olive oil and vinegar and some fresh lemon to use as dressing on salad, vegetables, or meat.

You'll likely have to skip all the sauces and dressings that come with your meal, as they all probably contain sugar. (That goes for ketchup, too!) Ask for fresh salsa, guacamole, olive oil, lemon, or lime if your food needs a little spicing up.

Order Up!

Keep a close eye on your meal as the waiter brings it to the table. Despite your clear communication, sometimes the waiter or chef gets it wrong. If it's something simple like croutons on your salad (and you're not highly sensitive to the food in question), just pick them off and enjoy your meal. If your plate arrives with rice, corn, or a side of bread, either politely send it back, or just eat around it as best as you can (unless you have an allergy, in which case you really have to send it back).

If you do have to send your meal back, don't assume it's your server's fault, and don't make a scene. Chances are your order wasn't simple, and your meal may have required a substitution or special request that the kitchen wasn't used to handling. Calmly and clearly explain what was wrong and thank your server for taking care of it. Treating restaurant staff with respect paints a great picture of our community (and is generally just the right thing to do).

Finally, remember that this social engagement is supposed to be fun. Do the best you can with the menu you have, don't stress about getting it perfect, and remember that even if your burger is plain or your garden salad is boring, you're there to commune with the people at your table. (You can always eat an Epic Bar from your "emergency stash" after the meal if you're still hungry.)

Dealing with Questions

If at any point your tablemates ask you about your meal preferences, don't panic. First, recognize that now is *not* the time to educate them about the benefits of the Whole30. Seriously. Look around. They're eating bread, onion rings, pizza, or sandwiches, and maybe having a drink. Do you really want to lecture them about inflammatory proteins and food-with-no-brakes?

We call that one, "How to lose friends and alienate people."

Remember that a shared dining experience isn't actually about the food—it's about the company, and the social interaction. If someone points out your preferences or order, you can simply say, "I'm doing a 'nutrition reset' this month, so I'm eating a little differently." If they ask for the details, enthusiastically offer to share more information via email, or when you get back to the office. Then, change the subject by posing a question to the group: "Did anyone see the game last night?" or "Anyone been golfing lately?"

If the whole table seems interested in your new healthy eating plan (and you feel comfortable sharing some of the details), focus on what you *are* eating, not what you're avoiding, and share something personal about your experience. "I'm eating nothing but whole, nutrient-dense, unprocessed foods for 30 days. It's kind of old-school—like what your great-grandparents would have eaten. I feel great, and it's really helping my energy levels." Then, offer to provide more details after your meal, and (again) change the subject.

If you're uncomfortably pressed or feel like your food choices have been thrown into a negative spotlight, fall back. A humorous but polite, "I hate talking about food over food. Let's just enjoy the meal, and we can make fun of my weird diet later." Then, change the subject or excuse yourself to use the restroom, to give the table a chance to come around to a new topic.

Check, Please

Whew—you made it! Your meal is over, and you're ready to show your appreciation for your hard-working waiter. When it comes to restaurant gratitude, money talks. Tip your waiter well, especially if this is a restaurant you plan to visit again. If you're splitting the check with the group, hand your waiter an extra few dollars and say, "Thank you for accommodating my special requests."

And with that, you're ready to take your happy, healthy self out on the town! Bon appétit.

travel

"My physical therapist, who was treating me for migraines with needling, recommended trying the Whole30. And it has been a miracle for me! My lifelong chronic migraines are almost completely gone as well as many other health problems. I have been able to reduce or eliminate my medications also." —GAYLE G., SUMMERVILLE, SC

Whether you're a frequent flyer, spend tons of time in the car, or are planning a family camping trip, staying Whole30 while traveling isn't as hard as you might imagine. The key, as you'll hear us say 172 times in this book, is planning and preparation.

In general, protein is going to be the hardest to get in good amounts when on the road. Plan ahead and stock up. Cook chicken or salmon the night before you travel, boil a dozen eggs, or whip up a batch of Protein Salad (page 161). Under normal climate-controlled temperatures, all of these will keep for hours without refrigeration, so they're perfect for a plane ride or road trip.

Smoked salmon is often overlooked, but the wild-caught stuff is a great source of omega-3 fatty acids and protein. Slice, roll around chunks of honeydew melon or mango, secure with a toothpick, and pack. It, too, will keep without refrigeration for up to three hours.

We'd avoid canned tuna, sardines, or anchovies, unless you're willing to endure hours of dirty looks from your fellow travelers.

Fruit is an easy carbohydrate source while you're traveling, but don't overlook your veggies! Carrots, celery, and bell pepper strips make for crunchy carbs, and are the perfect guacamole or salsa-delivery mechanism. If you're able, travel

TRAVEL CONSIDERATIONS

Here are some questions to consider when making your travel plans:

- What is the duration of my travel time? (Is it a 3-hour flight, or a 24-hour road trip?)

- Will I be eating in restaurants, from my own stash of food, or both?

- Are there healthy food stores near where I'm going, or do I have to bring everything from home?

- Will I have access to a refrigerator, or am I able to bring a cooler?

- Will I have a space to prepare food (like a kitchenette or camping stove) or does everything have to be grab-and-go?

- Can I pack a bunch of food to take with me, or is my capacity limited?

- Are there restrictions on what I can take with me (like liquids when flying)?

CAR CAMPING

If you're hitting the great outdoors on four wheels, bring a giant cooler and stock up on some Pre-Made Paleo (page 403). These are chef-prepared, Whole30 Approved, pre-cooked frozen meals perfect for reheating over an open flame or a small camping stove. Imagine dining on Pomegranate Pulled Pork, Grilled Creole Chicken, or Marinated Skirt Steak instead of charred hot dogs. Order vegetable sides to accompany your protein, or bring your own potato salad, roasted root vegetables, or soup to round out your meal. Bonus: bring pineapple chunks to roast over the open flames and you won't even miss those burned marshmallows.

with a flexible cutting board and sharp knife to assist you with food prep on the go. (And make sure you pack your own plastic silverware and napkins, in case you don't have time to stop while dashing through the airport or fueling up.)

Canned vegetables like sweet potato, pumpkin, or butternut squash are also a good idea, although you may have a hard time getting them through airport security. In that case, packets of baby food (100 grams or under) are your next best portable carbohydrate option.

Ignore the funny looks you'll get from the TSA when they inspect all your baby food, then notice you don't have a baby.

Finally, don't ignore the fat! It will help keep you satiated as you travel, and away from the candy aisle in the gas station. Nuts and seeds are an easy, portable fat source when traveling, but they are all too easy to overconsume. Try olives instead! They're portable, don't need refrigeration, and you can eat an awful lot for the same amount of fat as an ounce of nuts. Just drain the liquid and pack them in a plastic baggie before your air travel. You can also pack a can of coconut milk (or a few ounces if flying), coconut flakes, coconut butter, or a whole avocado.

Refer to our Travel Guide (page 195) for more detailed recommendations for on-the-go food and helpful hints.

BUSINESS TRAVEL, FROM MELISSA HARTWIG

We travel a lot for seminars and events, but we also do research ahead of time, and have been able to successfully manage many Whole30s while on the road. Before we even get on the plane, I know where the nearest grocery stores are located, and which restaurants in the area look like they serve food I can eat. (Yelp is great for this.) I always request a hotel room with a refrigerator, or a kitchenette if available. If we're cooking in a hotel room, I pack a small amount of coconut oil or other form of cooking fat, as we don't want to buy an entire jar every time we land somewhere new. Finally, we expect to eat boring-ish food when traveling—we often make do with a burger (no bun, no cheese, no bacon) and side salad in tight spots. As a result, we make sure our variety and food quality are fabulous at home, to make up for the lack of nutrition and flavor we get on the road. Finally, we always pack a stash of on-the-go foods like Primal Pacs, Chomps Snack Sticks, and Epic Bars for emergency situations like a delayed flight or being stuck in traffic. (See page 195 for details.)

treats, food fixations, and the scale

"Over the years I've gone from one diet or plan to another. This vicious cycle turned into major body issues and an eating disorder. The Whole30 has been a huge part of my transformation in the fact that it has changed my relationship with food. I no longer struggle with binging and this is no longer a diet to me but just the way I prefer to eat. My nasty sugar tantrums are gone as well! That was probably one of my biggest issues when I struggled with the eating disorder. I had so much trouble with sugar and now I don't want it at all."

—ELISE H., CITY/STATE WITHHELD

If the ingredients are all compliant, why can't I have baked goods or treats?

The short answer: because a cookie is a cookie, and cookies (or pancakes, bread, or brownies) have no place in the Whole30. The longer answer: The Whole30 is about changing the behaviors that led you to persistent cravings, unhealthy emotional relationships with food, and feeling out of control with your food choices. (We suspect that's a big part of why you're here.) Do you really want to spend the entirety of your Whole30 eating the same highly rewarding, nutrient-poor foods-with-no-brakes you've been eating all along? If you come out of your program with the same habits, cravings, and food choices you had when you started, your chances for long-term, life-changing success are slim. After all, those very same habits, cravings, and food choices are what got you into trouble in the first place! Use the Whole30 to change your habits, break unhealthy cravings, and create a new, healthy relationship with food. Follow this rule and you won't be sorry, as the new habits and patterns you create will stay with you for the rest of your life.

But my pancakes are just made with an egg and a banana.

Seriously, no pancakes. This is a rule. Please keep reading.

Shouldn't it be up to me to decide what's off-limits?

Well, technically, it is. You're all grown-ups, and we're not about to come into your kitchen and take away your pancakes. But we created the program rules, and those rules specifically state that certain foods are off-limits, and this is the program to which you committed. Signing up for the Whole30 and then complaining about the rules is like joining a soccer team and getting mad that you can't use your hands. If you want to reap the psychological and physical benefits of the program, follow it exactly as designed, including avoiding those baked goods or treats that we specifically list as off-limits. Remember, it's only 30 days. And we'd go so far as to say if you're getting anxious at the idea of not eating pancakes for a month, there's something there worth looking at.

⭐ TIP: *The trouble with these foods is that they're almost-but-not-quite as good as the stuff you used to eat. Pizza with an almond-flour crust and no cheese just isn't the same as the deep-dish pizza you love, but it's close enough that it keeps your brain thinking "I want pizza." If you keep eating these less satisfying knock-offs during your program, your brain will keep craving the reward that comes from junk food and treats. And one day, when you're stressed, upset, or lonely, you'll decide these poor recreations aren't going to cut it, and you're a grown-up, and if you want real pizza, you should have it . . . and before you know it, your Whole30 is over, and you're back to the same guilt/shame/reward cycle you've been desperate to break. It's just not worth it . . . and it's only 30 days.*

Besides bread, pancakes, and ice cream, what other foods are unacceptable under this rule?

A few off-limits foods that fall under this rule include: pancakes, bread, tortillas, biscuits, crepes, muffins, cupcakes, cookies, pizza crust, waffles, cereal, potato chips, French fries, and this one recipe where eggs, date paste, and coconut milk are combined with prayers to create a thick, creamy concoction that can once again transform your undrinkable black coffee into sweet, dreamy caffeine. However, while this list is off-limits for everyone (even those who don't

"have a problem" with bread or pancakes), your off-limits list may include other foods.

Wait, those aren't the only foods that fall under this category?

Not necessarily. These foods are expressly forbidden, but there are other foods that may be in that "gray area," and we ask that you take some personal responsibility with those. For example, Cashew Cookie Larabars are technically Whole30 Approved, and a great choice for those running a marathon or hiking the Appalachian trail. But if you're eating them as a substitute for your 3 p.m. candy bar, and find yourself slightly out of control when eating them (or after), we'd encourage you to identify that less healthy habit and say, "This food is not okay for me during my thirty days. It is a trigger food, and if I am trying to change my habits, I need to leave it off my plate."

Why are sweet potato "buns," kale chips, and zucchini noodles allowed on the Whole30? Aren't you recreating less healthy foods there too?

The real determining factor here is this: Are you attempting to recreate the exact look, texture, and flavor of the off-limits food? "Paleo" bread is designed to look and taste as much like real bread as possible; same with alternative-flour pancakes, brownies, or muffins. But sweet potato buns, kale chips, or zoodles are just a substitution for the bread, potato chips, or pasta they are replacing, not a recreation. Your brain isn't going to think it's still eating bread when it bites into a burger sandwiched between two sweet potatoes—which means you are effectively breaking your bread habit, not feeding it.

How do I know if a food should be off-limits for me?

First, ask yourself, "Am I trying to duplicate or recreate the exact look, texture, and flavor of something unhealthy I'm craving with approved ingredients, or am I merely looking for a healthier, more nutritious substitution for that food?" If it's the former, just say no. In addition, if the food in question is something you'd turn to after a hard day at work or stressful event, it's probably best to leave it out. While commercial mayonnaise isn't the healthiest choice (because of the vegetable oils and added sugars), rarely does someone come home after a tough day at the office and drown their sorrows in a jar of mayo, which means recreating it probably isn't an issue. Finally, when in doubt, leave it out. You can survive without this borderline food for 30 days—and if you feel like you can't or get angry just thinking about it, you may want to take a closer look at your relationship with that food.

But I don't have a problem with pancakes.

Still with the pancakes, huh? Here's the thing: this is just another rule of the program, like "no grains" or "no added sugar." You may or may not have problems with all of the foods we eliminate, but until you eliminate them for 30 days, you'll never know for sure. You also may be surprised at the hold some of these baked goods or treats have on you—something you never would have noticed until you told your brain "no." So please, just do the program our way for 30 days, and at the end, you can go right back to eating pancakes if you really want to. But we kind of suspect you won't.

I just started my Whole30, all I can think about is food. What to eat next, what to plan for tomorrow, what I can and can't have . . . is this healthy?

In the short term, yes. Eating this way is still new, so this is more an increase in awareness than an unhealthy obsession. You've jumped into a program that requires planning and preparation, detailed label reviews, and adherence to specific (unfamiliar) guidelines. It's natural to spend the first week or so thinking a lot about food, considering you have to eat three times a day, and your menus probably look a lot different than they used to. To combat this, meal plan (see page 26) and batch-prep your food twice a week so that you don't have to spend every day thinking about what you're going to eat; familiarize yourself with the rules to easily identify what's compliant and what isn't; and buy simple foods with few ingredients on the label—or no label at all. With this approach, you'll be cruising through your food choices with ease by Day 8.

If I feel like I'm not in control when eating certain "approved" foods like nut butter, dates, or frozen grapes, should I cut them out during the program?

Yes, yes, 100 percent yes. Sometimes program participants find that giving up brownies or pasta isn't as hard as they think, then find themselves elbow-deep in a jar of almond butter every night after dinner. Those compliant foods that cause you to binge eat, excessively crave, or eat when you're not hungry should be excluded from the program.

Won't restricting foods lead to cake-a-palooza after your Whole30 is over?

Junk food benders happen after many restrictive diets, but it's not common on the Whole30. First, our plan doesn't restrict calories—a common cause of the bounce-back effect of crash diets. Because you are full and satisfied every day of your Whole30, you're far less likely to actually feel restricted. Second, our plan focuses on changing your tastes and breaking cravings, so by the time the Whole30 is over, the junk foods you used to love are suddenly far less appealing. Finally, you came into this for the long haul, not a quick fix. You want to change your habits, so you won't spend all 30 days obsessing about what you're not eating—which means even if you *think* you'll be knee-deep in pizza, beer, and ice cream when your Whole30 is over, 76 percent of people* say they don't even want that stuff when Day 31 actually rolls around.

Why can't I weigh myself during my Whole30?

The Whole30 isn't a weight-loss diet. The program is designed to jump start optimal health for the rest of your life. The number on the scale says nothing about your overall health, and it's part of what is holding you hostage to your unhealthy relationship with food. So give yourself a long-overdue, well-deserved break from your preoccupation with body weight. You deserve it. At the end of 30 days, if the number on the scale is smaller, bonus! But during your Whole30, focus on getting healthier, not reducing the pull of gravity on your body mass.

*Per a 2014 survey of more than 1,300 Whole30 participants.

Doesn't some research show that the scale can be motivating in weight-loss efforts?

It does, but our research and experience shows that the scale is more likely to encourage our participants to second-guess the program, and renders them blind to their non-scale progress. One simple digital read-out can cause folks to shrink their meals to unhealthy portions, spend more time in the gym than their energy levels will support, beat themselves up with negative self-talk, or give up the program because "it's just not working." If you find motivation in seeing continual progress, that's fine—but let's find a non-weight-related motivator for you to track each day. Try your sleep quality, energy levels, mood, or self-esteem—things that actually make a difference for your health! (And if you happen to notice that your clothes are fitting better, you're allowed to give yourself a high-five.)

But will I lose weight on the Whole30?

Our nutrition plan will improve your overall health, and that is almost always reflected in an improvement in body composition. Meaning, if you focus on eating better, sleeping better, and making yourself healthier, your body composition *will* fall into line. So trust us, and be patient. We'll get you there the healthy way—the right way—in a manner that you'll be able to maintain for the rest of your life. Now, we'll actually answer your question. In a survey of over 1,600 Whole30 participants, 96 percent reported they lost weight and/or improved their body composition during their program. The majority lost between 6 and 15 pounds in 30 days. So, there you go—proof that weight loss is built right into the program, without you having to think about it.

I weighed myself. Does that count as breaking the rules? Do I need to start over?

Well, that's a tricky one. You see, our program guidelines are pretty darn clear. This is a big-picture, wide-reaching program designed to change many things at once. The goal is to increase your awareness of what you're eating and the habits that surround your food life, and change those that are detrimental to your body and brain. If you break a rule, we always recommend a full Whole30 restart. (Think about going all the way back to Day 1 the next time the scale calls your name! Is it worth it? Heck, no!) However, you're still a grown-up, and get to decide these things for yourself. We'll just ask you to be honest with yourself and work hard to break your dependence on the scale for validation.

Weight loss is important to me. How can I be sure I'm headed in the right direction?

For most people, weight loss happens effortlessly with improved health, so we encourage you to look for better health markers to make sure you're on track. A few things to notice: Are your cravings improving? Do you feel like you're more in control of your food choices? Are you able to better trust your body's "hungry" signal? Is your energy better, or steadier? Is your digestion improved, or have you lost some bloat? Are your symptoms decreasing? Are you happier, more self-confident, or better able to focus? Is your performance in the gym improving, or are you recovering faster? These are all signs that you're on the right track to changing your life and building new, healthy habits.

So I can't focus on scale weight—fine. what can I use to keep me motivated?

Focus on your accomplishments each day— what we call the "small wins." Did you make it through the day compliant? Great! Did you resist temptation, even though it was hard? Good for you! Did you make it through 3 p.m. without needing that extra coffee? Wonderful. Did you find a way to reward yourself without food? Amazing! Those are the victories we want you to celebrate throughout this process—and if you take the time to notice these small wins, you'll be amazed at how much you are actually accomplishing every day.

Am I allowed to track calories or macronutrients?

Technically, the admonition to avoid tracking calories or macronutrients is just a recommendation, not a rule. However, we'd caution you against it for the same reasons we caution against the scale. Your body knows how much you should be eating better than any calculator you'll find on the internet, and once you're eating Good Food, you'll be able to trust the signals your body is sending you. In addition, some of you have been so conditioned to restrict calories or macronutrients that even though you feel amazing eating as much as you are, you may still be tempted to cut back once you see the numbers add up. Don't let numbers on a spreadsheet mess with your head, or your Whole30 results. For now, just follow our meal template (page 194) and let your body's own cues (hunger, energy, cravings, mood, athletic performance, and recovery) be your guide to eating more or less.

medical conditions

"I have Hashimoto's thyroiditis, Raynaud's disease, psoriasis, asthma, and allergies. As a Physician's Assistant, I knew that my autoimmune disorders were progressing. At age 28, my energy was low, my symptoms were horrible, my hair was thinning, I had near-daily headaches, joint aches, frequent rashes, and poor digestion. My inflammatory blood markers were increasing, but I reached a dead end with my rheumatologist. During this time I did my first Whole30. I have since done two more, and have maintained this lifestyle for the past year and a half. I have the energy I never thought I would have again. My digestion is healthy. My hair is thick and my skin clear. My hands no longer look scalded, dry, or cracked. I do not take any prescription medications for the management of my diagnoses. I pass along the message of the Whole30 to patients, friends, and family almost daily. I share it because I know that living this lifestyle supports my health in a way I never could have imagined."

—MEGAN M., NEW YORK, NY

A brief reminder: We are not doctors, and this section is not an attempt to dispense medical advice. Everyone should always talk to their health care provider before beginning any new diet or supplement regimen. This goes double for those of you with medical conditions, especially if you are taking prescription medications to manage your condition.

We asked Luc Readinger, M.D. to help us answer some of these questions from his perspective, as a physician who has been successfully using the Whole30 to treat his patients' medical conditions since 2011.

Autoimmune or Chronic Diseases

The Whole30 is ideal to help normalize an overactive immune system, decreasing systemic inflammation and reducing or eliminating the symptoms of your autoimmune disease, chronic pain, or immune-related conditions (like Lyme disease). However, there are some Whole30 Approved foods that are healthy for most people, but might exacerbate your symptoms or fire up your immune system. The trouble is there isn't just one list of foods that negatively impact all chronic diseases.

You are a unique snowflake. That means foods that may be perfectly fine for someone else with your same condition may make your symptoms much worse, and vice-versa. This makes it incredibly hard to create one protocol that works well for everyone with an immune dysfunction. Eggs, tomatoes, peppers, eggplant, potatoes, instant coffee, nuts and seeds, beef, lamb, oranges, grapefruit, lemons, and limes . . . These are all foods that are either known to be commonly problematic for those with autoimmune conditions, or are common food sensitivities for those with increased gut permeability.

And that's not even the comprehensive list.

Continuing to eat stuff that is problematic for your body will lead to (you guessed it) systemic inflammation and an overactive immune system, which means your symptoms don't improve as much as you'd like them to.

So how do you know if some of these healthy Whole30 foods aren't so healthy for you? We wish there were an easy answer. It's hard to know whether these foods impact you without eliminating them, too, but that makes your Whole30 a ton more restrictive. Plus, simply adding these foods to your Whole30 "off-limits" list is a little like shooting at a target in the dark; you may end up restricting foods that you don't need to, and including foods that you are, in fact, sensitive to.

If you have an autoimmune disease, or a chronic pain or chronic fatigue condition, you have two options with respect to your Whole30:

OPTION 1: Complete the general Whole30 protocols exactly as written (optionally eliminating eggs and nightshades as well), then evaluate and make a decision as to where to go from there.

OPTION 2: Skip the Whole30 and go straight to a medical elimination diet, working with an experienced functional medicine practitioner who creates a specific plan just for you.

Let's discuss the pros and cons of each approach.

OPTION 1:
Start with the Whole30

There are a few benefits to this approach. First, compared to a medical elimination diet, the Whole30 requires far fewer changes to your overall diet, which means it's easier to follow and less stressful. You can also start making these changes immediately, bringing relief and results that much faster. It's also far cheaper—you could theoretically do the entire Whole30 for free, avoiding expensive fees for doctor visits and lab work.

The downside is that you may not experience all of the benefits you hope to see, because you may still be including some items in your diet that might be problematic for you. The Whole30 isn't a structured elimination approach based on your health history, symptoms, and lab results, which means it could be less effective in your specific context than it is for most people. You may get all the way through your program and think, "This isn't working!"

We assure you, it's working.

We're positive you'll experience other benefits from the program, and a calmer immune system is a huge step in the right direction, even if you're not all the way there. Just like a Whole30 that doesn't cause any weight loss, it is not a disappointment or a failure when you pay attention to all the changes in more subjective areas of your life. But the expectation of having "miraculous" results and not seeing them on

Day 30 can be pretty disheartening, which may prove to be the biggest risk of this approach.

All of that having been said, we still think this is where you should start.

Virtually every medical elimination program is going to exclude refined sugars, gluten, dairy, soy, and alcohol (on top of other specific foods), so you might as well get a head start before you begin working with a doctor. In addition, there's something to be said for gaining some confidence and feeling healthier before you take on something as rigid and restrictive as a personalized elimination diet. The improvements

---

EGGS AND NIGHTSHADES

You may improve your results by restricting eggs and nightshades, too. Egg whites contain proteins that can indirectly increase immune activity—a contributing factor in immune-mediated diseases. Nightshades are a group of plants that contain compounds that promote gut irritability, inflammation, joint pain and/or stiffness in sensitive individuals. Nightshades include potatoes (all varieties except sweet potatoes or yams), tomatoes, all sweet and hot peppers, eggplant, tomatillos, tamarios, pepinos, and spices like cayenne, chili powder, curry powder, paprika, pimento, and red pepper flakes. These two groups are the most commonly problematic in those with autoimmune conditions, chronic pain, and other immune-mediated medical conditions, so consider leaving these off your Whole30 if this is your context.

A WORD ON ANTI-INFLAMMATORY MEDICATIONS

There's something you should know about nonsteroidal anti-inflammatory drugs (NSAIDs) like aspirin, ibuprofen (Advil, Motrin), naproxen (Aleve), and Celebrex. This class of drugs has been shown to directly disrupt the lining of the gut, leading to intestinal permeability (leaky gut), a contributing factor in autoimmune disease and immune-mediated conditions. If you rely on a doctor-prescribed NSAID for pain control, remember that your doctor's orders always trump Whole30 recommendations. However, given the impact of these medications on gut integrity and immune function, we encourage you to talk with your health care provider about alternative methods for managing your pain. If you're unable to discontinue your NSAIDs at this time, that's okay—keep up with the rest of the Whole30 protocol, and work with your doctor to evaluate your symptoms along the way. You may find you're able to taper off the anti-inflammatory medication as your inflammatory symptoms start to decrease.

---

you see on the Whole30 (because you *will* see improvements!) will increase your self-efficacy, helping you feel more prepared and motivated to tackle a more restrictive approach, if that's where you decide to go.

If you choose to start with the Whole30, make sure you follow the standard protocol to the letter, and keep a journal of your auto-immune symptoms day by day. If you see an improvement in your symptoms by Day 30, you'll know you're on the right track! If your symptoms are resolved and you're happy with your progress, proceed with reintroduction as outlined on page 45. If you still aren't feeling as good as you had hoped, you can either extend your Whole30 for a longer period of time (for 60 or even 90 days, to see if the benefits keep coming), or start working with a functional medicine practitioner (see page 406) to see if you have other triggers in your diet.

OPTION 2:
Work with a doctor

The benefit of working with a doctor is that he or she will create an elimination plan specifically tailored to your health history, medical condition, and goals, which means you're likely to experience more successful management of symptoms long-term. You'll also have the benefit of expert guidance along the way, managing your condition with not only diet, but supplementation, medication, and/or other important lifestyle recommendations.

The downside is that this protocol may be considerably harder—you're left without many of the foods you would consider "staples" on a basic Whole30, and learning to cook without things like tomatoes or ghee may prove challenging. In addition, working with an experienced practitioner can be expensive—office visit fees, consultation fees, lab work, medication, and supplementation adds up fast.

If you decide to take this approach, use one of the resources listed on page 406 to help you find an experienced functional medicine practitioner, naturopath, or progressive medical doctor in your area. Also, feel free to start eliminating the most common dietary triggers now (like gluten, dairy, and soy), because that's probably the first thing they'll talk to you about.

Whichever approach you choose, we encourage you to be patient, and remember that when it comes to autoimmune disease, improvements don't happen overnight. When your immune system is this overworked and confused, it can take six months or more of dedication to a protocol like the Whole30 or a medical elimination diet to see results, so don't be discouraged if your symptoms aren't fully resolved in just a month. Focus on the improvements you *are* seeing, and let those motivate you to continue with your chosen regimen.

WHAT ABOUT A PALEO AIP?

A "Paleo Autoimmune Protocol" (Paleo AIP) is somewhere between a Whole30 and a medical elimination plan. It asks that you eliminate some Whole30 foods, plus many others that are commonly problematic for those with autoimmune conditions. This approach may be a good middle ground if you get done with the Whole30 and still haven't resolved all of your symptoms, but aren't ready to work full-time with a medical practitioner. Visit The Paleo Mom (www.thepaleomom.com) or Paleo AIP (www.autoimmune-paleo.com).

Diabetes

First, do not get discouraged from trying a Whole30 because you take insulin or diabetes medications. We believe the potential benefits far exceed the hassle of having a discussion with your health care provider and adjusting medication—and we've seen full reversal of type 2 diabetes in just 30 days.

That having been said, it is essential to talk with your doctor before doing the Whole30. Although not specifically meant to be low-carb, the Whole30 tends to be lower in carbohydrates than the standard American diet (SAD), and lower than what most people are eating on an otherwise unrestricted diet. If you're on insulin or insulin-sensitizing drugs and radically decrease the amount of carbohydrates you're eating without adjusting your insulin dose, your blood sugar could dip too low, with serious medical consequences.

This is especially true of type 1 diabetics—in fact, you and your health care provider might decide to ease into your Whole30 eating plan instead of jumping in cold turkey, so you can better monitor your blood sugar and adjust your long-acting and short-acting insulin dosages.

Discuss how to approach a Whole30 with your health care provider before you begin the plan, and schedule regular follow-ups to ensure blood sugars are staying within a reasonable range.

Irritable Bowel Syndrome (IBS) and Inflammatory Bowel Disease (IBD)

While the Whole30 is ideal for healing the gut and improving digestive conditions, we highly recommend those with IBS or IBD work with a qualified functional medicine practitioner (page 406), as your condition may also require targeted lab testing and probiotic supplementation. If you decide to try the Whole30 before seeking out professional help, please consider restricting high-FODMAP foods (page 130), known to impact gut bacteria and worsen IBS and IBD symptoms, in addition to the standard Whole30 eliminations.

Sorry.

We know this looks like a lot to take on. But remember, it's only 30 days, and you'll learn so much about yourself, your symptoms, and the triggers for your condition thanks to your short-term sacrifice—all information which will prove invaluable if you do choose to work with a professional during or after your Whole30. Here are some other recommendations to ensure your Whole30 is as healthy as possible, given your context.

Fiber-rich vegetables are good for your digestion, but they can also be hard for your body to process, especially if your gut is impaired. You can ease their trip through your digestive tract by cooking them thoroughly, and/or first breaking them down into smaller pieces manually. Try slow-cooking them as part of a stew, or using a food processor to turn your veggies into a soup or puree. Minimize your consumption of raw vegetables or big salads, especially if following the Whole30 means you are radically increasing your vegetable consumption.

Be careful with even low-FODMAP fruit, too, as there are strong links between fructose malabsorption and IBS. Make sure you peel all fruit, avoid what you can't peel (like grapes and cherries), and eat your fruit as ripe as possible, which makes it easier to digest. You should also avoid fruits that have seeds and a rough exterior (like berries), which can be tough on your digestive tract. Although no one knows why for sure, many IBS sufferers report increased symptoms after consuming citrus fruits, so you may want to avoid those as well. Finally, no dried fruits and fruit juices, which pack too much sugar into a small package for folks with serious GI disturbances.

And now the saddest news ever: avoid all forms of coffee, even decaf. We know, and we're sorry—we're really not trying to ruin your life. It's just that coffee is a powerful GI-tract irritant, and even decaffeinated coffee can trigger abdominal spasms and diarrhea in those with

IBS or IBD. In addition, caffeinated coffee is a double-whammy, as caffeine speeds up every system in the body (including the colon), which can lead to diarrhea, followed by constipation. (Double the fun!) Coffee can also increase stomach acid, which can contribute to inflammation in the GI tract. Try herbal tea instead, and drink plenty of water throughout the day—but not *with* your meals, as it can inhibit proper digestion by diluting stomach acid and digestive enzymes.

Finally, we'll caution that your digestion may get worse before it gets better. As your GI tract starts to heal, your mucosal layer will adjust, unhealthy gut bacteria will start to die off, healthy bacteria will begin to repopulate, and the intestinal lining will start to rebuild itself, plugging gaps and filling in holes. This can lead to gas, bloating, diarrhea, or constipation. In conditions such as IBD and IBS, it's not uncommon for digestive issues to continue for three to six months after making such radical dietary changes—but it is a necessary first step in restoring healthy gut integrity, so stick with it.

Download our Whole30 low-FODMAP shopping list at www.whole30.com/pdf-downloads.

Gallbladder

If you've had your gallbladder removed, you might be intimidated by the idea of taking on a "high-fat" diet like the Whole30. However, let us assure you that the Whole30 may be one of the healthiest things you've done for your digestion!

First, a little background. The gallbladder is a holding and concentration tank for bile (a fluid that aids in digestion), which is produced in the liver. The body likes having a concentrated reservoir of this fluid, because the liver produces it quite slowly, so it "trickles" instead of "gushes."

When you eat a meal with a decent amount of fat, your liver can't send enough bile out into the small intestine fast enough, so it sends a large amount from the reservoir stored in the gallbladder—enough to properly digest the fats you just ate.

When the gallbladder is removed, there is no longer a reservoir available for bile to be stored and called upon during a fatty meal. If you eat too much fat at once (requiring more bile than the liver can send), some of the fat remains undigested and passes through your system quickly, leading to loose, oily stools, diarrhea, and cramping. Thus, you may have been told by your health care provider to eat low-fat and whole grain, or eat only certain kinds of fat (generally avoiding animal fats), and above all, to stay away from "high-fat" diets like Atkins, Paleo, or the Whole30.

However, the Whole30 is not a high-fat diet. You may be eating more fat than you used to, but then again, you used to subsist on nothing but heavily processed, sweetened, low-fat foods, and how well did that work? Our added fat recommendations are actually quite moderate, which means your lack of gallbladder shouldn't affect your Whole30 strategy much.

First, you may need to switch from three big meals a day to four or five smaller meals, especially if you're large and active (and require more fat for energy). This will help you eat enough fat during your day without overly taxing your liver. Still, don't graze like an antelope, especially on high-fat foods like nuts and seeds, as that may tax your liver's capacity to send enough bile to get the job done.

And don't even *think* of intermittent fasting. There is no way you can eat enough calories in a shortened feeding window and still be able to properly digest all that fat without a gallbladder. (If you don't even know what intermittent fasting is, good. It's not for you.)

In addition, consume plenty of water during your day, but not during meals. Drinking water with your meal will dilute the small amount of bile available for digestion, making it even less effective.

You also may want to experiment with different kinds of fats. The medium-chain triglycerides found in coconut (oil, flakes, butter, or milk) are easier to digest, and coconut oil in particular digests without a need for bile. You may have an easier time with digestion by eating less animal fat, but adding more coconut oil to your meals or during cooking.

Finally, an ox bile supplement can often provide all the digestive help you need, even if you are eating bigger meals closer to our meal template recommendations. In addition, you may notice your capacity for digesting fats increasing after your surgery—the body has a remarkable ability to adapt to new conditions, and you may find a year post-surgery that you can enjoy bigger meals with more fat with little to no issue. As always, talk about doing the Whole30 with your doctor before you begin, and work closely with him or her when making these changes to your diet.

Other Conditions Requiring Prescription Medications

There are other medical conditions and prescription medications that may be affected by the dietary changes you're making on the Whole30—sometimes within just your first week on the program.

If you're taking medication for high blood pressure, consult your health care practitioner prior to launching your Whole30. Many have testified they no longer need their blood pressure medication after doing the Whole30, which means you and your doctor will need to monitor your blood pressure and medication dosage throughout the program. If your doctor agrees, you can purchase a blood pressure cuff and monitor your blood pressure twice a day for the duration of the Whole30. If your blood pressures fall below a certain level (as predetermined by your health care provider), or if symptoms of decreased blood pressure occur (light-headedness, especially when going from sitting to standing, generalized fatigue, etc.) then your doctor may decide it's time to back down on the amount of medication being taken. These changes tend to happen gradually, and not all at once, which makes it easier to monitor and adjust your medication.

As for thyroid conditions—chronic hypothyroidism (low thyroid) responds slowly to medication changes and dietary interventions. Check in with your doctor before embarking on the Whole30, and test thyroid hormone levels before and after the program. This is especially true if you have an autoimmune thyroid condition like Hashimoto's, which may respond well to this gluten-free, gut-healing diet.

Finally, if you're taking a statin medication like Lipitor, feel free to continue while on the Whole30. We don't know of any immediate or long-term dangers with the combination of a statin medication and a whole-foods based diet like the Whole30, but if you haven't had a discussion with your physician about *why* you're on a statin medication, it might be time to do so. We've had many testimonials of cholesterol levels and triglycerides dropping far beyond what their doctors told them was possible with dietary changes only, and many people are able to stop using their statins post-Whole30.

We haven't covered anywhere near the full scope of medical conditions and prescription medications that are affected by the Whole30— that would be impossible, as there appears to be no disease, condition, or symptom that isn't impacted in a positive way by a gut-healing, anti-inflammatory diet. In general, we encourage you to work closely with your health care provider before taking on the Whole30, and consult them throughout the program, especially if you observe a change in your health or symptoms.

Nervous about talking to your doctor about the Whole30? Follow Dr. Readinger's helpful tips at www.whole30.com/talktoyourdoc.

Eating Disorders

We admire your dedication in pursuing a healthy relationship with food, and do believe that eating real, nutrient-dense, unprocessed foods is the healthiest way to nourish your body and break unhealthy cravings and habits. However, if you have a diagnosed eating disorder (or a history of disordered eating), please use caution when taking on a program like the Whole30.

Some people with eating disorders (active or in recovery) have found amazing food freedom with the Whole30. The fact that we don't count or restrict calories, encourage you to eat healthy foods to satiety, and take the scale and body measurements out of the equation may prove to be the paradigm shift that you need to get back to a healthier relationship with food.

However, there are probably just as many people who have found the rigidity, rules, and structure of the Whole30 program too reminiscent of their disorders. For these people, the Whole30 "as prescribed" is actually a trigger for disordered eating behavior, hurting their progress more than it helps. The restrictions may carry over to calorie or macronutrient restriction in anorectics, or may trigger a binge in those with a history of compulsive overeating.

If you have a history of disordered eating and are wondering if the Whole30 is right for you—we simply can't answer this question for you. In fact, you shouldn't try to figure it out on your own, either. If this is your context, you *must* work with a qualified counselor or mental health professional to determine whether the Whole30 is right for you before you begin the program.

If you and your counselor do decide the Whole30 is appropriate for you, you may also decide together to modify the rules or relax the restrictions. We know—that basically goes against everything we've written about the program and the need to follow it to the letter, but this is not your normal scenario. While we insist the Whole30 must be completed exactly as written to obtain the full benefit, we didn't write the program with eating disorders in mind. That language was written to discourage people from thinking they can have a bite of this here and a glass of that there and it really won't make a difference. However, in your context, if you and your counselor need to adjust the rules, duration, or structure of the program to make it work for you, by all means do so. If following just a select portion of our healthy eating program helps you make progress in your recovery, we're happy to have you on board.

However, even if you're working with a trusted counselor, it's possible your commitment to the Whole30 will cross into dangerous psychological territory. The signs are different for everyone, but you can use these simple questions to help determine if your Whole30 is going to an unhealthy place:

- Does the idea of accidentally eating an off-plan food or "cheating" literally keep you up at night?

- Do you feel you have to measure, track, and analyze every bite of food (and does being unable to do so make you anxious)?

- Are you hyper-selective with respect to food quantity or food choices simply in an effort to be "more strict"? (Carrots are too sugary, fruit and nuts are off-limits?)

- Have you deliberately changed the program (by eliminating calories, fat grams, carbs, or food choices) to the degree that it is no longer optimally healthy?

- Do you feel compelled to make alterations to the program for any reason other than health?

If you answer yes to any one of these questions, take some time to seriously think about your motivation for doing this program and whether you want to proceed. If you answer yes to more than one, take a time-out from the program, and speak with a trusted counselor before returning to the Whole30.

For more information on the Whole30 and eating disorders, including reader stories and testimonials, visit www.w30.co/w30ed.

pregnancy and breastfeeding

"I am a doctor of chiropractic and mother of two. The Whole30 saved me from post-partum depression. About four months postpartum, I was exhausted from sleep deprivation, and really depressed about still being 20 pounds overweight. My diet was out of control. The final straw was one morning when my 3-year-old son came into my room excited for the day and I snapped at him because I felt so awful. I felt like such horrible mom and I knew something had to change. My husband and I started the Whole30 the next day and it changed our lives! We both noticed our increase in energy, stable energy all day, better sleep, and no cravings or desire for the 'bad' foods. My joints are not inflamed and I am able to exercise. I fit in all my pre-pregnancy clothes; we both lost 13 to 15 pounds. The Whole30 also got me out of my depression so I can show up in this world like the mom, wife, and doctor I want to be. In addition, my patients' recoveries have been quicker and long-lasting with the added focus on diet. Doing the Whole30 has taught me that it really does start with food."

—DR. MICHAELA MCCLURE, WATERLOO, ON

I f you are pregnant or breastfeeding, you know how important mom's nutrition is to her baby's health and development. The diet that's healthiest for you is also going to be the healthiest for your baby—the more nutrition you receive from your diet, the more you are able to pass along to the little one. We can't imagine your doctor coming up with a diet more nutritious than one that focuses on whole, unprocessed meat, seafood, and eggs, lots of vegetables and fruits, and natural fats—but always speak with your health care provider when making dietary or lifestyle changes when pregnant or nursing.

We consulted with Registered Dietician and pregnancy expert Stephanie Greunke to design healthy Whole30 recommendations for this special time in your life.

Pregnancy

While our program doesn't need to be modified to accommodate your growing baby, you will want to take care with a few of our general recommendations. First, a very-high-protein diet isn't the healthiest thing for your baby, so pregnant women should limit protein consumption to no more than 20 percent of total calories.

If you follow the lower-protein end of our meal template (page 194) you'll fall well within the safe range. (Nature usually helps us out here—many women report an aversion to, or loss of appetite for, protein during pregnancy, especially during the first trimester.) However, if you naturally tend toward a higher-protein diet, you'll have to consciously eat more carbohydrates and fat to make up for the calories you're missing. In addition, if you're one of the lucky women who don't have protein aversions, you may find you have to consciously reduce the amount of meat, seafood, and eggs you eat. Tracking and logging your calories and macronutrients may prove helpful here, just until you get the hang of what your new lower-protein diet should look like.

In addition, though you're not really "eating for two," it's critical for you to consume enough calories. During the first trimester, you really don't need to eat any more than you were before you got pregnant. In later months, an extra 300 calories a day is sufficient to feed you and your baby—the equivalent of eating an extra avocado. Incorporating more starchy vegetables and slightly more healthy fats into your diet is an easy way to make sure you're not underfeeding yourself or your baby. Now is not the time to be limiting your carbs or trying to follow a very low-carbohydrate diet—your baby needs the calories and nutrients coming from the fruits and vegetables you're eating, and going very low-carb is too stressful during pregnancy. If you're coming to the Whole30 from a low-fat diet or have a history of dieting in general, you may have to work harder to consciously eat enough healthy fats with every meal. If you're exercising during pregnancy, make sure you purposefully include enough potatoes, winter squashes, plantains, or other fruits to support your activity level.

Finally, you may have to ditch our "no snacking" recommendation, especially as your pregnancy moves into the third trimester. As any pregnant woman can tell you, it gets a little crowded in there as your baby grows, and you may not have the physical space in your stomach to eat big meals. You may have to resort to smaller, more frequent meals throughout the day, but try to avoid constant grazing. If possible, allow 3 to 4 hours between your smaller meals to give your hormones a chance to do their job.

Foods to avoid

Some of the nutrient-dense foods we recommend as part of a healthy Whole30 diet may not be the healthiest during pregnancy. Experts generally recommend avoiding fish containing mercury like tuna, swordfish, and marlin; raw eggs or fish (like sushi), and raw or undercooked meat. This means avoiding Whole30 staples like homemade mayo, and cooking all your burgers and steaks to well-done.

Ultimately, these are personal decisions best made between you and your health care provider—we can't tell you whether your pastured, organic, local eggs are really unsafe to eat raw. (The good news? If you do choose to abstain, you can still make our Egg-free Mayonnaise on page 180!)

Morning sickness and food aversions

Another Whole30 challenge during pregnancy may be that you just cannot stomach the thought of eggs, meat, certain spices, or the vegetables you used to love. Morning sickness (which can happen any time of day, unfortunately) and food aversions may make your Whole30 more challenging, so here are our strategies for managing to stay Whole30-compliant during this difficult time. (And keep your chin up, because most women find these symptoms improve tremendously after the first trimester.)

- **BRING THE WHOLE DARN GROCERY STORE HOME.** Your aversions may vary from week to week, but if you can go "shopping" for Whole30-compliant foods in your own fridge or cabinet, you'll eventually settle on something you want to eat. This does require more frequent trips to the grocery store— but it's only three months, and this is what husbands/partners/family members are for.

- **BE FLEXIBLE.** You may discover that eggs aren't okay when you first wake up, but by around 11 a.m. they become palatable again. So, find something else to eat for Meal 1 (a burger, canned tuna, smoked salmon—you may be surprised what you're craving these days!) and eat the eggs later. Be methodical about your food evaluations—just because you passed on the chicken sausage at noon doesn't mean you won't want to eat it at 3 p.m. Get used to planning meals at the last minute (and warn your family this is coming, too), because there's a good chance you won't know what you want to eat for dinner until ten minutes before you start making it.

- **RELAX ON PERFECT PORTIONS.** At this stage in the game, it's not about creating balanced meals three times a day—it's about getting calories into mom so she doesn't get run down and even more exhausted. If every meal doesn't have a palm-sized serving of protein, don't worry. If carrots are your only veggie for three days in a row, that's fine. If you need food-in-a-blender just to get something into you, fire it up. Do the best you can with what you have, and remember that everything you're eating is nutrient-dense and healthy for your baby, which is the most important thing.

- **KNOW WHEN IT'S TIME TO TAKE A WHOLE30 BREAK.** If you're having terrible morning sickness or if your food aversions are so severe that you're under-fed and exhausted, it may be time to take a break from the Whole30. Find whole, unprocessed, nutrient-dense foods you can eat (ideally, things like gluten-free grains; full-fat, pastured dairy; and whole, unprocessed foods you know from experience won't mess you up), and get your energy and strength back. Then, as soon as you are able and your health care provider approves, return to the Whole30.

Pregnancy supplementation

First, it's important to talk to your health care provider before taking any new supplement, especially if you are pregnant. However, we feel there are a few supplements that may be of benefit to your health, and your baby's health, during these special times.

PRENATAL VITAMINS. The problem with most prenatal multi-vitamins is that they contain too many potentially harmful nutrients (like iron and folic acid) and not enough of what a pregnant woman really needs (like vitamins D_3, folate, and K_2). It's best to meet as many of your nutritional needs as possible with food, even while pregnant or nursing. That said, the recommended amounts of certain nutrients, like folate, vitamin K_2, and vitamin D_3, during pregnancy may be difficult to obtain solely through diet. For this reason, taking a prenatal vitamin with the appropriate nutrients in the right dosages and forms may be a good insurance policy. You want at least 1,000 IUs of vitamin D_3, 500 mcg of vitamin K_2 (MK-4 form), and 800 mcg of folate (not folic acid). See page 404 for our recommendations.

OMEGA-3 FATTY ACIDS. The anti-inflammatory fatty acids EPA and especially DHA provide excellent benefits for your baby's neurological and early visual development, and may reduce the risk of pregnancy complications like preeclampsia, gestational diabetes, postpartum depression, and pre-term delivery. If you're eating lots of fatty, cold-water fish (like wild-caught salmon, mackerel, sardines, or herring), you may not need to supplement at all. If not, however, we recommend supplementing with 300 mg of DHA per day while you are pregnant, but do not exceed a total of 1 gram of EPA and DHA combined. The easiest way to supplement with EPA and DHA is with a high-quality fish oil; your label will detail the amount of EPA and DHA per pill or teaspoon.

FERMENTED COD LIVER OIL. This healthy source of omega-3 fats also contains vitamins A, K_2, and D, helping you meet some of your other nutritional requirements. Alternate supplementing with 300 mg of DHA from fish oil with 1 to 2 teaspoons of fermented cod liver oil. (Remember, regardless of the source, keep total omega-3 intake to under 1 gram a day. See page 404 for our fish oil and fermented cod liver oil brand recommendations.)

VITAMIN D₃. Vitamin D_3 is really not a vitamin at all—it's actually a hormone, and plays a huge role in your health, especially in pregnancy. Studies show that mothers who supplement with vitamin D_3 have a reduced risk of gestational diabetes, preterm birth, pregnancy-related complications, and postpartum depression. Normally, vitamin D_3 is produced by exposing your skin to the sun, but the further you live from the equator and the darker your skin, the harder this is during the early and later parts of the day and in winter. During fall and winter in climates north of Atlanta, Georgia, the angle of the sun means the UVB rays don't penetrate the earth's atmosphere, so your skin won't produce enough, if any, vitamin D. (A good rule of thumb is if your shadow is longer than you are tall, you're not making vitamin D.) During these months, supplementation is your only option to keep levels adequate for you and your baby. Doctors say pregnant women can take up to 10,000 IU (international units) of vitamin D safely, although the Vitamin D Council recommends between 4,000 and 6,000 IU per day while pregnant. (On summer days when you get full-body sun exposure, however, you can skip the supplement.) Refer to page 404 for our vitamin D supplement recommendations.

BONE BROTH. You may not think of homemade bone broth (page 176) as a supplement, but it's a great source of calcium,

> **PREGNANCY EXTRA CREDIT**
>
> We recommend getting vitamin D levels tested before pregnancy, during the first trimester, and at the beginning of the third trimester, when the fetal skeleton is rapidly developing and mom's need for vitamin D is the highest. You should be roughly in the range of 40 to 70 ng/ml; if you're low, work with your health care provider to supplement with the appropriate amount.

magnesium, phosphorous, collagen, and amino acids not found in muscle meat. As 25 to 30 grams of calcium are transferred to the fetus in the last trimester of pregnancy, adding a cup or two of bone broth a day to mom's diet can help ensure her baby grows strong and healthy without leaving her mineral-deficient.

VITAMIN B-COMPLEX. The eight B vitamins are critical for baby's growth and brain development, but pregnant mommas may also find taking a complex helpful for morning sickness and fatigue, especially in the first trimester.

LIVER PILLS. There are enormous benefits to eating organ meats while pregnant. Liver in particular is a dense source of vitamins like A, D, and E, iron, and choline, all of which are essential for a healthy pregnancy. If you can't source or stomach the idea of eating actual liver, taking a grass-fed, freeze-dried liver supplement will provide you with all the benefits without the gag factor. Aim for an ounce (six capsules) a few times a week. (See page 404 for our recommendations.)

Finally, understand that during pregnancy, high-quality supplementation takes precedence over Whole30 rules, especially if your supplements are doctor-prescribed. Some of the best supplements out there unfortunately include traces of soy or dairy in the capsule. It's up to you and your health care provider to decide whether the benefits of taking any supplement or medication outweigh the benefits of avoiding these less-healthy ingredients. (In this case, we believe they do, and are only recommending supplements with trace amounts of these ingredients in forms that are not generally problematic.)

Breastfeeding

The Whole30 is one of the best things nursing moms can do for their baby's health and happiness, but it also keeps you healthy, energetic, and sleeping well (as well as can be), and keeps your immune system strong. When you're nursing, your baby's health is your body's top priority. This means that micronutrients stored in your body and found in the food you eat are passed along in your breast milk to your baby. This is so important that your body will sacrifice its own health and micronutrient stores to make sure your baby has enough. Keeping your diet high in vitamins, minerals, phytonutrients, and healthy fats with the Whole30 ensures there is enough to keep both you and your baby well nourished.

In addition, if mom isn't eating potentially inflammatory foods, that means baby isn't, either! Mothers report their babies are less fussy, nurse better, have fewer digestive issues and skin conditions, and sleep longer when they're on the Whole30.

That last one alone should convince you to give it a try. Trust us—as the mother of a

BREASTFEEDING SURVEY

The most common question we receive from nursing moms is, "Will I be able to maintain my milk supply during the Whole30?" In fact, in a 2014 survey of 600 women who started the Whole30 while nursing, 90 percent said their milk supply either remained stable or increased during the Whole30!

two-year-old, Melissa remembers exactly what those days of round-the-clock nursing and sleep deprivation feel like. In fact, she did a Whole30 herself when her son was four months old, and found that not only did her milk supply stay plentiful, she and her baby slept better—which meant less stress on mom, and an even easier time maintaining a healthy breast milk supply.

Maintaining breast milk supply on the Whole30

The main thing needed to maintain an ample milk supply is simple—the more often and effectively your baby nurses, the more milk you will have. During pregnancy and the first few days postpartum, milk supply is hormonally driven, meaning you produce milk based on the hormonal changes following birth. Your milk supply regulates between six and twelve weeks, and by three months, it's basically set based on prior demand.

So, the best advice we can give you for maintaining supply on or off the Whole30 is feed on demand right from day one! Don't stick to a pre-determined "schedule"—let your baby decide when and how often to nurse. In addition, an empty breast means faster milk production, so make sure you empty each breast either by nursing, pumping, or a combination of both every time your baby feeds.

Calories, macronutrients, and nutrition also play a major factor in your breast milk supply. A sudden drop in caloric or carbohydrate intake may put your milk supply at risk. It's easy for those new to the Whole30 to under-eat. Your meals are more satiating, you may be a little fat-phobic, and you may be eating so many leafy greens that you forget to include some starchy vegetables and fruit. This may be one context in which tracking your calories and macronutrients for a few days is actually recommended, especially if you're new to the Whole30. Consuming fewer than 1,800 calories per day may put your milk supply at risk, so make sure you're eating enough, and don't go below 100 grams of carbohydrate a day.

Hydration levels can also significantly affect milk supply. You may notice you are abnormally thirsty while nursing, but even if you're not, have a large water bottle on hand and sip on it throughout the day.

In addition, eating just three meals a day per our meal template (page 194) may be impossible with your nursing and sleep schedule, so plan on eating four, five, or six smaller meals whenever it's convenient. Make sure each meal includes a chunk of protein, a healthy amount of fat, and carbohydrates. Remember, there is no need to limit protein once your baby is born; in fact, a growing baby needs the protein you secrete in your breast milk, so don't skip your meat, seafood, and eggs! Follow the lower end of our fat recommendations (at a minimum) to ensure you're getting enough, and be sure to purposefully include some starchy vegetables like potatoes and winter squash and a variety of fruit to ensure you're eating enough carbohydrate.

Finally, understand that there are a huge number of factors that contribute to your baby nursing well and your milk supply staying abundant, including sleep, stress levels, other medications you may be on, how well your baby or pump empties each breast—even things like sleeping on your stomach or wearing a bra that's too tight can inhibit milk supply. With so many issues at play, it's best to work with an experienced lactation consultant and your health care provider to arrive at a comprehensive strategy to keep you healthy (and keep your milk supply plentiful) while nursing and pumping on the Whole30.

Supplementation while breastfeeding

First, it's important to talk to your health care provider before taking any new supplement, especially if you are pregnant or nursing. However, we feel there are a few supplements that may be of benefit to your health, and your baby's health, during these special times.

OMEGA-3 FATTY ACIDS. It's important to keep supplementing with DHA in particular after delivery, as breastfeeding transmits mom's reserves of DHA to the baby through your breast milk. (DHA remains critical for your baby's brain development.) Continue supplementing with 300 mg of DHA per day from fish oil or cod liver oil, but still do not exceed a total of 1 gram of EPA and DHA combined.

VITAMIN D$_3$. Continue with 4,000–6,000 IU per day while nursing, so you are able to pass a healthy amount of vitamin D along to your baby in your breast milk. (On summer days when you get full-body sun exposure, however, you can skip the supplement.)

BONE BROTH. While nursing, bone broth can help keep you healthy by supporting your immune system, and keeping your mineral levels high. Drink a cup or two a day as part of your healthy eating plan.

FENUGREEK. This spice used as flavoring in curry powders or processed maple syrup is a low-risk way to boost or maintain your milk supply. (Melissa had great results with fenugreek during her Whole30.) Fenugreek can boost your milk supply in as little as 24 hours, and once you've reached your desired supply, you may be able to discontinue supplementation without a drop. However, some studies show that taking less than 3.5 grams a day may not provide benefits, and lactation experts recommend a daily intake of six grams, which may mean you're taking 12 capsules a day—far more than the supplement label recommends. Higher doses may lead to hypoglycemia or gastric distress, so you and your health care provider will have to decide the dose that's right for you.

OTHER GALACTAGOGUES. Other supplements thought to increase breast milk supply or stimulate let-down include fennel, Rescue Remedy, Motherlove More Milk Plus, and Mother's Milk herbal tea. Work with your lactation consultant or health care provider to create a customized, safe lactation plan, especially when including supplements.

Visit the special Pregnancy and Breastfeeding section of our Whole30 Forum (www.w30.co/w30forum) for support during your program.

kids

"The Whole30 transformed my life—no more high blood pressure or sleep apnea, and I lost over 100 pounds! It also changed my wife's life; she reversed her type 2 diabetes and lost a great amount of weight. But most important, it set my children up for a solid nutritional and health foundation that will benefit them for the rest of their lives. That's something I can't put into words."
—STEPHEN S., DUNNE, NC

Is the Whole30 healthy for kids?

First, we're not doctors, so we encourage you to speak with your child's pediatrician or family care practitioner before changing their diet, especially if they have medical conditions, behavioral disorders, or sensory processing disorders. But since you asked us, we think the Whole30 is optimally healthy for kiddos! Just think about all the nutrient-dense foods they'll be eating: They'll get protein, vitamin B_{12}, and heme iron from quality meats, and take in vitamins, minerals (like calcium and magnesium), antioxidants, and fiber from fruits and veggies; while natural fats like avocado, coconut oil, and ghee promote brain development and steady energy. Our program eliminates the calorie-dense, nutrient-poor foods that fill their bellies but don't nourish their bodies, the sugars that keep energy fluctuating and tantrums alive, and potentially problematic foods that may be contributing to their asthma, skin conditions, allergies, or attention disorders. If the plan is approached as a family experiment rather than restriction or punishment, it can actually become a bonding experience for you and your kids.

Don't kids need milk?

Kids need nutrient-dense foods to grow and be healthy, but there is nothing in cow's milk that kids can't get in more biologically appropriate forms from meat, vegetables, fruits, and fats. Yes, calcium is a key factor in building strong, healthy bones, but it's important to remember that it's not the only factor. Other vitamins and minerals play a big role in bone development, as do lifestyle choices like activity levels and stress. Your entire family will get enough calcium and the other vitamins and minerals you need from a wide variety of Whole30-compliant foods.

What benefits can I expect to see with my kids?

As with adults, your child's Whole30 results will vary, but parents have reported some very consistent results in some areas. Generally, kids on our plan have more stable energy, fewer tantrums (especially in kids with hyperactivity), focus better in school, take fewer sick days, and sleep better. Digestion improves tremendously, too—fewer reports of gas, bloating, or bellyaches. We've also had many testimonials of dramatically improved medical conditions like asthma, allergies, type 1 diabetes, and attention deficit disorders. Kids also experience all of the less-visible benefits of the program, like regulated hormones and stable blood sugar.

Should you go cold turkey or ease them into the Whole30?

There is no simple answer to this question. Every child is different—some respond well to change, some love a challenge, some are born experimenters, and some just want to be left well enough alone. To answer this question, you have to know your child, but we'll offer you one of three approaches. The first is an "all or nothing," where you say, "This is what we're eating—deal with it." After a brief rebellion, the kids usually come around, and boom—you're all on board. This approach is rough for a week or so, but it accomplishes your goal fast, and it's most likely to produce dramatic results. Plus, we promise your kids won't starve, even if they do refuse to eat for a meal or two. The second approach is a gradual but firm transition, where off-plan foods just aren't restocked when you run out. Your confrontation level is much lower with this strategy, although it will take you much longer to gear up for the actual Whole30, and longer to see improvements. Finally, you can baby step it, offering your kids better choices but not fighting with them if they refuse. This probably won't get them on board with a by-the-books Whole30 or our dramatic results, but there won't be any battles, and if they do make self-directed changes, they'll likely stick. Choose the approach that's right for your kids, your family, and your stress levels.

Should kids follow the same meal template?

Your child's plate should look like yours—some protein, some natural fat, lots of veggies, and some fruit. You can use our meal template (page 196) as a jumping off point, but don't stress if your kids don't want to eat exactly according to plan. Offer plenty of good food at each meal, let your kids help decide what goes on their plates, and their bodies (which are still very good at communicating things like hunger and satiety) will work it out in the end. However, kids probably need more than three meals a day—their stomachs are small, and metabolisms are humming! Be willing to offer snacks (which should look like small meals) in between breakfast, lunch, and dinner, but don't allow them to graze all day long.

My kids are picky eaters. How can I get them to eat their vegetables?

Research shows most children need five to ten exposures to a new food before giving it a thumbs-up, so keep offering those beets, and be patient. In addition, colorful food fare is more appealing to children than adults, so put lots of different foods (in lots of different colors) on your kid's plate. Don't be afraid to use the dressings or sauces starting on page 302 to make their greens more appealing, and remember—they watch every move you make, so make sure you're eating your veggies with a huge smile and a big, "yum!"

My kids still want pancakes.

This is a tough one. Ultimately, it's your decision whether or not to stick to our baked goods or treats rules with your children. On one hand, it's more important for you to discover whether the foods they used to eat are responsible for their skin condition, tantrums, allergies, or asthma than it is to address their emotional relationship with food, especially if they're young. In that case, do whatever you need to do to get them to stick to the program, even if it means making egg-and-banana pancakes on Sunday morning. On the other hand, older kids may already have a really unhealthy association with sweets and treats, and you may want to tackle all of these factors (the emotional and the physical) with your family's Whole30. Ultimately, make your decision based on the age of your kids, the reason they're on the Whole30 in the first place, and your goals for your family's program. Just know that if you do make your kids pancakes, we're still going to insist that *you* not eat them.

What if they eat off-plan foods when they're away from home?

Holding kids to a strict Whole30 can be difficult for many reasons. Schoolteachers, loving relatives, strangers at the bank, and playmates will likely offer your kids "treats." Before you begin your Whole30, inform your caregiver, teachers, and play group parents of your family's new food boundaries. Be polite, offer to bring in alternatives for your kids, and ask for their help in keeping your child compliant. Food restrictions may be inconvenient, but if you're trying to improve a medical issue, behavioral issue, or digestive issue, the next 30 days are important. That having been said, unless there's a significant sensitivity or an allergy involved (or you're medically testing for one), don't get too bent out of shape if it happens. Talk to your kids about the experience and how you saw it affect their health, behavior, or mood; remind them that some foods are more healthy (anytime) choices and some foods are less healthy (sometimes or never) choices; and see if you can get them on board to make these short-term changes as part of a family experiment. Then, just keep on going with your Whole30.

Can I help my kids understand how less-healthy foods affect their health or behavior?

That depends on the child's age and level of awareness. A two-year-old will have difficulty verbally acknowledging the connection between their food and their health, behavior, or mood, but older children should be able to make those associations. Reintroduce foods in a casual but controlled environment when you'll be able to observe your child for a few hours afterward. Make mental notes of any changes you observe in your child's digestion, energy, mood, temper, attention span, or medical condition. Then, draw a connection between the off-plan food and the less-than-desirable outcome you observed. Help your children see that the healthier foods they've been eating help them behave better, play longer, and feel better, and they're more likely to make better choices going forward.

See page 406 for more resources on the Whole30 for kids.

vegetarians and vegans

"During my first vegetarian Whole30, I started to view food differently for the first time in my life. I was breaking away from old habits of wanting to eat to celebrate or chase away every emotion. I saw how what I was eating was playing a huge role in my depression. In my first 30 days my mood was steadily lifting and more stable than ever. My food cravings actually diminished and I couldn't believe the freedom I was feeling. Prior to my vegetarian Whole30, I was dealing with cystic acne, but during the program, my facial acne completely cleared. I also lost 15 lbs." —LAURICE B., LONG BEACH, CA

We welcome vegetarians and vegans to our program, and want you to reap many of the benefits of our healthy-eating plan while still honoring your ethical or religious obligations. In fact, we've had a loyal vegetarian/vegan following for several years now, and we created a special section of our Whole30 Forum just for you. Despite the fact that these lifestyle choices seem in conflict with our healthy eating recommendations (which include a moderate amount of animal protein), please don't rule our program out! We think the Whole30 has a lot to offer you, even if you choose to avoid animal products, or limit their inclusion in your diet.

In fact, let's talk about all of the things the Whole30 has in common with health-conscious vegetarians and vegans. We are all concerned with sourcing our food ethically, responsibly, and healthfully. We embrace a diet that includes copious amounts of nutrient-dense plants. We avoid fake processed foods with little nutrition but lots of sugar, fat, and salt.

Honestly, our approaches have an awful lot in common—and it's that spirit of positivity and connection that we focus on here.

Are You Ready for a Change?

If your primary reason for becoming vegetarian or vegan was for health, we invite you to reconsider your approach for the next 30 days. We believe the inclusion of some animal protein (dairy doesn't count) in your daily diet is necessary for optimal health, and we've provided well-reasoned, well-sourced arguments (in *It Starts With Food*) to back up our position. So if this is where you are coming from, give our plan a try! Consider it a self-experiment: Go back to eating high-quality animal protein as part of your Whole30. We'd be shocked if your health, body composition, and quality of life did not improve, but if you don't experience the benefits you hope to see, you can simply return to your vegetarian or vegan lifestyle having learned a bit more about how certain foods work for you.

If your concerns are largely ethical—animal welfare, sustainability, your local economy, or global economic factors—know that there are ways to responsibly, ethically source meat, seafood, and eggs. In fact, supporting those efforts sends a strong message (financial and otherwise) to the large corporations invested in factory farming; you'll have more of an impact voting with your dollar than you will opting out of the system altogether. See page 404 for more information on sourcing responsible animal protein options.

For those of you who have texture or conceptual issues with meat, but want to try to incorporate it back into your diet, here are our best tips for the "meat challenged":

First, choose meats or cuts of meat that aren't as "fleshy" or fatty in texture or format. Lighter, flakier fish are often a good, neutral texture choice. Ground beef may be easier to stomach than a steak. Lean cuts of meat may also smell (and taste) better to the meat-shy.

Avoid meat on the bone, like ribs or chicken wings—the bone only serves to remind you of exactly what you're eating. When preparing chicken breasts, pound them with a meat tenderizer so they're thinner and more tender. Cut your meat into small pieces or chunks before cooking, but don't over-cook it; that makes it taste rubbery and tough and may prove even harder to get down.

You can also play little tricks on yourself to sneak more meat into your diet. "Hide" your meat in other parts of your meal, like mixed up into a soup, stew, curry, slow-cooker dish, or salad. This technique works especially well with slow-cooker meals, as your meat will be both hidden in the mix, and very tender.

Finally, start off with smaller portions at first—a 16-ounce rib eye may prove too overwhelming, but a ¼-pound burger may seem manageable.

If you'd rather proceed with the Whole30 using your vegetarian or vegan preferences as a framework, here are some tips to help you make the most of your experience.

Pescetarians and Vegetarians

If you'll eat some animal products (like eggs or fish), we recommend getting the bulk of your protein from these sources and supplementing with plant-based sources as little as possible. Yes, you'll get tired of eggs, salmon, and cod, but remember, this is just a 30-day experiment. Remember that the information you'll gain at the end of this experiment is worth a week or two of food boredom.

If dairy is a viable source of protein for you (not causing digestive distress, skin break-outs, or other obvious negative consequences) we recommend putting pastured, organic, fermented sources like yogurt or kefir at the top of your list. You could also use a whey protein powder from grass-fed, organic sources, which would provide the protein you need with fewer downsides than other dairy products (including all forms of milk and cheese).

Unless you're really active in the gym or in your sport, aim for the lower end of our protein recommendations (page 194). There's no need to shoot for some arbitrary number like "1 gram per pound of body weight" with such limited protein sources, unless your context and activity level truly demands that much food. Make up for the calories you may be missing from protein by adding a little more fat to your meals. Studies show a higher-fat diet can be muscle sparing, and you need to make sure you're eating enough calories in general to support your activity levels.

Vegans

If this is your context, it's important for us to be clear in our expectations. We can get you to *better* health with our Whole30 framework, but not *optimal* health. The inclusion of plant-based protein sources known to have detrimental effects on hormonal balance, the digestive tract, and the immune system, and the lack of nutrients (like vitamin B_{12} and heme iron) found only in animal protein sources means, in our experience, that your health potential is limited. In this chapter, we'll do our best to help you implement the Whole30 framework in a way that makes the most of your dietary choices, but we caution you not to expect the same stunning, dramatic results that omnivores commonly report.

That wasn't meant to sound harsh or judgmental. Please know that even if we disagree on what's "healthy," we respect and honor your choice, and will work with you to find a way to become the healthiest version of you. Since you're coming to us for healthy eating advice, though, we'd be remiss not to share what we believe to be true. So please, keep reading, because we think you'll like our plan to fine-tune your plant-based diet.

First, the idea of "protein combining" (specifically pairing two plant-based protein sources in a meal to achieve a "complete" amino acid profile) is outdated—your body has the capacity to store amino acids from the food you eat over the course of a day or two. Just eat a wide variety of plant-based protein sources, and don't worry about making a "complete" protein in any given meal. Your best choices are minimally processed, fermented soy products like tempeh or natto, or organic edamame (soybeans). You can also include non-fermented, organic soy (like extra-firm tofu) and various legumes in rotation. Pseudo-cereals like quinoa are another gluten-free protein source, and are less likely to cause disruption to the gut or immune system than other grains.

A hemp- or pea-protein powder is also an option for you, although you'd have to include quite a lot of it in your diet to get any substantial amount of protein at all. (Read your labels carefully to make sure these protein powders include as few inflammatory ingredients as possible.)

We still highly encourage you to avoid all gluten grain, including seitan (which is made from wheat gluten), non-organic soy, processed soy products (like soy-based "burgers" and "cheese"), and peanuts. The good news? You can still make our Egg-free Mayonnaise (page 180), which opens you up to a world of dressings and sauces to top your veggies.

One last thing—aim for as little protein as possible, as we don't want you eating any more plant-based protein sources than you have to. If you have to track your intake for a few days to see where your numbers fall, that's okay. Shoot for the recommended amounts as detailed in the United States Recommended Daily Allowance (USRDA): 46 grams a day for women, 56 grams a day for men. You're probably not going to become a power lifter on these amounts, but it will keep a moderately active vegan as healthy as we can get you.

You'll also need to eat more carbohydrates and fat, to cover the missing calories from your relatively low-protein diet. (The extra carbohydrates should actually come naturally via the plants you're eating, many of which contain far more carbohydrate than protein.)

You can download a free copy of our shopping list for vegetarians and vegans on our website, www.whole30.com/pdf-downloads. For support, visit the vegetarian and vegan section of our Whole30 Forum at www.w30.co/w30forum.

troubleshooting your whole30

"About eight months ago, my husband's health began to falter. At first, it was just super-ficial with skin inflammation and hair loss, but after a number of biopsies, cultures, and blood tests, the dermatologist uncovered extremely elevated liver enzymes, and non-alcoholic fatty liver disease. By this time, his ALT level was over 600. Three months of a low-fat diet did not help. After doing some research, we started the Whole30. We were hopeful that we'd see some improvement in his liver enzymes at his next doctor's appoint-ment, but we had no idea his ALT level would drop from 660 to 106 after only 23 days on the program! Even the doctor was surprised at the dramatic drop. This has saved my husband from a life of likely liver failure." —REBECCA C., CITY/STATE WITHHELD

I have some food allergies. How do I work around these in the Whole30?

Simple! Just take our shopping list on page 192 and cross off the foods to which you are allergic. Now, just meal plan from what's left, choosing dishes that don't use those ingredients, or recipes where it would be easy to leave that particular ingredient out. (For example, if you're allergic to nuts, Melissa's Chicken Hash on page 228 would be delicious even without the walnuts.) The good news is that some people have reported a reversal of food allergies by healing their gut and calming their immune system with the Whole30. (Don't try this at home, though—always reintroduce allergenic foods under the supervision of your health care provider.)

I feel like I've been hit by a truck (the first week). Is this the "carb flu" everyone is talking about?

The "carb flu" (a period of headaches, fatigue, cravings, light-headedness, and "brain fog")

isn't really a flu—it's actually an energy issue. Your old diet included lots of carbohydrates from grains, legumes, added sugar, and processed foods. That carbohydrate digests into sugar in the body, and your body then used that sugar for energy. In fact, you got so good at using sugar to keep you running that your body became wholly dependent on it. Now, you start the Whole30. Your carbohydrate (sugar) intake is naturally lower because you're eating vegetables and fruit instead of bread and cookies. Your body is no longer getting all that sugar it's used to running on. So what happens? You run out of gas. Without all that sugar (energy), you get tired, you get headaches, your brain is foggy, and you're hungry. So. Hungry. Mostly for sugar. Some describe it as "withdrawal," and that wouldn't be far off.

You now have another excellent energy source available to you—fat! Fat from your diet and body fat can also fuel you as you work, play with your kids, study, or run errands. The trouble is, your body doesn't know how to use it, because you've been giving it so much sugar all the time. (Think of your body's mitochondria—the powerhouses of your cells—like six-year-olds. If you give your six-year-old the choice between a candy bar and an avocado, which one will they pick? Candy, every single time.) If your body has sugar all the time, it's going to preferentially run on sugar all the time. Only in the relative absence of all that sugar will it start running efficiently on fat as fuel.

In summary, your body isn't getting the energy source it's used to depending on, and not very good at running on the more stable energy source you're giving it now. So for a few days (or maybe even a week), you're stuck in this no-man's land that feels like you've got the flu.

The good news is that this passes fast. The process of "fat adaptation" (being able to use body fat and dietary fat as fuel) begins in just a few days, although it will take a few weeks to fully ramp up. The good news is that you'll start to feel better really soon (usually by Day 14), and those headaches will be a thing of the past.

⭐ TIP: *Have a good plan for these first few days, because they can be rough. Take time off from the gym or your longer runs, go to bed early, make sure your pantry is clean (because you will be craving), and don't skimp on the fat! Use our meal template (page 194) to make sure you're giving your body enough of the energy source it's now being primed to use.*

Why did my digestion get worse during the Whole30?

Any significant change to your diet can cause short-term changes to your digestive function. You can easily imagine how eating foods that harm your gut could mess up your digestion, but even *removing* these problematic foods can create issues, temporarily. It's impossible to know for sure which dietary changes are responsible for

which symptom during your Whole30, but it's common to have periods of constipation, bloating, and/or diarrhea as your body adjusts to its new diet.

These short-term changes are *not* indications that eating nutrient-dense food is harmful to you! The vast majority of the time, these transitional issues sort themselves out within a few weeks, as your body adapts to the absence of problematic and/or inflammatory food components.

Chronic stress also has direct effects on your digestion and can contribute to indigestion and bloating, especially if you are eating more nutritious protein sources and natural fats than you historically have. The great news is that eating nutritious foods during your Whole30 and the benefits that provides (sleeping better, having more energy, and feeling more self-confident) is a big step toward reducing a chronic stress response, and helping your digestion get back on track.

⭐ TIP: *There is a small subset of people who, due to the consequences of their long-term dietary choices and the current condition of their digestive tract, may not tolerate even "healthy" foods very well. These mostly involve fiber-rich and/or starchy foods, typically vegetables and fruit. Cooking your vegetables well and introducing new foods in small amounts over time often helps. In addition, as we already mentioned, nutrition is not the only factor in digestive health. If you continue to struggle with your digestion even after your Whole30 is over, it's time to recruit a professional to evaluate your diet in conjunction with your lifestyle and current health markers. (See page 406.)*

Why are my symptoms and/or medical condition getting worse?

This answer largely has to do with how your immune system works, and how your immune system "learns" from repeated exposure to potentially problematic foods (or in the case of leaky gut, foods that cross the gut barrier when they shouldn't). If your immune system has formed antibodies against certain foods, it will take several weeks with no exposure to those foods to allow the levels of antibodies to significantly decrease.

If you've "dosed" yourself with a lot of foods that trigger these immune system antibodies just prior to your Whole30, there's often a worsening of inflammatory symptoms between weeks two and three of your program. (Yes, there's a bit of a delayed response here—it has to do with the way these antibodies and their "triggers" bond and stimulate an immune response over time.) That means your pizza-beer-ice-cream bender the night before your Whole30 could come back to bite you in the gut (and everywhere else in the body) halfway through your program.

As the timeline on this type of a reaction is fairly consistent person-to-person, the good news is that symptoms almost always improve around the third or fourth week, but *only* if you've maintained *zero exposure* to potential triggers (that is, stayed 100 percent committed to the Whole30 guidelines). We told you to take this whole "no slips, no cheats, no excuses" advice seriously.

In summary, going on a binge with unhealthy foods right before your Whole30 may seriously hamper how good you feel once you're on the program, and may actually make the symptoms or condition you are hoping to improve worse before they get better. Please, don't go junk-food-crazy the day before you begin. (And if you do, don't say we didn't warn you.)

I was feeling great earlier in my Whole30; now I'm exhausted. Why?

This can tie in with the previous "medical symptom" question, since inflammation directly contributes to fatigue and malaise. However, a more common explanation is that you are simply not eating enough nutritious food—particularly carbohydrates. We see this especially with active individuals (those who exercise or participate in sports). You're taking our "fill your plate with veggies" to heart, and those veggies are nutrient-dense for sure, but broccoli, spinach, asparagus, and kale won't effectively fuel those exercise sessions. Eventually, your low-carb choices catch up with you, and you start to slow down. A lot.

The good news is that it's easy to tell if this is your situation. Eat more carbs! Immediately make it a point to add carb-dense vegetables and fruit to every meal. Have a bowl of berries and a banana with your frittata for breakfast, a baked sweet potato and an apple with your protein salad for lunch, and butternut squash soup and a salad with sliced pears as your dinner sides. You should feel better immediately, and be back to your Tiger Blood self by tomorrow. (Now, keep it up! Your body obviously needs more carbohydrates than you've been giving it.)

This may also happen if you're hesitant to add enough natural fats to your meals. (Not enough fat means not enough calories, which means not enough energy.) Review our meal template on page 194 and make sure you are getting enough energy from nutrient-dense food (protein, carbohydrate, and fat) to fuel your everyday activities and exercise.

Finally, if you're trying to implement other high-tech nutrition strategies into your Whole30 (like intermittent fasting or carb-cycling) please, just stop. Changing too many things at once means you'll never know what behavior is responsible for which result, and the Whole30 is meant to stand alone as a learning experience and an elimination protocol. Save the other experiments for after your Whole30 is over, when you'll be better able to evaluate their impact on your health, energy levels, and body composition.

⭐ TIP: *This is more a reminder than a tip: the Whole30 is not a quick-fix weight-loss program. If you're purposefully restricting calories, carbo-hydrates, or fat during your Whole30, you will (ironically) only make it harder for you to achieve success with your Whole30 and with long-term body composition management. Just follow the plan and trust that it will work for you, as it has for hundreds of thousands of people just like you.*

Why has my sleep quality diminished during my Whole30?

Having trouble falling asleep is typically a dif-ferent issue than waking up in the middle of the night, which is different than waking up very early in the morning and not being able to go back to sleep. The issue most likely to be directly related to your Whole30 is waking up in the middle of the night. If you were sleeping fairly well before your Whole30, but during the program find yourself popping your eyes open at 2 a.m., it's most likely due to blood sugar volatility. (Your body's still not very good managing your blood sugar, leading to blood sugar highs and lows, even in the middle of the night.) Eating a snack-sized portion of protein like eggs, chicken, or salmon about an hour before bed helps to stabilize blood sugar levels over the nighttime hours. (While we don't typically recom-mend eating shortly before bed, this is a strategy that helps during your transition period.) Try it consistently for a week, then see if you're able to sleep more restfully without your pre-bed snack.

If this doesn't help, or if your sleep issues involve being "tired but wired" in the evenings or waking up too early in the morning, here's some bad news: We're going to take away your coffee. If you are still consuming any caffeine, these sleep troubles are a good indication that it's time give it up, at least for a few weeks. Stubborn sleep issues can be exacerbated by even small amounts of caffeine many hours before bed. While it's not an official Whole30 rule, you asked us how you could sleep better, so we're telling you. (Are you sorry you asked?)

⭐ TIP: *Nutrition is not the only factor in determining sleep quality. In fact, poor sleep during your Whole30 isn't necessarily because of your current nutrition choices. Are you worried about finances or an upcoming work project? Do you do intense exercise or run late in the evening? Are you on your computer or smartphone just before bed, or watch TV as you fall asleep? These things can all negatively impact sleep quality. Visit www.w30.co/w30sleep for suggestions on how to improve your sleep.*

Why is my athletic performance decreasing?

This is common in the first week for reasons we've already explained. If you're in your first ten days of Whole30, don't expect to set any personal bests or enter any big races. In fact, now may be a good time to take a week off, or spend a week focusing on low-intensity activity, skill work, and recovery.

If your energy has improved overall but you still struggle with your runs, workouts, or games, we bet you're not eating enough carbohydrate (or simply enough food overall). We love that you're eating so much broccoli, asparagus, and spinach, but that's not going to fuel those hard runs very effectively—high-intensity exercise demands carbohydrates. If you're very active, you have to purposefully incorporate starchy vegetables (potatoes, winter squashes, taro, or yuca) and a variety of fruits into your daily diet to ensure your energy stores are well maintained.

In addition, you may notice other benefits before you notice performance gains. Keep an eye on other fitness-related happenings and know that more restful sleep, less muscle sore-ness, greater mobility, less joint pain, and faster recovery from a tough workout is the Whole30 working its magic, and will translate into improved performance soon enough.

I'm a week or two into my Whole30 and I haven't lost any weight. Why isn't this working?

Before we answer this, we have a question for you: *Why are you on the scale?* The Whole30 rules explicitly state that you are not to step on the scale during your program, and this is exactly why! You become so focused on that numerical read-out that you don't pay attention to any other aspect of your program. Scale weight tells you almost nothing about your overall health, and the Whole30 isn't a weight-loss diet—it's designed to jump-start optimal health for the rest of your life. So please, give yourself a much-needed, long-overdue, well-deserved break from a preoccupation with body weight and focus on health instead. Turn to page 43, take note of the things that are working better, and trust that with improved health comes natural, sustainable, effortless weight loss. (Now please get off the scale.)

⭐ **TIP:** *In a recent survey of more than 1,600 Whole30 participants, 96 percent reported having lost weight and/or improved their body composition. The majority lost between 6 and 15 pounds in just 30 days. So there you go—proof that weight loss is built right into the program, without your having to think about it.*

I can't afford to lose any weight.

If this is your context, our first tip may seem obvious, but we really do need to explain this—eat more. You may think you're eating plenty, but you could still be under-fed. Swapping out grains and sugary refined foods for vegetables and fruits puts you at a serious caloric deficit. You've got

to make those calories up somewhere—namely, healthy fats and starchy vegetables. But if you've been a little fat-phobic, adding as much fat as you need to maintain a healthy body weight may be scary. On the other hand, if you're a little carb-phobic (because someone told you consuming carbohydrates would make you fat and diabetic), you may be limiting potatoes, winter squashes, and fruit on purpose. If you're already at the lean or downright skinny end of the body composition spectrum, you can't afford to subsist on leafy greens and low-carb veggies alone.

Make sure you're eating at least three meals a day, even if you feel like skipping meals. If you find you're hungry between meals, have a snack—ideally including a decent amount of protein and fat. (Snacking on just an apple isn't doing much for your cause.) Eat more fat, meeting or exceeding the higher end of the fat recommendations in our meal template. Eat more carbs; don't fill up on bowls of salad and platefuls of broccoli, leaving less room in your belly for meat and fat. Eat more protein, prioritizing protein-dense meat like steak over lower protein items like eggs. And don't even think about intermittent fasting. Do we really need to explain this one?

Other lifestyle factors, like training, recovery, and stress, also play directly into your ability to maintain or gain weight. If you're running ten miles a day, sleeping six hours a night, and are chronically stressed with work, school, family, or financial worries, your diet may not be the biggest factor in maintaining muscle mass. (Plus, again . . . coffee. Caffeine is an appetite suppressant, so it is not your friend if getting enough nutritious food into your body is a challenge.) Consider asking a functional medicine practitioner to analyze factors like your stress hormones, thyroid function, and gut health to help you address your weight management from a big-picture perspective. (See page 406 for resources.)

Is it normal to be very thirsty?

It can be, especially in the beginning, but it's hard to say exactly why. Could be sodium-related: When you cut out all the processed foods, you also cut out a significant amount of sodium from your daily diet. Sodium helps your body retain water, so moving to a whole foods–based low-sodium diet may cause your body to make some adjustments to your intake. It may be that you've eliminated non-compliant beverages from your diet (like juices or soda) and haven't replaced those liquids with water. In addition, changes in both dietary intake and metabolism of carbohydrates and fats may lead to a short-term drop in how much water your body is storing. Oh, and if you're not eating as many vegetables and fruit ("wet" foods) as we encourage, you may be missing out on hydration there, too. Regardless of why it's happening, listen to your body here. Make a conscious effort to drink more water and compliant beverages (see page 70) throughout the day, eat your veggies, and please add some table salt and/or sea salt to your cooking or food. And don't worry—the body will generally sort its water balance out quickly, so you shouldn't have to carry that gallon jug around for long.

My sugar cravings are killing me! What do I do?

Step one: take a deep breath. First, let's figure out if you're craving, or just hungry. Here's our favorite trick: Ask yourself, "Am I hungry enough to eat steamed fish and broccoli?" (If that would never sound appealing, pick another straightforward protein source, like hard-boiled eggs.) If the answer is yes, then you are legitimately hungry! Time to eat your next meal, or grab a snack to tide you over.

If the answer is, "No, but I'd eat (fill in crunchy/salty/sweet food here)" then it's confirmed: you're having a craving—but there is no need to panic. Based on studies of smokers resisting the urge to light up, the average craving lasts just three to five minutes. Your brain will be screaming that you really need sugar, but if you can distract yourself briefly, you'll find that craving will pass. So go for a quick walk, phone a friend, check the sports scores, or throw in a load of laundry—whatever it takes to get you through. Whew.

Here's what not to do: reach for a Whole30-compliant sweet treat to satisfy your sugar craving. If you're used to something sweet every day at 3 p.m., your brain has come to expect that reward. But your brain doesn't know the difference between a candy bar and a dried fruit-and-nut bar. All your brain knows is that it's 3 p.m., and here comes the sweet reward! This behavior doesn't help you change your habits—it actually reinforces them. Remember, every time you resist a craving, your Sugar Dragon gets a little less fiery, so don't use fruit or nut butters as a sugar crutch.

> ⭐ TIP: *Do you find yourself prowling through your pantry after dinner looking for "a little something?" We've been so conditioned to eat dessert, and while subbing your ice cream for a bowl of blueberries in coconut milk is a healthier choice, you're still giving your brain that after-dinner treat. One lovely post-dinner ritual that won't feed your Sugar Dragon is brewing a cup of rooibos herbal tea. It's naturally decaffeinated, has a naturally sweet taste, but isn't anything like the treats you're craving, so it won't act as a "sugar crutch."*

I finished my Whole30 and my digestion is still unhappy.

There are other food groups that may potentially be inflammatory or digestively disruptive. Two of the most common are high-FODMAP foods and high-histamine foods.

FODMAPS: This stands for Fermentable Oligosaccharides, Disaccharides, Monosaccharides, and Polyols—a collection of fermentable carbohydrates and sugar alcohols found in various foods, like grains, beans, vegetables and fruits. FODMAPs include fructose (found in various amounts in all fruit), lactose (found in dairy), fructans (found in wheat, garlic, onion, artichoke, asparagus, and the sweetener agave), galactans (found in legumes, cabbage, and Brussels sprouts), and polyols (found in many fruits like apples, pears, and peaches; and sweeteners like sorbitol or xylitol). These FODMAPS are not well absorbed, and can "feed" bacteria in the intestinal tract when eaten in excess. In sensitive individuals, this fermentation causes gas, bloating, cramping, and digestive distress, unbalances your gut bacterial population, and promotes systemic inflammation.

HIGH-HISTAMINE FOODS: Certain foods either contain a naturally occurring chemical called "histamine," or stimulates the body's own natural release of the chemical. Histamine is also released in the body as part of an allergic reaction, causing the typical allergy symptoms, like itching, sneezing, wheezing, and swelling. (Many over-the-counter allergy medications contain an antihistamine.) When sensitive people eat too many histamine-rich foods, they may suffer allergy-like symptoms such as headaches, rashes, hives, itching, gastro-intestinal upset, asthma, or eczema. This is called histamine intolerance.

Your digestive distress may also be the result of an undiagnosed food sensitivity (or multiple sensitivities) not included on this list. If you've been following the Whole30 protocol for 60 days and are still experiencing digestive issues or other immune-related symptoms, it's time to work with a functional medicine practitioner (page 406) to help you build a treatment plan (including diagnostic lab work and supplementation) that will work for your particular condition or symptoms.

⭐ TIP: *A food journal can also help you identify potentially "healthy" foods that may be triggering unpleasant symptoms. Write down all the foods in your meals and snacks for a week, and note the severity and type of symptoms you experience after each to try to pinpoint the culprit(s). This information will be especially helpful if you choose to work with an expert. If you want to experiment with a low-FODMAP or low-histamine diet on top of your Whole30 elimination, you can download customized shopping lists at www.whole30.com/pdf-downloads.*

What if the Whole30 doesn't work for me?

You may have wanted to see improvements in a particular area (a medical condition, athletic improvement, a specific area of your body composition, or your hot flashes), but on Day 30, you're just not seeing it, and you're really disappointed. We understand, and we're really sorry. While the program works amazingly well for the vast majority of people who take it on, the Whole30 isn't perfect (no diet is, universally), and it doesn't fix everything for everyone.

The one thing we want you to take away from this experience is that if the Whole30 didn't work for you, you are not a failure, and there is nothing wrong with you. We hope by now you recognize the other benefits of the program (the things that did improve for you), and can see all the progress you've made over the last 30 days. Take a minute to be proud of yourself, and celebrate how far you've come!

Now, let's talk about why the Whole30 may not have worked as well for you as you had hoped, in whatever area you hoped to see improvements:

- **YOU DIDN'T DO IT RIGHT.** Tough love time: this is the hardest one to hear, but also the most common reason for the failure of elimination diets like the Whole30 to provide results. You followed the technical letter of the rules, but didn't embrace the spirit or intention of the program. You "slipped" or "treated yourself" or modified our rules because you had to/wanted to/figured it wouldn't really matter. You adjusted the program to suit your cravings, your social life, your idea of "healthy." You only gave it two weeks before deciding it wasn't working.

- **THIRTY DAYS WASN'T LONG ENOUGH.** While radical health improvements can take place in just a month, when you put it into context, decades of less-than-healthy behavior often can't compete with 30 days of Whole30. Overcoming chronic stress, medical issues, and years of unhealthy cravings, habits, and emotional ties to food are often the longest battles. Many Whole30ers with this history report that they didn't feel or see "the magic" until day 45, 60, or beyond.

- **YOU STILL HAVE FOODS IN YOUR DIET THAT AREN'T HEALTHY FOR YOU.** It's possible that some "healthy" foods included in the Whole30 aren't right for your context. Undiagnosed food sensitivities or a FODMAP or histamine intolerance may require you to eliminate even more foods to identify the triggers for your symptoms. Now is the time to work with a functional medicine practitioner (see page 406) to help you create a specific plan for you and your individual health situation.

- **YOU AREN'T PAYING ATTENTION TO THE RIGHT STUFF.** You really wanted to lose weight on your Whole30, but you didn't (or you didn't lose as much as you had hoped), so you deemed the program a failure. But were you paying attention to what else happened during your program? Did your sleep, energy, athletic performance, recovery, medical symptoms, cravings, mood, or self-esteem improve? A smaller number on your scale's digital read-out isn't the only measure of Whole30 success—in fact, we'd venture to say it's pretty far down the list of potential life-changing results. (See page 43 for our very long list.)

- **YOU'VE GOT OTHER LIFESTYLE FACTORS IMPEDING YOUR PROGRESS.** Not even a Whole365 will completely resolve your issues if you've had years of physical, mental, or emotional chronic stress. Under-sleeping, under-eating or being undernourished, over-exercising (or not exercising at all), a chronic medical condition, financial stress, marital stress, job stress, unresolved trauma . . . they all take a massive toll on your hormones, your gut, and your immune system. If the Whole30 didn't take you as far as you hoped to go, then diet may not be your biggest issue. As we have said at dozens of seminars, "don't look for a nutrition solution to a lifestyle problem." It's time to work with a professional (see page 406) to see what other lifestyle factors and/or medical issues you need to prioritize to get things moving in the right direction. (But please, continue with your Whole30—the first thing any good functional medicine practitioner is going to talk to you about is your diet, and they usually love our program.)

whole30 reintroduction FAQ

"When I started the Whole30, I weighed 415 pounds. I couldn't walk longer than five minutes without my lower back cramping and feeling like it was on fire. For as long as I can remember my body has hurt with the lightest pressure. I had many other issues such as PCOS, irregular periods, bloating, and constant fatigue and headaches. I started my Whole30 on May 5, 2014. Just four months later, I can walk more than five miles with no pain at all. I have even started jogging in 15–20 second spurts during my walk. I have lost 65 pounds and have more energy than I've had in twenty years! I feel alive today. This has changed my life!" —ANN MARIE L., FREDERICK, MD

I've just spent 30 days without some of my favorite foods. Now you're telling me I need to continue eating (mostly) Whole30 for another ten days?

Yep. You'll thank us for it, too. The point of the Whole30 is to figure out how the foods you used to eat are actually affecting you—your digestion, energy, sleep, mood, focus, cravings, athletic performance, and the symptoms of your medical condition. If you stuff your face with pizza, beer, and ice cream on Day 31, how will you know what food caused what symptoms later on, when you feel like junk? (And you will feel like junk.) Careful, systematic reintroduction is the key to identifying which specific foods aren't okay for you (and the effects they have on your body and brain), so don't skip this step, or try to speed it up. You've spent this long working so hard to change your life—what's another ten days?

⭐ TIP: *Reintroduction is actually a lifelong process. The more you pay attention to how you look, feel, perform, and live after eating certain foods, the more you'll notice their subtle effects. For some, gluten makes them sad. For others, dairy makes them break out—but not until two or three days after exposure. In other cases, eating one piece of bread has few discernable side effects, but eating bread three days in a row makes people look three months pregnant. You should continue to pay attention to your body, brain, and symptoms when you eat off-plan foods, even after your official reintroduction period is over.*

Do I have to reintroduce food groups in the order you've outlined?

You don't have to, but we recommend it. We've arranged your reintroduction food groups in the order of least likely to be problematic to most likely, per the scientific literature and feedback from thousands of Whole30 participants. Gluten comes last because it tends to have the most serious and long-lasting effects on your body and brain. If you start with gluten grains, you may have to wait a few extra days to let your system settle back down before reintroducing your next food group.

It's three days later, and I'm still feeling like junk from my last reintroduction. Should I wait even longer before eating my next food group?

Yes, you should. The point of reintroduction is to carefully evaluate the effects of one food group at a time. If you still have hives, allergies, or stomach bloating three days after exposure to dairy, that means your gut and immune system are still fired up—and dumping even more potentially inflammatory foods on top of an already inflamed system isn't a good idea. Stick to Whole30 eating until you no longer have symptoms, then wait one more day and reintroduce your next food group into a "clean" environment. You only get one shot to reintroduce and evaluate the effects, so be patient and do it right.

What about reintroducing sugar?

This is a tough one, because many of the foods in the other food groups will also contain sugar. If you choose to reintroduce pancakes on your gluten day, for example, you may have a hard time knowing if the lethargy, crankiness, and brain fog are from the pancake, the maple syrup, or (most likely) the combination of both. It's safe to say that reintroducing sugar in significant quantities usually brings back cravings and energy slumps—but you probably won't notice the three grams of sugar in your ketchup at all. If you want to specifically evaluate sugar by itself, do this first, and add a step (and another three days) to your reintroduction schedule. Keep the rest of your food Whole30-compliant, but add sugar to your morning coffee, drink a sugary fruit juice mid-morning, top your lunchtime sweet potato with ghee and honey, and pour a generous amount of maple syrup over poached peaches after dinner. See how the added sugar

makes you feel—evaluate energy, mood, hunger, and especially cravings.

Going forward in your reintroduction schedule, don't stress about a few grams of sugar here or there (like in your condiments, chicken sausage, or salad dressing). However, it's still good to be aware of how often companies add sugar in places you wouldn't suspect, so continue with your label reading.

TIP: *If adding sugar back into your coffee makes you want to drink a lot more coffee, ask yourself, is that a good thing?*

What kind of alcohol can I reintroduce in the first stage?

First, if you're not missing it, feel free to skip this step—many Whole30ers have commented how little they actually missed drinking. If you choose to reintroduce alcohol, avoid gluten-containing alcohols (like beer, rye, scotch, or whiskey) during this stage, as your goal is to evaluate the alcohol, not the gluten, and experts aren't sure whether distilled grain-based drinks are really gluten-free. Save those other drinks for your gluten reintroduction days, if you choose. (You'll already know how the alcohol makes you feel, so if you get a new symptom, like bloating, digestive upset, or skin breakouts, you'll know to blame the gluten and not the alcohol.) You can drink things like wine, tequila, or potato-based vodka in this stage to evaluate how the alcohol makes you look, feel, and live. Pay extra attention to whether you're tempted to make poor food choices under the influence. The "reduced inhibition" that alcohol promotes is important to recognize!

TIP: *If you drink wine, you are also getting a dose of sulfites, unless you specifically choose wine that is organically produced. If you end up with a headache, flushed skin, or other unpleasant effects, it may be difficult for you to tell whether it was the alcohol or the sulfites responsible. You could always test this further by drinking a non-sulfite beverage (like 100 percent agave tequila) and comparing effects. Just be sure to wait at least three days between experiments.*

Can you separate these foods out further, like breaking out soy from the rest of the legumes?

You don't have to, but the more carefully and systematically you approach reintroduction, the more you'll gain awareness of an individual food's effects. If you already suspect you have a sensitivity to a particular food (like corn, soy, peanuts, etc.), consider breaking that food out and adding one step to the standard reintroduction schedule. That would alter the original schedule to look like this if you were evaluating corn on its own:

DAY 1: Evaluate non-gluten containing alcohol (optional), while keeping the rest of your diet Whole30-compliant.

DAY 4: Evaluate legumes, while keeping the rest of your diet Whole30-compliant.

DAY 7: Evaluate corn, while keeping the rest of your diet Whole30-compliant.

DAY 10: Evaluate other non-gluten grains (rice, certified gluten-free oats, quinoa, etc.) while keeping the rest of your diet Whole30-compliant.

DAY 13: Evaluate dairy, while keeping the rest of your diet Whole30-compliant.

DAY 16: Evaluate gluten grains, while keeping the rest of your diet Whole30-compliant.

You can also "test" certain foods later if you continue to eat mostly Whole30 meals, just by paying attention when you eat them. (This doesn't work so well if you've gone back to eating meals with gluten, dairy, soy, etc. on a regular basis, however.)

I've had allergic reactions to a particular food (like oranges, avocado, or eggs) before. Can I try to reintroduce these foods now that my gut and immune system are healthier?

First, before reintroducing any food to which you have had an allergic reaction in the past, you must consult with your health care provider. Allergies are not to be taken lightly, so don't go this alone. Second, 30 days probably isn't long enough for your immune system to have calmed down enough to reintroduce a food to which you have had a serious allergic response. Our general rule of thumb is that you must go one full year without any exposure to that food before you can even consider reintroduction. (And we do mean zero exposure—don't eat even a tiny bite of that troublemaking substance all year long.) If you've been working hard to heal your gut and avoid the trigger for a full year, only then is it time to talk with your doctor about reintroducing, if it's that important to you.

⭐ TIP: *If you don't have a diagnosed allergy but have experienced negative effects when eating certain foods (like bloating when eating certain fruits, or hives when eating eggs), your health care provider may decide there is more leeway to re-test these foods. Note, however, that it still might require more than 30 days of gut healing to notice a difference, and you still may find that large quantities or repeated exposures to that food is not okay.*

What kinds of things should I be looking for when I reintroduce foods?

It's hard to come up with a comprehensive list, because everyone has a different experience when eating foods that their bodies don't tolerate well. However, here are some general things to look for when you reintroduce off-plan foods:

DIGESTION: Are things moving too fast or too slow? Do you have gas, bloating, pain, or cramping? Has your heartburn or GERD returned?

ENERGY: Are you back to a 3 p.m. slump, dragging yourself out of bed in the morning, or just feeling lethargic? Are your workouts suffering, or have you lost motivation to exercise?

SLEEP: Are you sleeping more restlessly? Do you have a hard time falling asleep? Are you waking up in the middle of the night, or too early in the morning?

CRAVINGS: Is your Sugar Dragon back in full effect? Are you having a hard time resisting the pull of sugar or carbs? Are you now eating foods just because they're in front of you?

MOOD AND PSYCHOLOGY: Are you cranky, moody, or otherwise less happy than you've been? Have your anxiety, depression, attention deficit, or compulsive habits returned?

BEHAVIOR (ESPECIALLY IN KIDS): Do you notice more tantrums, talking back, inability to control emotions or behaviors, or a lack of focus or shortened attention span?

SKIN: Did you break out, get a rash or hives, or see a reappearance of eczema, psoriasis, or other skin conditions?

BREATHING: Are you congested or having sinus pain? Have your "seasonal allergies" reappeared? Are you experiencing shortness of breath or asthma?

PAIN AND INFLAMMATION: Have you triggered a migraine or headache? Has your chronic pain, fatigue, tendinitis, or arthritis returned? Are joints more sore, stiff, or swollen? Do you have other tangible symptoms of inflammation?

MEDICAL CONDITIONS: Have your symptoms reappeared or gotten worse?

Some effects will be impossible to ignore, while others are subtle and may require a few more "tests" before you can reliably attribute the cause with the effect. Awareness is key—make sure you actually pay attention to all of these areas immediately after eating the food, later on that day, and in the days to come.

I used to eat (fill in food) just fine, but now it makes me feel terrible. Did the Whole30 create a sensitivity?

The Whole30 will not create a sensitivity. There are a few reasons why this food may bother you now in ways (you think) it never did before. First, after 30-plus days on the program, you have so much more awareness about how food affects you. It's highly likely that this food used to upset your digestion, make you break out, or bring on sinus issues, but you just didn't notice it. (It's like a smoker asserting he feels great. Is he *really* feeling great, or have the effects of the smoking on his lungs become his new "normal," where he doesn't even notice them anymore?) You've been feeling so good these last few weeks that any disruption to your system is a definite diversion from your new normal—one that cannot be ignored. So when reintroducing this food upsets your digestion, skin, or sinuses, you really notice, because you've been without these effects for some time now.

Second, when you're eating foods your body doesn't like, it creates all kinds of defense mechanisms to help protect you. Your gut bacterial population changes, you build up a bigger mucosal lining (a "buffer zone") in your gut, and your immune system goes on high alert. When you remove these triggers, the body adapts again. It no longer needs to protect you from the food you've been eating, so your gut and immune system are able to "relax" and begin to recover. This is a healthier state of being, but it also means these same defenses aren't in place when you reintroduce the food. It's like this: If someone kicked you in the shins every time they saw you, you'd probably put on some shin guards, right? But if they stopped kicking you for a month straight, you'd probably relax and think, "Great, I can take these shin guards off now." Imagine how much more it would hurt if they came along the very next day and kicked you again, after your shins had time to (partly) heal from the damage!

In summary, the Whole30 only showed you what was already there, magnified so you'll really pay attention. If a reintroduced food negatively impacts you now, you can be sure it was doing that all along to some degree.

I've noticed when I eat (fill in food), I get (fill in negative side effect). Does this mean I can't eat this food anymore?

We can't answer that for you—that's something you'll have to decide for yourself. We will say that if your body is clearly telling you, "I don't like this food!" you'd be wise to listen, and leave that food off your everyday plate. After all,

ignoring these signals is what led you toward all the symptoms and conditions you're now trying to reverse with the Whole30. However, if you discover ice cream gives you gas and bloating, but you really love ice cream, you're free to eat it anyway. Only you can make that call—but remember, you also have to own the consequences.

I've noticed when I eat (fill in food), I get absolutely no negative side effects. Does this mean this food is healthy for me?

Maybe. Remember, reintroduction isn't just a ten-day process, and sometimes it takes more time (or more exposure) for us to notice the negative effects foods have on our system. For example, Melissa can eat a small piece of bread with dinner and not notice any issues, but if she has three pieces of bread, she gets lethargic and kind of depressed. In other instances, the negative effects of these foods are cumulative—you don't notice their effects on the first day, but by the fourth day in a row, you've got symptoms. You may also experience "silent" consequences (at first)—nothing noticeable on a moment-by-moment basis, until one day a week later you wake up and you realize your energy levels are in the tank and your knee hurts again. The lesson? Continue to pay attention to how off-plan foods make you feel (both physically and psychologically), and err on the side of caution when it comes to reincorporating these foods into your everyday routine.

TIP: *The scientific literature against gluten, peanuts, and added sugar (specifically) is so convincing that we think these should be off your everyday plate whether you notice symptoms or not. You don't have to stress about a few grams of sugar in your ketchup or the once-a-year Christmas cookies your mom bakes, but in general, we believe these items make everyone less healthy—so read your labels even after your Whole30 is done, and indulge with caution (if at all).*

Can I include "paleo" foods desserts or treats in my reintroduction too?

Absolutely, although we'd encourage you to separate these foods from the rest of your reintroduction schedule, and pay just as much attention to how these make you feel. For example, when your general reintroduction is over, go ahead and have pancakes made from bananas and egg for breakfast and almond flour cookies after dinner, but be just as rigorous about evaluating how you look, feel, and live after eating these sweet treats. For many, they'll reawaken your Sugar Dragon in a major way, leading you to crave off-plan foods that you've already decided aren't good for your everyday plate. Others find the extra sugar in their day (even if it is from a "natural" source) negatively impacts hunger, mood, and energy levels.

I'm leaving for vacation/getting married/on my honeymoon on Day 31. How do I handle reintroduction?

This is a tricky one, because we would have wanted you to plan your Whole30 a little differently from the get-go. (Go back to page 17 for help with planning your Whole30 start date.) Ideally, you'll have time to get through both the program *and* your reintroduction before you are thrown into a situation where you'll be tempted to Eat All the Things. However, that's not what happened, so now we have to deal with the situation at hand.

If we're being honest with ourselves, you're not going to complete the reintroduction as outlined while traipsing through Italy. You're just not. And that's okay. We would never want you to miss out on a once-in-a-lifetime experience for your Whole30 reintroduction—but that doesn't mean you have a free pass to mindlessly inhale gelato. If you eat everything you haven't been eating all at once, you will likely ruin your vacation (at least for that day), so tread with caution. Try to keep treats to one food group at a time, if possible, and only eat as much as you need to satisfy your taste buds. (You don't have to eat four slices of freshly baked bread if one will do.) Pay attention to how foods make you feel, and choose your next meal based on the consequences of the last. If gelato makes you feel like junk, there's no need to retest that particular experiment. Finally, plan on getting back on the Whole30 (even if it's just for a week or two) as soon as you get home, because your brain will probably be back in full-on "old habits" mode—and you don't want your "vacation" from healthy eating to continue months after your trip is over.

TIP: *Many people report the bread in Europe isn't as disruptive to their systems as the bread in the U.S. Some theorize that the strains of wheat overseas aren't as hybridized, which makes the gluten less troublesome in our guts. We don't have any scientific evidence of this, but take heed—just because you eat bread in Italy with little consequence doesn't mean you'll have that same experience when you're back in the United States.*

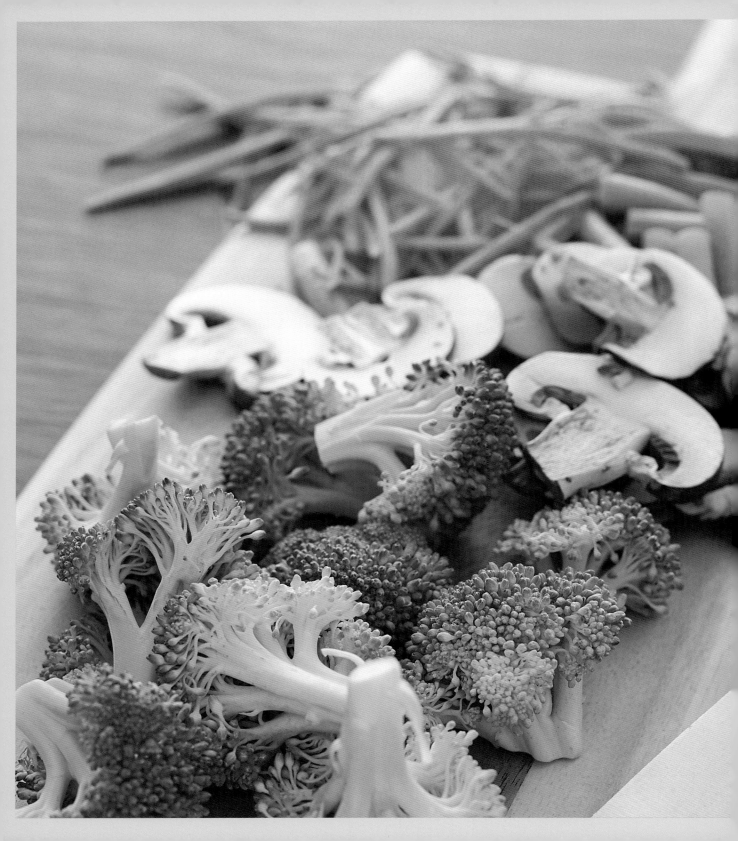

whole30 kitchen fundamentals

One of the founding principles of Whole30 cooking is this: You don't need to cook complicated meals from fancy recipes—all you need are fresh ingredients and basic kitchen techniques. In fact, some of the most delicious Whole30 dishes we've ever made were simple "ingredient meals," no recipe required.

Think of a burger topped with a fried egg, roasted sweet potato spears, and a garden salad; grilled chicken, peppers, and onions smothered in salsa and guacamole with a side of sliced mango; or canned tuna on top of fresh greens, topped with jicama, blueberries, and sliced almonds, drizzled with a homemade creamy vinaigrette.

We can hear your stomach growling from here.

If the idea of following a recipe makes you nervous, you could legitimately cook your way through your entire Whole30 just using this Kitchen Fundamentals section. (Although you might want to try your hand at a few Dressings and Sauces on page 302 just to keep things interesting.) This is where we teach you all of the basic cooking skills—how to cook meat, seafood,

and eggs, four different techniques for cooking vegetables, Whole30 staples like homemade broth and condiments, and helpful cooking and kitchen tips.

If this isn't your first Whole30, you'll still find this section helpful. We'll give you guidelines for cooking times and temperatures, detailed charts to help you make the most of your meat thermometer, and a few (simple) recipes that an experienced cook will easily be able to customize dozens of different ways.

Plus, you've probably been cooking bacon wrong, and that alone is worth the read.

Let's begin this section with a tour of your Whole30 kitchen, and the tools that will make the next 30 days an estimated 72 percent more fun.*

*No actual scientific studies were completed, but we're pretty sure this is true.

essentials for your whole30 kitchen

"I am 50 years old, and was treated for hormone imbalance, hypothyroidism, and Ankylosing Spondylitis. I had been dealing with AS since 1998, and on a drug called Enbrel that I desperately wanted to discontinue. I was convinced it was the reason for my fatigue, weight gain, grey complexion, insomnia, uncontrollable appetite, loss of endurance, muscle loss, and body aches. I did my first Whole30 in February 2013. After 30 days, my cholesterol and triglycerides were better than normal, I had lost weight (20 pounds), my skin wasn't grey, I could exercise longer and feel good afterward, and I was sleeping better. All wins, so I stuck with it! About 90 days in, I went off the Enbrel. So here it is—you changed my life!" — DIANE W., EVANSVILLE, IN

We're starting things off with what we consider the necessities. You *should* already have most of these things in your kitchen, unless you've been living off nothing but take-out and microwave meals for the last decade. Which, thanks to today's fast-food, convenience-food, eat-it-in-your-car culture, isn't actually uncommon. So if that's the case, we're not judging.

But we're awfully glad you're here.

If you're ready to invest in your Whole30 experience now, but aren't sure what you need, this is a detailed list of our essentials and "nice-to-haves." However, we understand you may not be able to purchase a bunch of new kitchen tools before you start your Whole30, and *that's totally okay*. You can cook your way through the book by getting creative with the tools you have on hand, and skip the recipes requiring something specific (like a food processor) that you're missing. We purposefully made these recipes simple to prep, cook, and serve so that no one would be left out. That one cutting board you have will be working hard, but the point is, it *will* work.

So don't stress about this stuff, okay? You're here, you're committed, and we're about to walk you through the basics in a way that (we hope) leaves you as excited about getting into your kitchen as we are to get you there.

POTS AND PANS

You'll use a variety of pots and pans throughout your Whole30, but while they make a pan for every occasion, you just need a few of the most versatile. As for pots, buy a set of three or four—something that ranges from a small (1 to 2 quart)

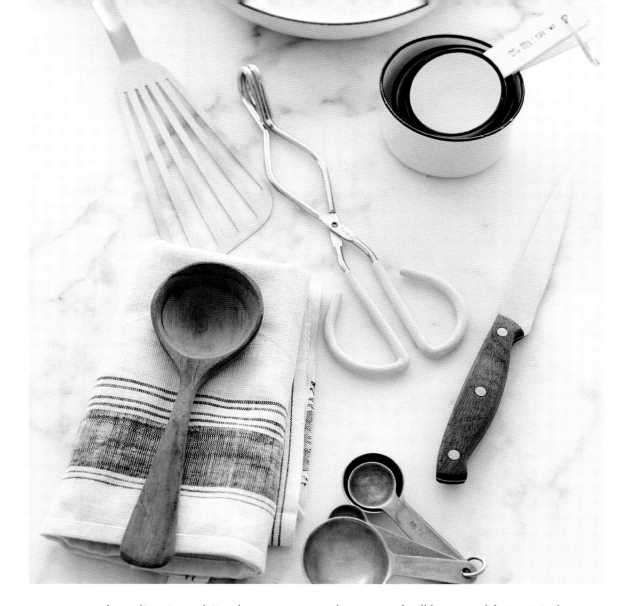

saucepan to a large (3 to 4 quart) Dutch oven. This should cover everything from sauces (like our Balsamic Glaze on page 361) to a larger dish (like the Pulled Pork Carnitas on page 254).

You'll want two frying pans (also called *skillets*): one should be a cast-iron or oven-safe skillet. These are great for taking dishes like our Frittata (page 206) straight from the stovetop to the oven, and will last you a lifetime. It's also nice to have one non-stick pan for eggs, and if you're only buying two, get them both in a large size. (It's better to have the versatility of two big pans.)

If you can buy one more pan, a large high-walled sauté pan with a cover is an excellent choice for things like Cauliflower Rice (page 272) or our Chicken Cacciatore (page 334).

STRAINER

A strainer serves double-duty, allowing you to drain water from boiled vegetables or broths (like our Bone Broths on page 176), and functioning as a steamer when placed inside a large stockpot. (You could also buy one large pot with a steamer/strainer insert, if you want to be really fancy.)

It's nice to have two strainers—one fine mesh hand-held strainer to filter out smaller particles of food, and a larger one with bigger holes for straining out larger pieces and steaming.

MEASURING CUPS AND SPOONS

You'll need at least one basic set of measuring cups and spoons, but we highly recommend doubling up, especially if you aren't comfortable eyeballing measurements. You'd be surprised how many times you'll need a teaspoon as you cook your way through this book.

It's also a good idea to have at least one larger glass measuring cup with a pouring spout—something that can handle three or four cups at a time. You'll use this for things like our Basic Mayonnaise (page 179), or any recipe that calls for more than a cup of broth.

BAKING SHEETS

You won't be making chocolate chip cookies on the Whole30, but you *will* be roasting and baking lots of meat and vegetables in the oven. Make sure you have at least two baking sheets, so you don't crowd your sweet potatoes when they're roasting. (See page 166 for our vegetable roasting tips.)

CUTTING BOARDS

We'll be up front about this: there is a lot of chopping in your future. (Just take Melissa's lead and think of it as stress relief.) To ensure you aren't constantly running between the counter and the sink, you should have at least three cutting boards—different sizes are also really nice. (Why break out your largest board just to mince a clove of garlic?)

We're generally not fans of plastic cutting boards, even though they're cheap and easy to wash. One recent study found more bacteria are recovered from plastic surfaces than wood, and the plastic is easy to mar with your knife, which means plastic gets into your food. *No bueno.* However, if you want a cheap cutting board for car camping or as backup, plastic will do the trick.

Bamboo is a good option, and relatively inexpensive, but they're so hard they tend to dull knives fast. (We'll get to that.) Maple is a splurge, but boy will it look pretty sitting on your kitchen counter, and it's kind to knives. Our favorite cutting boards are made from recycled wood fiber—they're eco-friendly, a snap to clean, and dry super fast.

KNIVES

We know you have knives, but do you have Whole30-worthy knives? Investing in a few good, sharp knives will make your Whole30 experience more enjoyable than eating almond butter straight off the spoon.

And that is pretty enjoyable.

Your knife options are even more complicated than your pot and pan options, so let's just talk about the basics. You'll want to get three knives—a paring knife for small cuts (like dicing an apple), an 8-inch chef's knife designed for chopping, and a long, thin slicing knife for carving things like Braised Beef Brisket (page 214) and the turkey from our Holiday Dinner (page 388).

Look for knives that are all one piece (not a blade and handle joined together), and spend some money here. Trust us, this is one investment that will pay you back every single time you cook.

Oh, and don't forget the knife sharpener. If you're like us, you'll become slightly obsessed with making sure your knives slice through tomatoes like butter.

FOOD PROCESSOR

We know this sounds like an expensive tool, but there are a number of excellent products to fit any budget. But first, what's the difference between a food processor and a blender?

Blenders only blend if the food is soft and there's enough liquid in the mixture; for many of our sauces (like the Romesco Sauce on page 318) or mashes (like the Cauliflower Mash on page 270), there just isn't enough liquid to work. You *could* use a hand-held immersion blender—those are incredibly versatile, make small jobs like Basic Mayonnaise (page 179) a snap, and clean up in five seconds flat—but those don't chop anywhere near as finely as a food processor, sometimes leaving you with chunks of ingredients in what should be a smooth final product.

A food processor is designed to take solid ingredients and chop, shred, or mix them to a perfect consistency. You can use them to finely chop cilantro or parsley for our Chimichurri (page 306), dice tomatoes for our Salsa (page 319), or smooth out our Tangy BBQ Sauce (page 322).

If you're cooking for one, you may be able to get away with a mini-food processor for around $25. However, these only process foods in small batches (usually just two or three cups at a time), and if you're doubling our Cauliflower Mash recipe for a family of four, that small motor will be working awfully hard. However, that doesn't mean you need a $400 professional-grade appliance; there are plenty of seven-to-ten cup food processors available for between $40 and $100—some are even combination blenders/food processors, saving you money and counter space.

MEAT THERMOMETER

This is one of the most important tools for the budding chef. Cooking meat and poultry to just the right degree—not too raw, not overdone, just right—takes time, attention, and lots of practice, but using a meat thermometer is like cheating in a good way. We've given you the perfect cooking temperature for dishes like Perfect Whole Roasted Chicken (page 157), Perfect Grilled Steak (page 154), and Walnut-Crusted Pork Tenderloin (page 252). By taking the guesswork out of when your meat is ready to remove from the oven, you're far more likely to nail the perfect level of doneness on the first try, and avoid having to choke down expensive meat that you accidentally overcooked.

Make sure you get a meat thermometer (designed to tell you the internal temperature of meat) and not an oven thermometer (designed to tell you how hot your oven really is on the inside). Look for something that says "instant read" (though these actually take about 20 seconds to get up to the right temperature)—you should be able to find one for around $10.

PARCHMENT PAPER

You're probably used to lining your baking sheets and dishes with aluminum foil—which means you're also used to your more delicate meats and veggies sticking to the foil like crazy. This is where parchment paper comes in. It's a moisture-resistant paper specially treated for oven use, keeping your dishes clean and your No-Fuss Salmon Cakes (page 346), Chicken Meatballs (page 226), or Balsamic Roasted Sweet Potatoes (page 262) sliding onto the spatula with ease. At about $3 a roll, this is a great investment for easy Whole30 kitchen clean up.

whole30 really-nice-to-haves

Technically, these kitchen tools aren't absolutely necessary for your Whole30 kitchen, but they sure will cut your prep time and expand your range of cooking techniques. Plus, most of these cost under ten dollars—a steal, given how easy they make so many of your Whole30-related kitchen tasks.

GARLIC PRESS

Mincing garlic is one of our least-favorite tasks; it's a challenge to get the pieces small enough before you're bored out of your mind with chopping. However, mincing by hand is only one option—there's also the garlic press. Peel the clove, put it in the press, squeeze the handle, and you've got perfectly minced garlic in ten seconds. They key to this tool is making sure you rinse the leftover garlic pulp out of the press as soon as you're done (before it dries and hardens), and use a kitchen brush or toothbrush to keep the holes clean.

Or, just buy minced garlic in a jar and call it good. It's more expensive, but it's definitely got the convenience factor going for it.

JULIENNE PEELER

Vegetable noodles are an easy way to add variety to your Whole30 meals in a way that's fun for the whole family. Our Roasted Spaghetti Squash (page 294) is naturally spaghetti-like, but for vegetables like zucchini or cucumber, you need a way to turn them into noodles.

Enter the julienne peeler.

It looks just like a normal peeler (and works the same way), but its special grooves turns vegetables into long, thin strings, just like noodles. You can find them for under $10 at any kitchen store, and it only takes about a minute to julienne an entire zucchini.

If you want to splurge a bit here, you could also buy a fancy tool called a spiral slicer for about $40. This nifty gadget slices, grates, or juliennes any vegetable in a way that basically guarantees your kids will help with your dinner prep, and makes things like Melissa's Chicken Hash (page 228) a breeze to prepare.

CITRUS JUICER

Trust us on this one—squeezing lemons and limes by hand is messy, and doesn't ever get all the juice out. Buy a hand-held combination lemon/lime squeezer for around $10. The end.

ZESTER

Many of our recipes call for citrus zest—that is, tiny pieces of the lemon, lime, or orange peel mixed right into the dish. You'd be surprised at how much flavor a small amount of zest can add, but getting to it can be a pain without the right tool. You could use a vegetable peeler to remove strips of the skin, then tediously chop them into skinny strips or tiny pieces.

Or, you could use a $5 zester and do the same job in three seconds.

A zester has tiny holes designed to remove long, skinny pieces of skin as you scrape it down the outside of your citrus fruit, no extra chopping required. Or, for about $15, buy a Microplane—a multifunctional miniature grater perfect for zesting fruit or grating spices (like nutmeg) or roots (like ginger).

MEAT TENDERIZER

This handy and inexpensive kitchen tool looks like a hammer of sorts, with a long handle, one flat end, and one texturized end. It's pretty literal in name—you essentially whack your steak, chicken breast, or pork shoulder to break up the muscle fibers.

It's been described as "pre-chewing the meat," only less messy.

This is one easy way to make tougher cuts more tender, or to ensure those who prefer well-done meat aren't chewing for hours. It's also a great way to speed up cooking times, and get more consistent results. You know how there's always one end of the chicken breast that's thicker than the other? Without pounding it flat, you'll end up with the thin end overcooked by the time the thicker end is cooked through. Use a meat tenderizer to make the chicken from our Perfect Seared Chicken Breasts (page 157) or Harvest Grilled Chicken Salad (page 232) uniform in thickness so it cooks faster and more evenly all around.

To minimize mess, place a sheet of plastic wrap or wax paper over your meat before you start hammering away, and make sure you properly clean and sanitize your meat tenderizer immediately after use.

GRILL BASKET

Our final recommendation isn't a necessity—we give you two other ways to grill vegetables and fruit starting on page 163—but none as easy as using a basket. Chop your veggies up, toss them in some oil, throw them in the basket, and leave them on the grill while you tend to the rest of your food.

Every once in a while, give them a shake. Yep, that's it.

You can buy a grill basket for around $20; some even have heat-proof handles to make taking it on and off the grill easier. One tip to make the most of this kitchen tool—put it on the grill while you're preheating. A warmed grill basket will cook your vegetables faster and with less "stick" than a cold one.

We may mention other kitchen items, like cheesecloth for straining Clarified Butter (page 183) or a basting brush to use with our Baby Back Ribs (page 256), but there are easy workarounds if you don't have these. We also mention some pretty specific tools with our Fancypants Meals on page 354—these are important for this particular dish, even though you may only use them once a year.

In summary, there are more kitchen gadgets, appliances, and tools than you could ever hope to use in a single year, and it's up to you to decide what's important to you, and what fits your budget. (We love our avocado saver, although even we think it's a little silly.) Make notes as you work your way through these recipes of tools you're missing, or tools that might make your prep a little easier. Then, figure out what's most important to you, and add to your collection over time, as you can.

Don't stress about outfitting it all at once.

You have the rest of your life to build your kitchen, because the Whole30 is just your first step in a long, rewarding, delicious journey of cooking (and eating) real food. So now that your kitchen is well stocked with the basics, it's high-time you start cooking!

For our kitchen tool recommendations, including brands and models we like, visit www.whole30.com/whole30kitchen.

whole30 cooking fundamentals

" I had always been a terrible cook. Cooking totally stressed me out, and I was envious of people who loved it. The Whole30 forced me to seek out recipes I could make. I started following Whole30 food bloggers and bought new cookbooks. I started cooking most days of the week. Now, meals for me and my family are healthy and delicious! I am definitely better at cooking and much more kitchen-confident as a result of my Whole30."
— ANDREA R., NASHVILLE, TN

In this section, we're going to teach you how to cook meat, seafood, eggs, and vegetables, and make some Whole30 fundamental ingredients like bone broth, mayonnaise, and clarified butter.

We'll also walk you through some basic knife cuts, because boy, will you be chopping.

This section is where you build your kitchen confidence, perfecting your techniques for roasting, baking, steaming, searing, and grilling. You'll learn how to cook your steak to the perfect temperature, how to keep your chicken breasts juicy and tender, and discover you actually *do* like mayonnaise. (You do. Trust us.) You'll experiment with four different ways to cook your vegetables, (quadrupling your chances of falling in love with Brussels sprouts), discover making bone broth is actually *really* easy, and learn which grilling technique is right for those pineapple slices you've been craving. Consider this section the perfect prep for the more than one hundred recipes to follow in the fourth part of this book.

We could go on, but we won't, because you look hungry.

Bon appétit.

Knife Cuts

CHIFFONADE (RIBBON CUT)

The French word *chiffonade* means "little ribbons," referring to leafy greens like spinach, lettuce, kale, and herbs like basil that have been cut into long, thin strips.

To chiffonade, stack your greens or herbs from large (on the bottom) to small (on top) and roll into a cigar shape. Then, cut thin slices perpendicular to the roll to make ribbons.

DICE

To *dice* means to cut food into small blocks of a specific size. Dicing creates evenly sized pieces so they'll all cook at the same rate. You'll see

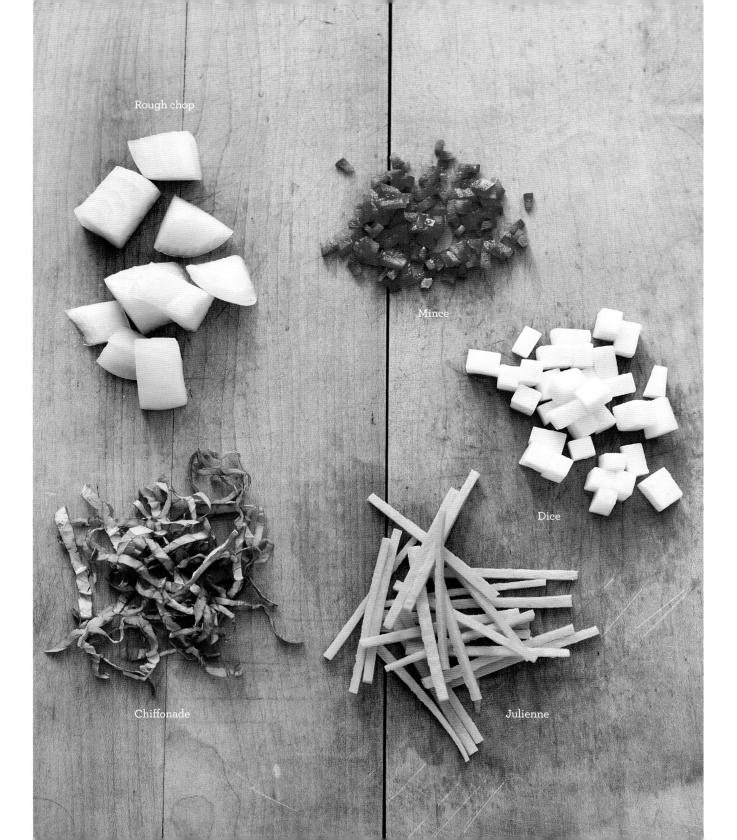

three sizes mentioned here: large dice (1-inch cubes), medium (or unspecified) dice (½-inch cubes), and small (or fine) dice (¼-inch cubes).

To dice, slice the vegetable into rectangular strips that are ¼ inch thick (small dice), ½ inch thick (medium), or 1 inch thick (large). Line the strips up together and cut across at the same size to create cubes. Don't bust out the ruler here—it's less important that your dice are *exactly* the right size, and more important that all your cubes are similarly shaped.

JULIENNE

This knife cut makes long, thin strips (like matchsticks) on longer vegetables like carrots, potatoes, jicama, and bell pepper quarters. Technically, a proper julienne will measure ⅛ inch square and 2 inches long.

To julienne, trim off the sides of the vegetable (if necessary), creating a flat surface on each side and turning it into more of a rectangle shape. (You can still use the ends for salads, soups, or other meals.) Slice the vegetable lengthwise into ⅛-inch slices. Stack the slices and cut again lengthwise at ⅛-inch increments to create matchstick-size strips. Again, don't worry about the exact size—just cut them thin and uniform in thickness.

MINCE

The word *mince* just means to very finely chop. It's usually used with garlic, onions, and chile peppers like jalapeño.

To mince, slice the vegetable into very thin strips. Line the strips up together and cut across in very thin slices to create tiny pieces. To mince garlic, you can also use a garlic press—it's much faster than cutting by hand.

We may also ask you to "finely chop" ingredients like celery, mushrooms, or other vegetables. That's somewhere between a small dice and a mince—just chop until the pieces are small, and don't worry about their shape or size.

ROUGH CHOP

This is the easiest knife cut, because it's nowhere near as precise as a dice or julienne. A rough chop is perfect for soups, stews, or vegetables headed for the food processor—where it doesn't matter how pretty the vegetables look.

To roughly chop, cut the vegetable in half horizontally and vertically. Slice in half a few more times until the pieces are in large chunks. Don't overthink this! Just take those veggies and chop 'em up.

perfect boiled eggs

SERVES 2

PREP TIME: 5 minutes

COOK TIME: 7 to 10 minutes

TOTAL TIME: 12 to 15 minutes

---

4 eggs, large

This technique and cook times are the same whether you boil 2 eggs or a dozen. We like boiling a large amount at once for on-the-go protein or to include in a Protein Salad (page 161).

PREPARE a small bowl half-full with ice water.

FILL a small saucepan halfway with water. Bring the water to a rolling boil, then add the eggs by sliding them gently into the pan with a wooden spoon.

FOR soft-boiled eggs, cook on high heat for 7 minutes. (This will leave your eggs truly soft-boiled, with very runny yolks.) For soft but not runny yolks, cook for 9 minutes. For true hard-boiled eggs, cook for 11 minutes.

REMOVE the pan from the heat, and immediately transfer them to a bowl of ice water for 5 minutes to prevent them from cooking further and make them easier to peel.

TO peel your eggs, crack the shell at the very bottom of the egg. Then, peel under cool running water, using the shell membrane to guide the removal of the shell pieces.

⭐ PRO TIP *Use the oldest eggs you have for hard-boiling, as they'll peel more easily.*

perfect fried eggs

SERVES 2

PREP TIME: 3 minutes

COOK TIME: 2 to 5 minutes

TOTAL TIME: 5 to 8 minutes

---

2 tablespoons cooking fat

4 eggs, large

Salt and black pepper

HEAT the cooking fat in a medium skillet over medium heat and swirl to coat the bottom of the pan. When the fat is very hot, crack the eggs one by one into the pan. Step back, as these eggs will sizzle! Do your best not to break the yolks—but if they do, just keep going with the instructions.

IF you really like runny yolk, carefully scoop some of the cooking fat from the pan over the egg yolks with a spoon. Repeat 5 or 6 times, helping the yolks cook faster. When the egg white is just barely opaque, slide a spatula under the egg and transfer yolk-side up to a plate.

IF you prefer your yolks cooked a bit more, skip the spoon part; when the egg white is just barely opaque, carefully slide a spatula under the eggs and flip them over. Cook for 1 to 2 minutes for "over easy," 3 to 4 minutes for "over medium." If you prefer your yolks "over hard" (not soft at all), carefully flip the eggs over again and cook for an additional 30 seconds to 1 minute.

REMOVE the eggs from the pan, transfer them to a plate yolk-side up and serve hot with a sprinkle of salt and pepper.

⭐ PRO TIP *You could use a cast-iron pan for fried eggs, but it's hard to keep them from sticking. This is where it's nice to have at least one non-stick pan.*

perfect poached eggs

SERVES 2

PREP TIME: 3 minutes

COOK TIME: 3 to 5 minutes

TOTAL TIME: 6 to 8 minutes

2 teaspoons white vinegar

1 teaspoon salt

4 eggs, large

FILL a large skillet with 2 to 3 inches of water and add the vinegar and salt. Bring the water to a boil over high heat.

WHILE waiting for the water to boil, carefully crack each egg into separate small bowls.

WHEN the water comes to a boil, gently pour each egg into the water. As soon as all of the eggs are in the pan, remove the pan from the heat, cover, and let sit for 3 minutes (for very soft yolks), or 5 minutes (for firm yolks).

REMOVE the cooked eggs from the pan with a slotted spoon, allowing any excess water to drain. Serve warm.

⭐ PRO TIP *Use the freshest eggs you have when poaching, as the egg white is thicker when fresh. You can also use poaching cups or a poaching tray; both are inexpensive kitchen tools that make the process a bit more foolproof. (Cooking times may vary from above when using these gadgets.)*

perfect scrambled eggs

SERVES 2

PREP TIME: 3 minutes

COOK TIME: 8 to 10 minutes

TOTAL TIME: 10 minutes

4 eggs, large

1 tablespoon coconut milk (optional)

½ teaspoon salt

¼ teaspoon black pepper

2 tablespoons cooking fat

CRACK the eggs in a small bowl, add the coconut milk if using, and the salt and pepper. Mix together with a whisk or fork until the eggs are uniform in texture and appear fluffy (from all the air you've whipped into them).

MELT the cooking fat in a medium skillet over medium heat and swirl to coat the bottom of the pan. When the cooking fat is hot, pour the eggs into the pan. Use a spatula to fold the cooked eggs from the outer edges into the middle. Then scrape the cooked eggs from the bottom of the pan, so the uncooked portion can flow into contact with the hot pan. Repeat every minute or so while cooking.

COOK until the eggs look slightly shiny (but not runny), 5 to 7 minutes, and serve warm.

⭐ PRO TIP *Your eggs will continue to cook after you remove them from the heat, so transfer them out of the pan just before you think they look done.*

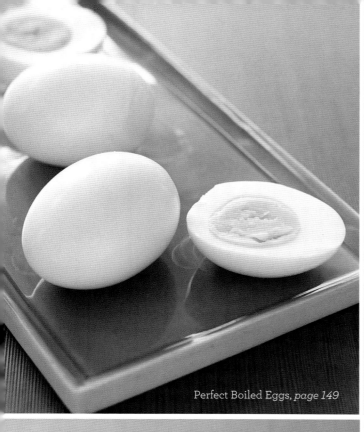
Perfect Boiled Eggs, *page 149*

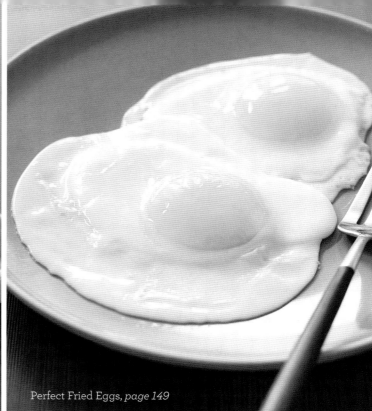
Perfect Fried Eggs, *page 149*

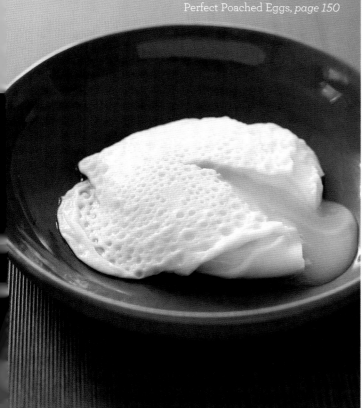
Perfect Poached Eggs, *page 150*

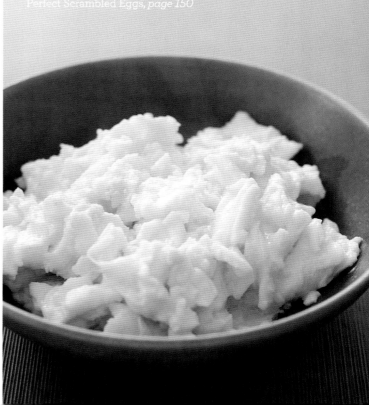
Perfect Scrambled Eggs, *page 150*

perfect ground meat

SERVES 2

PREP TIME: 5 minutes
COOK TIME: 5 to 10 minutes
TOTAL TIME: 10 to 15 minutes

Cooking fat, as needed

1 pound ground meat

Ground meat (beef, bison, buffalo, lamb, chicken, or turkey) is one of the easiest proteins to whip up in a hurry, and it's incredibly versatile. The trick is using the right amount of cooking fat in your pan, and experimenting with different seasoning combinations to change the flavor of your meal so you don't get bored.

PLACE a large pan on medium heat. Add the cooking fat to the pan, if necessary, and swirl to coat the bottom of the pan. Add the ground meat to the pan, breaking it up into large chunks with a spatula or wooden spoon. As the meat starts to brown, continue to break the meat up into smaller and smaller pieces, stirring so the meat cooks evenly. Cook until the meat is browned through and no pink remains, 7 to 10 minutes.

REMOVE the meat from the pan with either a slotted spoon (to leave some fat in the pan), or a large spoon (to enjoy the added fat with your meat).

⭐ GENERAL RULE OF THUMB: *The leaner the meat, the more cooking fat you want to use in the pan.*

GROUND BEEF, 80 PERCENT LEAN: *no cooking fat required*

GROUND LAMB: *no cooking fat required*

GROUND BEEF, 85 TO 90 PERCENT LEAN: *1 tablespoon of cooking fat per pound*

GROUND CHICKEN THIGH: *1 tablespoon of cooking fat per pound*

GROUND BEEF, 95 PERCENT LEAN: *2 tablespoons of cooking fat per pound*

GROUND BISON/BUFFALO: *2 tablespoons of cooking fat per pound*

GROUND CHICKEN BREAST: *2 tablespoons of cooking fat per pound*

GROUND TURKEY: *2 tablespoons of cooking fat per pound*

It's also a good idea to double the amount of ground meat you cook with dinner and transfer half (unseasoned) to a storage container to refrigerate, so you can make a totally different lunch or dinner tomorrow with the leftovers! For example, you could use half the ground beef to make our Stuffed Peppers (page 222) for dinner tonight, then reheat the rest of the ground beef and top with Salsa (page 319), Guacamole (page 308), and a drizzle of Ranch Dressing (page 316) for an easy lunch tomorrow.

You can also make your ground meat an easy one-pot meal by cooking the meat, transferring it to a holding dish when it's browned, then cooking a mix of vegetables in the fat that's left in the pan. When the vegetables are done, return the meat to the pan, stir to reheat and combine, and serve, topped with your favorite dressing or sauce (starting on page 302).

PRO TIP *Try a variety of seasonings to change the flavor of your dish.*

MEXICAN: *½ teaspoon chili powder, ¼ teaspoon cumin, ¼ teaspoon salt, ¼ teaspoon pepper, ⅛ teaspoon crushed red pepper flakes, ⅛ teaspoon paprika, and sprinkle with minced cilantro.*
ASIAN: *2 minced garlic cloves, 1 tablespoon sesame oil, 1 teaspoon rice vinegar, ½ teaspoon ground ginger, and sprinkle with sesame seeds.*
ITALIAN: *Our Tomato Sauce (page 324), or add 1 tablespoon pre-mixed Italian seasoning, 1 teaspoon of freshly minced herbs (oregano, thyme, or basil), ¼ teaspoon salt, and ¼ teaspoon pepper.*
THAI: *Our Curry Sauce (page 307)*
BBQ: *Our BBQ Sauce (page 322)*

perfect burger

SERVES 3

PREP TIME: 5 minutes

COOK TIME: 15 minutes

TOTAL TIME: 20 minutes

---

1 pound ground meat

1 teaspoon salt

½ teaspoon black pepper

½ teaspoon mustard powder

¼ teaspoon garlic powder

PREHEAT the oven to 350°F.

IN a large mixing bowl, combine all of the ingredients. Form into 3 equal-sized patties. Chill in the freezer for 15 minutes.

TRANSFER the patties to a baking sheet lined with parchment paper if desired and roast in the oven until the internal temperature reaches 145°F, about 15 minutes.

⭐ CHEF TIP *For extra flavor, grill the patties over high heat for 4 minutes on each side, then remove from grill and finish in a 350°F oven for 4 to 5 minutes.*

TEMPERATURE GUIDELINES FOR BEEF STEAKS AND GROUND BEEF, BISON, BUFFALO, AND LAMB

RARE: *120° to 125°F*

MEDIUM RARE: *130° to 135°F*

MEDIUM: *135° to 140°F*

MEDIUM WELL: *140° to 150°F*

WELL DONE: *155°F +*

To achieve the perfect temperature, remove the meat from the heat when it is 5°F less than the desired temperature, as it will continue to cook while it rests. For example, if you want your steak medium, remove it from the heat at 130° to 135°F.

NOTE: *For safety reasons, the United States Department of Agriculture recommends cooking ground beef to a minimum temperature of 160°F and steaks and roasts to a minimum temperature of 145°F.*

perfect grilled steak

SERVES 2

PREP TIME: 3 minutes

COOK TIME: 16 to 22 minutes

TOTAL TIME: 19 to 25 minutes

---

2 portions (5 ounces each) steak (sirloin, strip, rib eye, tenderloin)

½ teaspoon salt

¼ teaspoon black pepper

REMOVE the steaks from the refrigerator at least 30 minutes before cooking. Preheat the grill to high, preheat the oven to 350°F, and line a baking sheet with foil.

SEASON the steak evenly on both sides with the salt and pepper. Lay the steaks on the hot grill at a 45-degree angle to the grate. Let the steaks sear for 2 to 3 minutes. Use tongs to peek at the grill marks—your steak should pull off easily once you have a proper sear. When ready, don't flip the steaks yet, but turn them 90 degrees to create crosshatch grill markings. Sear in this position for just 2 minutes. Flip the steaks and repeat the double searing process on the other side.

REMOVE the steaks from the grill, place them on the prepared baking sheet, and put them in the oven. Bake for 8 to 12 minutes, depending on the thickness of the steak and your desired temperature (see chart). Be sure to use a meat thermometer as you learn this technique.

ALLOW the steaks to rest for 5 minutes before serving.

⭐ PRO TIP *To achieve a proper sear, don't peek at the halfway mark! Just let the steaks sit on the grill grates for the allotted time, then gently pull with tongs to test if they're ready to move.*

TEMPERATURE GUIDELINES FOR STEAK:

RARE: *120° to 125°F*

MEDIUM RARE: *130° to 135°F*

MEDIUM: *135° to 140°F*

MEDIUM WELL: *140° to 150°F*

WELL DONE: *155°F+*

To achieve the perfect temperature, remove your steak from the oven 5°F early, as it will continue to cook while it rests. For example, if you want your steak medium rare, remove it from the heat at 125° to 130°F.

NOTE: *For safety reasons, the United States Department of Agriculture recommends cooking all steak to a minimum temperature of 160°F.*

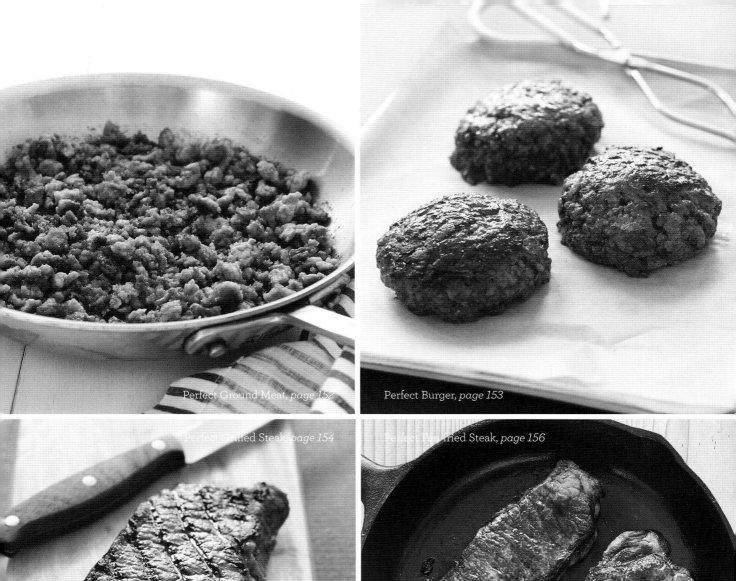

Perfect Ground Meat, *page 152*

Perfect Burger, *page 153*

Perfect Grilled Steak, *page 154*

Perfect Pan-fried Steak, *page 156*

perfect pan-fried steak

SERVES 2

PREP TIME: 3 minutes

COOK TIME: 11 to 16 minutes

TOTAL TIME: 14 to 19 minutes

---

2 portions (5 ounces each) steak (sirloin, strip, rib eye, tenderloin)

½ teaspoon salt

¼ teaspoon black pepper

2 tablespoons cooking fat

PREHEAT the oven to 350°F.

SEASON the steaks evenly on both sides with the salt and pepper. In a large oven-safe skillet, melt the cooking fat over medium-high heat, swirling to coat the bottom of the pan. When the fat is hot, place the steaks in the pan and sear for 3 to 4 minutes. The steak should pull off the pan easily once you have a proper sear. Using tongs, turn the steak over and put the entire pan in the oven to finish cooking.

BAKE for 8 to 12 minutes, depending on the thickness of the steak and your desired temperature (see chart). Be sure to use a meat thermometer as you learn this technique.

AFTER removing the steaks from the oven, allow them to rest for 5 minutes before serving.

PRO TIP *If you don't have an oven-safe pan, transfer the seared steak to a foil-lined baking pan before placing in the oven.*

TEMPERATURE GUIDELINES FOR STEAK:

RARE: *120° to 125°F*

MEDIUM RARE: *130° to 135°F*

MEDIUM: *135° to 140°F*

MEDIUM WELL: *140° to 150°F*

WELL DONE: *155°F*

To achieve the perfect temperature, remove your steak from the oven 5°F early, as it will continue to cook while it rests. For example, if you want your steak medium rare, remove it from the heat at 125° to 130°F.

NOTE: *For safety reasons, the United States Department of Agriculture recommends cooking all steak to a minimum temperature of 160°F.*

perfect seared chicken breasts

SERVES 2

PREP TIME: 3 minutes

COOK TIME: 13 to 19 minutes

TOTAL TIME: 16 to 22 minutes

---

2 portions (5 ounces each) skinless boneless chicken breasts

½ teaspoon salt

¼ teaspoon black pepper

2 tablespoons cooking fat

PREHEAT the oven to 350°F.

SEASON the chicken breasts evenly on both sides with the salt and pepper. In a large oven-safe skillet, melt the cooking fat over medium-high heat, swirling to coat the bottom of the pan. When the fat is hot, place the chicken top (rounded) side down in the pan and sear for 3 to 4 minutes. Your chicken should pull off the pan easily once you have a proper sear. Using tongs, turn the chicken over, then put the entire pan in the oven to finish cooking.

BAKE for 10 to 15 minutes, depending on the thickness of the chicken, until the internal temperature reaches 160°F. Be sure to use a meat thermometer as you learn this technique. Let the chicken rest for 5 minutes before serving.

⭐ PRO TIP *If you don't have an oven-safe pan, transfer the seared chicken to a foil-lined baking pan before placing in the oven.*

perfect whole roasted chicken

SERVES 2 (WITH LEFTOVERS)

PREP TIME: 10 minutes

COOK TIME: 1 hour 30 minutes

TOTAL TIME: 1 hour 40 minutes

---

1 whole chicken (4 to 6 pounds)

3 tablespoons cooking fat, melted

1 teaspoon salt

1 teaspoon black pepper

PREHEAT the oven to 425°F.

IF necessary, remove the giblets from inside the chicken and discard. Rinse the chicken inside and out under cool running water and place breast-side up in a roasting pan. Rub the cooking fat evenly over the skin of the chicken and season with the salt and pepper. (If you'd like to add fresh herbs, garlic, etc., run your fingers under the skin to loosen, then place the seasonings between the skin and the meat.)

ROAST the chicken uncovered for 1 hour and 30 minutes. Check the temperature by placing a meat thermometer in the thickest part of the chicken (without touching bone); it should read 160°F.

LET the chicken rest for 5 minutes before serving.

⭐ PRO TIP *Be sure to save the carcass to make a batch of our Chicken Bone Broth (page 177).*

perfect grilled shrimp

SERVES 2

PREP TIME: 10 minutes
COOK TIME: 5 minutes
TOTAL TIME: 15 minutes

1½ teaspoons garlic powder

1½ teaspoons garlic salt

1½ teaspoons dried oregano

¾ teaspoon paprika

¾ teaspoon black pepper

2 tablespoons extra-virgin olive oil

1 pound large shrimp, peeled and deveined

Shrimp may seem intimidating, but they're actually fast and easy to cook. Our recipes all call for large shrimp—these are the kind most commonly found in your supermarket's seafood section, and usually come about 25 to 35 to a pound.

Before you cook shrimp from this book, you'll peel and devein them—a process that's also easier than it sounds. To peel, just use your fingers to pull off the outer shell, starting at the top and working your way down to the tail. Remove the tail itself by pulling on it gently while holding the shrimp. (Don't be too aggressive here, or a good chunk of meat may get stuck in the tail.) Then, using a sharp paring knife, carefully cut into the back of the shrimp, starting at the top, until you see the black thread running down toward the tail. Using the knife or your fingers, remove the vein and discard. Now you're ready to cook!

PREHEAT the grill to high heat (500°F). If using wooden skewers, soak them in water for 30 minutes to 1 hour to prevent them from burning on the grill.

TO make the rub, combine the garlic powder, garlic salt, oregano, paprika, and pepper in a plastic bag or a large bowl with a lid. Mix the spices together, then add the olive oil and the shrimp. Close the bag or cover the bowl and toss until the shrimp are well coated.

REMOVE the shrimp and thread them onto metal or soaked wooden skewers. Place the skewers on the grill and grill until the shrimp are seared, 2 to 3 minutes. Flip the skewers and cook for an additional 2 to 3 minutes.

REMOVE the skewers from the grill and serve hot.

⭐ PRO TIP *Your shrimp is done cooking when it's curled into the shape of the letter "C." If it's curled over itself into a tight "O" shape, it's overdone, and is likely to be tougher in texture.*

⭐ CHEF TIP *If you don't have a grill, roast your shrimp in the oven. Preheat your oven to 400°F. Make the rub and toss the shrimp as instructed, then lay them in a single layer on a baking sheet. Bake for 6 to 8 minutes, until the shrimp turn opaque and are curled into a "C" shape.*

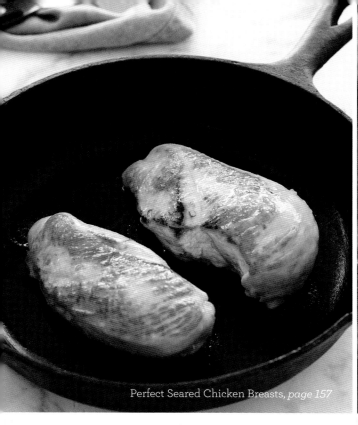

Perfect Seared Chicken Breasts, *page 157*

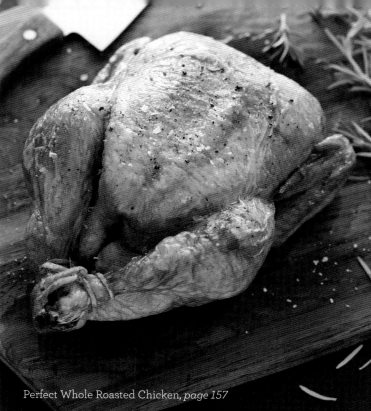

Perfect Whole Roasted Chicken, *page 157*

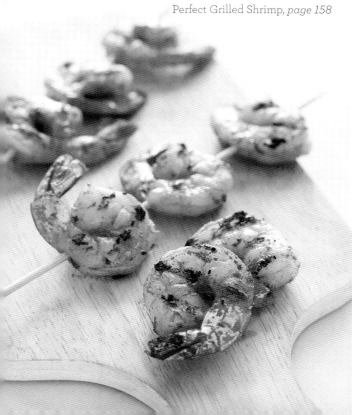

Perfect Grilled Shrimp, *page 158*

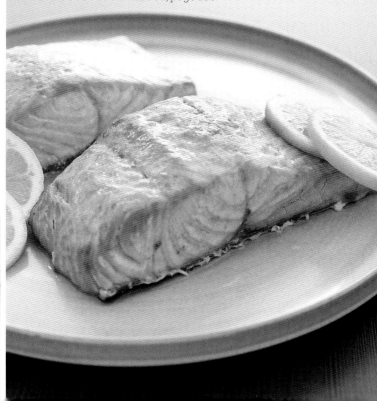

Perfect Oven-baked Salmon, *page 160*

perfect oven-baked salmon

SERVES 2

PREP TIME: 5 minutes
COOK TIME: 12 to 15 minutes
TOTAL TIME: 17 to 20 minutes

---

1 tablespoon cooking fat, melted

2 salmon fillets (5 ounces each)

½ teaspoon salt

¼ teaspoon black pepper

1 lemon, cut into wedges

PREHEAT the oven to 450°F. Line a baking sheet or glass baking dish with parchment paper. Drizzle the cooking fat over the paper and spread with a brush or your fingers to coat the paper.

PLACE the salmon skin-side down on the lined baking sheet. Season the salmon evenly with the salt and pepper.

BAKE the salmon for 12 to 15 minutes. White "curd" (protein) will show on the sides of salmon when fully cooked, and the thickest part of the fish will no longer look raw, wet, or feel spongy when you try to flake it with a fork. Remove the salmon from the oven and transfer to a serving dish or individual plates. Serve with the lemon wedges.

⭐ PRO TIP *You can adjust this technique to cook white fish (like cod, haddock, halibut, etc.) by reducing the oven temperature to 350°F, basting the fish with an additional tablespoon of cooking fat, and baking for 10 to 12 minutes. You want to pull the fish out of the oven when it's opaque in color, but doesn't easily flake with a fork—if it's flaky, it's likely to be too dry when served.*

Perfect Protein Salad

There are a few things you should always have on hand in your Whole30 kitchen: Basic Mayonnaise (page 179), Bone Broth (page 176), Perfect Boiled Eggs (page 149), and some kind of Protein Salad. Why are we focused on portable protein? It's easy to grab-and-go with vegetables, fruit, and healthy fats, but protein can be tough when you're in a hurry. And we *really* don't want you to skip protein—it's the most satiating of all the macronutrients.

Translation: It's what keeps you full between lunch and dinner, and less likely to dip into your office-mate's candy jar.

This is where an easy, versatile protein salad comes in. Use leftover chicken, tuna, salmon, or eggs, and stock your pantry with canned chicken or fish so you'll always have some at the ready. Hold all the ingredients (and flavors) together with a creamy base and an acid. Store the salad in the fridge and you'll always have some quick and easy protein on hand, or something to take to the office for lunch. Depending on your ingredients, a Protein Salad will keep for up to 3 to 5 days, so make a big batch and vary what you add so you'll never get bored.

Also, use a big bowl. Bigger than you think you need. We know this from experience—sometimes we get a little out of hand with our protein salad additions.

Mix and match your additional ingredients, using whatever you have on hand—any combination of fruit, vegetables, nuts and seeds, and fresh herbs and spices is fair game. Here are some of our favorite salad combinations:

TRADITIONAL: *Take a traditional approach with sliced grapes, celery, onion, and slivered almonds.*

GREEK: *Go Greek with Kalamata olives, roasted tomatoes, pine nuts, and basil, using red wine vinegar as your acid.*

ASIAN: *Get Asian-inspired with mandarin orange slices, celery, chopped kale, and cilantro, and using rice wine vinegar or lime juice.*

SUMMER: *Focus on fruit with sliced strawberries, blueberries, green onion, pecans, and fresh parsley.*

FALL: *Think fall with diced apples, roasted sweet potato or butternut squash, sweet onions, a handful of raisins, and toasted walnuts, with apple cider vinegar as your acid.*

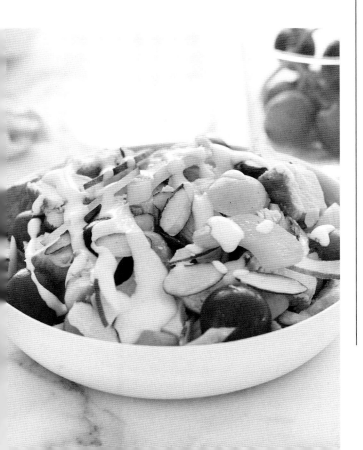

protein salad

SERVES 2 (WITH LEFTOVERS)

PREP TIME: 10 to 15 minutes

---

1 pound cooked or canned chicken, salmon, or tuna, or 8 hard-boiled eggs

¼ cup creamy base, such as Basic Mayonnaise (page 179)

2 tablespoons acid, such as lemon juice

¼ teaspoon salt

⅛ teaspoon black pepper

Additional ingredients of choice

If you're using canned chicken, tuna, or salmon, you'll need 3 cans (5 to 6 ounces each). Start the salad off with just ¼ cup mayo and the juice of 1 lemon or lime (or 2 tablespoons vinegar). You can always add more if you want your salad creamier or tangier. Serve on its own, over a bed of lettuce, in a hollowed-out tomato or bell pepper, or inside ribs of celery.

IF necessary, chop or shred the protein into large chunks. Combine the protein and mayo in a large mixing bowl and mix thoroughly. Add the lemon juice, salt, pepper, and any additional ingredients, and stir to combine.

PRO TIP *The creamy base can be Basic Mayonnaise, Egg-free Mayonnaise (page 180), or mashed avocado. The acid can be lemon juice, lime juice, apple cider vinegar, white vinegar, red wine vinegar, or rice wine vinegar.*

perfect sausage

SERVES 2

PREP TIME: 10 minutes
COOK TIME: 11 to 13 minutes
TOTAL TIME: 21 to 23 minutes

---

2 tablespoons cooking fat

½ cup minced white onion

1 pound ground meat (pork, chicken, turkey)

½ teaspoon dried sage

½ teaspoon salt

¼ teaspoon black pepper

¼ teaspoon garlic powder

PREHEAT the oven to 350°F. Line a baking sheet with parchment paper.

HEAT 1 tablespoon of the cooking fat in a heavy skillet over medium heat. When the fat is hot, add the onion and cook, stirring, until softened, about 2 minutes. Combine the sautéed onions, ground meat, sage, salt, pepper, and garlic powder in a large mixing bowl and blend well with your hands. Form into 8 equal patties about 1-inch thick.

HEAT the remaining 1 tablespoon of fat in the same skillet over medium heat and swirl to coat the bottom of the pan. When the fat is hot, add the sausage patties and brown for 2 minutes on each side. Transfer the sausage to the baking sheet and finish cooking them in the oven for 5 to 7 minutes, until no pink remains in the middle of a patty.

⭐ PRO TIP *These freeze beautifully—just stack them in a covered container between sheets of wax paper so they don't stick together. Defrost them the night before making our Diner Breakfast (page 208) to cut your prep time in half.*

perfect bacon

SERVES 2

PREP TIME: 2 minutes
COOK TIME: 15 to 20 minutes
TOTAL TIME: 17 to 22 minutes

½ pound **Whole30-compliant bacon**

While it's challenging to find Whole30-compliant bacon, we've given you a list of approved brands on page 404. You won't find these brands at your local grocery store, though, so unless you're willing to order in bulk or can find them in a local health food market, you may be out of bacon luck for 30 days. The good news? No one ever died from lack of bacon. (Science.) And if you're craving that salty, fatty, crispy flavor, you do have some alternatives. You may be able to find pork belly at your local butcher shop—ask them how to bake or roast it so it's crispy on the outside, soft on the inside.

PREHEAT the oven to 375°F. Line a baking sheet with foil.

SPREAD the bacon slices evenly on the sheet in a single layer. This method will leave the bacon slightly chewy in the center and crisp around the edges. If you prefer your bacon crispy all the way through, place a wire baking rack on top of the foil-lined sheet and lay the bacon evenly on the rack. Be careful not to overlap—use two baking sheets if necessary.

BAKE for 15 to 20 minutes, depending on the thickness of the bacon and desired level of crisp. Transfer to a paper towel–lined platter and serve immediately. Leftover bacon will last about a week in the fridge.

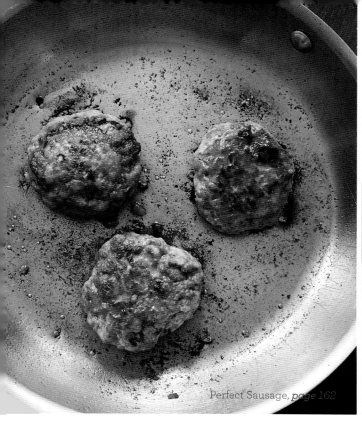

Perfect Sausage, *page 162*

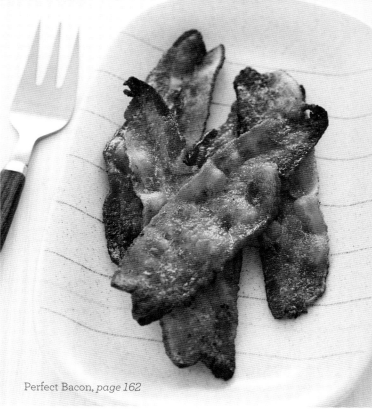

Perfect Bacon, *page 162*

⭐ PRO TIP *It's also not that hard to find Whole30-compliant prosciutto, which bakes up crunchy just like bacon. Line a baking sheet with parchment paper and preheat the oven to 375°F. Lay the prosciutto flat and bake for 12 to 15 minutes, until the meat darkens. Set aside for 5 minutes—it will continue to crisp up as it cools. Crumble and sprinkle on salads, soups, or over a baked sweet potato for a salty crunch similar to bacon.*

If you're able to find Whole30-compliant pastured, organic bacon (lucky ducks), after frying it up, you can pour the warm bacon fat into a glass storage jar and refrigerate for later use, either as a cooking fat or a recipe ingredient.

Grilled Vegetables and Fruit

Grilling is the most effective way to impart a sweet, smoky, caramelized flavor to vegetables and fruit. There are three ways to prepare produce for grilling—long slices that sit right on the grill, large cubes or chunks that you thread onto skewers, or large cubes or chunks placed in a grill basket.

You can grill just about any vegetable, except leafy greens. Favorites include bell peppers, chile peppers (poblano or hatch), onions, cherry tomatoes, zucchini, summer squash, radishes, eggplant, asparagus, Brussels sprouts, mushrooms, and butternut squash. You can also add fruit to your grill grate or on your skewers—think pineapple, mango, peaches, apples, pears, cantaloupe, and grapes. (Don't put fruit into your grill basket, however—their juices will release over the vegetables, making them soggy.)

perfect grilled vegetables

SERVES 2 (WITH LEFTOVERS)

PREP TIME: 10 minutes
COOK TIME: 4 to 20 minutes
TOTAL TIME: 14 to 30 minutes

---

1 pound mixed vegetables and/or fruit

2 tablespoons extra-virgin olive oil

Salt and black pepper

PREHEAT the grill to high heat (500°F).

TO GRILL DIRECTLY ON THE GRILL GRATE: Cut the vegetables into large, flat pieces, so they won't fall through the grate. (Avoid small vegetables like cherry tomatoes, radishes, mushrooms, and Brussels sprouts with this method.) Specifically, cut pieces into relatively flat strips, 2 inches wide, and ½ inch thick. (If grilling asparagus, simply trim the ends and leave them whole; for onions, apples, or pears, cut into six equal wedges)

PLACE the cut vegetables in a large bowl and drizzle with the olive oil. Toss or mix the vegetables with your hands until they are well coated. Place on the grill at a 45-degree angle to the grate to prevent them from falling through.

GRILL the vegetables according to the chart. (Cooking times are highly variable based on your grill, too—so experiment, and check your vegetables often as they cook as you become familiar with this technique.) When you're ready to flip, turn them with grill tongs, peeling them off along the axis of the grill grate to prevent them from sticking or tearing. Cook the veggies or fruit until lightly charred on the outside and fork-tender on the inside.

TOSS with your favorite dressing or sauce (starting on page 302), or sprinkle with salt and pepper and our seasoning suggestions and serve warm.

TO GRILL ON SKEWERS: If using wooden skewers, soak them in water for 30 minutes to 1 hour to prevent them from burning on the grill.

CUT the vegetables or fruit into 1-inch chunks or cubes. Leave whole smaller vegetables and fruits like cherry tomatoes, smaller mushrooms, radishes, and grapes.

PLACE the cut vegetables in a large bowl and drizzle with the olive oil. Toss or mix the vegetables with your hands until they are well coated, then alternate them on the skewers. Place the skewers on the grill at a 45-degree angle to the grate to prevent some of the smaller items from sticking.

GRILL the vegetables for 10 to 15 minutes, turning the skewers every few minutes so all sides make contact with the heat. Cook until the most hearty vegetables (like peppers, onions, and mushrooms) are charred on the edges and tender enough to eat, but not so long that more delicate vegetables (like zucchini and summer squash) are burned or dried out.

TOSS with your favorite dressing or sauce (starting on page 302), or sprinkle with salt and pepper, drizzle with a tablespoon of extra-virgin olive oil, and serve warm.

TO GRILL IN A GRILL BASKET: Cut the vegetables or fruit into 1-inch chunks or cubes. Leave whole smaller vegetables and fruits like cherry tomatoes, smaller mushrooms, radishes, and grapes.

PLACE the cut vegetables in a large bowl and drizzle with the olive oil. Toss or mix the vegetables with your hands until they are well coated, then place in a grill basket.

PLACE the basket on the grill and grill for 15 to 20 minutes, shaking the grill basket occasionally. Grill until the most hearty vegetables (like peppers, onions, and mushrooms) are charred on the edges and tender enough to eat, but not so long that more delicate vegetables (like zucchini and summer squash) are dried out.

TOSS with your favorite dressing or sauce (starting on page 302), or sprinkle with salt and pepper, drizzle with a tablespoon of extra-virgin olive oil, and serve warm.

Grilling Fruits and Vegetables

VEGETABLE OR FRUIT	GRILL TIME	SEASONING SUGGESTIONS
Asparagus	4 to 6 minutes (no need to flip or turn)	squeeze of lemon juice and sprinkle of zest
Bell peppers	5 to 6 minutes per side	splash of balsamic vinegar
Butternut squash	7 to 8 minutes per side	dried thyme
Eggplant	6 to 7 minutes per side	fresh chopped tomatoes, dried oregano
Hatch or poblano peppers	5 to 6 minutes per side	keep it simple with salt and pepper
Onion	8 to 10 minutes per side	squeeze of lemon juice and sprinkle of zest
Summer squash	4 to 5 minutes per side	lemon zest, dried chives
Zucchini	4 to 5 minutes per side	lemon zest, dried chives
Apple	6 to 8 minutes per side	squeeze of lemon juice, dash of cinnamon
Cantaloupe	2 to 3 minutes per side	perfect as-is, no seasoning needed
Mango	2 to 3 minutes per side	perfect as-is, no seasoning needed
Peaches (halved)	3 to 4 minutes (no need to flip or turn)	perfect as-is, no seasoning needed
Pear	3 to 4 minutes per side	drizzle of melted ghee, dash of cinnamon or vanilla bean
Pineapple	5 to 8 minutes per side	perfect as-is, no seasoning needed

Roasted Vegetables

Roasting is one of the easiest ways to cook vegetables, and also one of the most flavorful. For those of you who say, "I don't like broccoli/Brussels sprouts/asparagus," we'd encourage you to give them another shot with roasting—we're pretty sure you'll change your tune.

Roasting allows the vegetables' natural flavors to thoroughly develop, delivering a nicely browned crispiness on the outside and sweet tenderness on the inside. Plus, roasting requires very little hands-on cooking time, allowing you to batch-prep a bunch of veggies for the week while you're doing other stuff around the house.

Roasting means to cook in dry heat at a high temperature—we use 425°F. You'll want to use a baking sheet lined with parchment paper to keep the vegetables from sticking. Don't use a pan with high sides, as that will trap some moisture, and your veggies will steam instead of roast.

perfect roasted vegetables

SERVES 2 (WITH LEFTOVERS)

PREP TIME: 10 minutes

COOK TIME: 15 to 50 minutes

TOTAL TIME: 25 minutes to 1 hour

---

1 pound vegetables

2 tablespoons cooking fat, melted

Salt and black pepper

You can roast just about any vegetable, even some hearty greens. Vegetables well suited to this technique include starchy roots like carrots, potatoes, parsnips, and beets; hearty vegetables like Brussels sprouts, broccoli, cauliflower, onions, fennel, bell peppers, and eggplant; and squashes like butternut, acorn, or spaghetti. You can even roast more delicate vegetables like green beans, tomatoes, and kale!

PREHEAT the oven to 425°F. Line 1 or 2 baking sheets with parchment paper.

IF necessary, peel and trim the vegetables. Cut each vegetable into even-sized pieces if necessary (refer to the chart for our recommendations). Place the vegetables in a large mixing bowl and drizzle with the melted fat. Toss or mix thoroughly so the vegetables are evenly coated.

SPREAD the vegetables evenly on the prepared baking sheet(s). Do not crowd or overlap the veggies, as they'll steam instead of roast. Season with salt and pepper.

ROAST the vegetables in the oven according to the chart, flipping or stirring once to ensure all sides are cooked evenly. (Cooking times are variable, so experiment and check often as the vegetables cook as you get familiar with this technique.) Cook until the vegetables are lightly browned and crispy on the outside and fork-tender on the inside.

IF the vegetables are browned to your liking before they've reached your desired tenderness, turn the heat down to 350°F and continue roasting, checking for doneness every 5 to 7 minutes.

TOSS with your favorite dressing or sauce (starting on page 302), drizzle with balsamic glaze (page 361), or use our serving suggestions.

Roasting Vegetables

VEGETABLE	PREP	ROAST TIME	SEASONING SUGGESTIONS
Acorn squash	halved	45 to 50 minutes	drizzle of ghee, dash of cinnamon
Asparagus	whole	25 minutes	drizzle of extra-virgin olive oil, squeeze of lemon juice and sprinkle of zest
Beets	1-inch pieces	35 to 45 minutes	squeeze of orange juice and sprinkle of zest and fresh thyme
Bell pepper	1-inch pieces	25 to 35 minutes	splash of balsamic vinegar
Broccoli	1-inch florets	20 to 25 minutes	squeeze of lemon juice and sprinkle of zest
Brussels sprouts	halved	35 to 40 minutes	squeeze of lemon juice and sprinkle of zest
Butternut squash	1-inch pieces	45 to 50 minutes	drizzle of ghee, sprinkle of thyme or rosemary
Cabbage	8 wedges	25 to 30 minutes	squeeze of lemon juice, dried chives
Carrots	1-inch pieces	20 to 25 minutes	squeeze of lemon juice, fresh minced parsley and mint
Cauliflower	1-inch florets	20 to 25 minutes	squeeze of lemon juice, dried chives
Eggplant	½-inch slices	20 to 25 minutes	splash of balsamic vinegar, fresh chopped tomatoes, dried oregano
Fennel	1-inch pieces	30 to 40 minutes	squeeze of orange or lemon juice and sprinkle of zest
Green beans	whole	12 to 15 minutes	splash of balsamic vinegar
Kale	2-inch pieces	10 to 12 minutes (kale chips!)	drizzle of extra-virgin olive oil, minced garlic
Mushrooms	halved	30 to 35 minutes	splash of balsamic vinegar, chives
Onion	8 wedges	20 to 25 minutes	squeeze of lemon juice and sprinkle of zest
Parsnips	1-inch pieces	20 to 25 minutes	sprinkle of dried thyme
Potatoes (all varieties)	1-inch pieces or ½-inch spears	35 to 40 minutes	drizzle of ghee, sprinkle of fresh rosemary
Radishes	halved	15 to 20 minutes	squeeze of orange juice, sprinkle of fresh parsley
Spaghetti squash	halved	1 hour	drizzle of ghee, coarse salt
Tomatoes	quartered	30 to 40 minutes	drizzle of extra-virgin olive oil, coarse salt
Turnips	1-inch pieces	45 to 50 minutes	drizzle of extra-virgin olive oil, dried chives

Sautéed Vegetables

To *sauté* means to cook, stirring or tossing, in a small amount of fat in a pan over relatively high heat. This technique releases flavor and moisture from vegetables, and concentrates their sweetness through caramelization (although nowhere near as much as roasting).

The benefits of sautéing are that it is much quicker than roasting, and can be done with just one pan on the stovetop. The down side is that it requires more attention than roasting, as you're generally adding vegetables to the pan one at a time, and you must stir or mix your vegetables often while they are cooking. (The word *sauté* comes from the French word for "jump," so remember to keep those veggies jumping in the pan!)

perfect sautéed vegetables

SERVES 2 (WITH LEFTOVERS)

PREP TIME: 10 minutes

COOK TIME: 5 to 20 minutes

TOTAL TIME: 15 to 30 minutes

---

1 pound vegetables

2 tablespoons cooking fat

Salt and pepper

---

*The key to successful sautéing is to prepare all the ingredients *before* the first one hits the pan, so you can time the cooking of each ingredient perfectly. As all vegetables have different cooking times, make sure vegetables that take longer to cook are added first.*

PREPARE each vegetable by peeling and trimming, and cutting into uniform size, if necessary. (Refer to the chart for recommendations.) Heat the cooking fat in a large skillet over medium-high heat, swirling to coat the bottom of the pan. When the fat is hot, add the vegetables in the order of longest to cook to shortest to cook.

COOK the vegetables according to the chart, stirring often to ensure all sides are cooked evenly and nothing sticks to the pan. (Cooking times are variable, so experiment and check often as the vegetables cook as you become familiar with this technique.) Cook the veggies until they are slightly browned on the outside and fork-tender inside.

IF the vegetables are browned to your liking before they've reached desired tenderness, turn the heat down to medium and continue to cooking, stirring.

TOSS with your favorite dressing or sauce (starting on page 302), our seasoning suggestions, or sprinkle with salt and pepper, drizzle with a tablespoon of extra-virgin olive oil, and serve warm.

Sautéing Vegetables

VEGETABLE	PREP	SAUTÉ TIME	SEASONING SUGGESTIONS
Asparagus	whole	5 to 10 minutes	squeeze of lemon juice and sprinkle of zest
Beets	1-inch pieces	15 to 20 minutes	squeeze of orange juice and sprinkle of zest
Bell pepper	1-inch pieces	5 to 6 minutes	splash of balsamic vinegar
Broccoli	1-inch florets	5 to 7 minutes	squeeze of lemon juice and sprinkle of zest
Brussels sprouts	halved	6 to 8 minutes	dried thyme and lemon zest before cooking
Butternut squash	1-inch pieces	7 to 9 minutes	dried thyme before cooking
Cabbage	8 wedges	8 to 10 minutes	squeeze of lemon juice, dried chives
Carrots	1½-inch pieces	6 to 8 minutes	squeeze of lemon juice, minced fresh parsley and mint
Cauliflower	1-inch florets	5 to 7 minutes	squeeze of lemon juice, dried chives
Eggplant	1-inch pieces	6 to 8 minutes	fresh chopped tomatoes, dried oregano
Fennel	1-inch pieces	8 to 10 minutes	squeeze of orange or lemon juice and sprinkle of zest
Green beans	whole	5 to 6 minutes	splash of balsamic vinegar
Kale	2-inch pieces	6 to 8 minutes	squeeze of lemon juice and sprinkle of zest
Mushrooms	halved	4 to 5 minutes	splash of balsamic vinegar, chives
Onion	½ inch slices	5 to 7 minutes	squeeze of lemon juice and sprinkle of zest
Parsnips	1½-inch pieces	6 to 8 minutes	sprinkle of dried thyme
Potatoes (all varieties)	1-inch pieces	12 to 15 minutes	drizzle of ghee, sprinkle of rosemary
Spinach	2-inch pieces	4 to 6 minutes	squeeze of lemon juice and sprinkle of zest
Sugar snap peas/ snow peas	whole	4 to 5 minutes	splash of sesame oil, chopped green onions
Tomatoes	1-inch pieces	3 to 4 minutes	drizzle of extra-virgin olive oil, coarse salt
Zucchini/summer squash	½-inch-thick rounds	5 to 6 minutes	lemon zest, dried chives

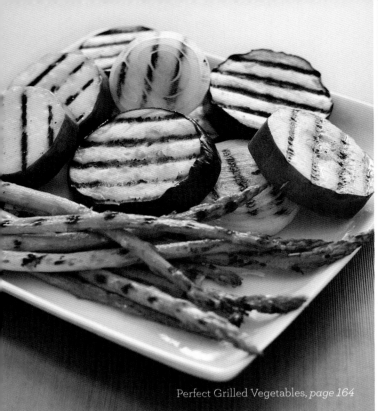

Perfect Grilled Vegetables, *page 164*

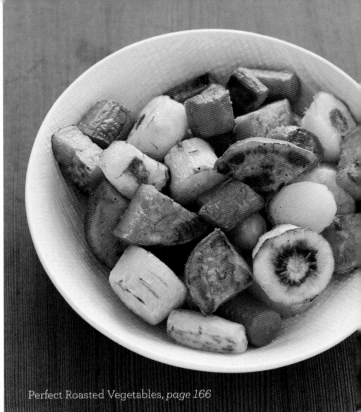

Perfect Roasted Vegetables, *page 166*

Perfect Sautéed Vegetables, *page 168*

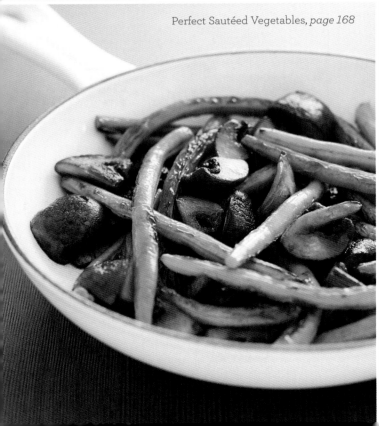

Perfect Steamed Vegetables, *page 171*

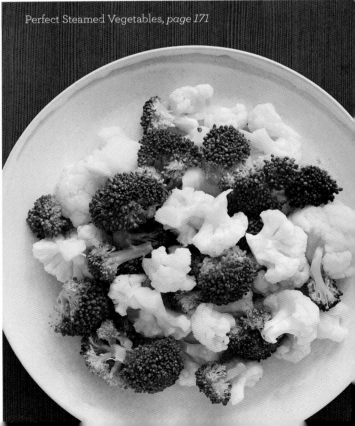

Steamed Vegetables

Steaming vegetables is practically synonymous with "healthy," but unfortunately, it's also commonly synonymous with "boring."

We are going to bust that myth right now.

Steamed vegetables *are* healthy, but they're also intensely flavorful, preserving the fresh, bright, crisp tastes without imparting any smokiness or browning. This makes steamed vegetables the perfect vehicle for any number of our dressings and sauces (see page 302), or the perfect light, fresh side dish with a squeeze of lemon or lime juice and a dash of salt and pepper.

You can steam just about any vegetable, but keep in mind that tomatoes, mushrooms, bell peppers, eggplant, and garlic have much better flavor when roasted or sautéed.

Our two go-to methods for steaming vegetables are stovetop steaming and oven steaming. While stovetop is generally our preference, it's nice to have the second method when the stove burners get crowded.

perfect steamed vegetables

SERVES 2 (WITH LEFTOVERS)

PREP TIME: 10 minutes

COOK TIME: 3 to 50 minutes

TOTAL TIME: 13 minutes to 1 hour

---

1 pound vegetables

Juice of ½ lemon or lime

Salt and black pepper

While you can steam a mix of vegetables all at the same time, they all have different densities and steam at different rates. Root vegetables like potatoes, winter squash, and turnips take longer to steam than lighter vegetables like broccoli and summer squash. You want each vegetable fork-tender when you're done steaming, so either group like vegetables together and steam in batches, or place the vegetables requiring the most time in the pot first, adding faster-cooking vegetables a few minutes later. As steaming requires no added cooking fat, remember to add fat into your meal elsewhere, either in the form of a dressing or sauce or with added fat elsewhere in the meal.

PREPARE each vegetable by peeling, trimming, and cutting into uniform size, if necessary. (Refer to the chart for recommendations.)

TO STEAM IN THE OVEN: Preheat the oven to 350°F. Bring 2 cups water to a boil in a small pan, an electric kettle, or microwave. Place the vegetables in a casserole dish large enough to easily accommodate them—you don't want your vegetables stacked to the very top. Make sure the dish has a well-fitting lid.

ADD 1 inch of the boiling water to the bottom of the dish. Add the vegetables, cover, and place in the oven to steam until fork-tender. (Refer to the chart for general time guidelines.) Check the vegetables often by tasting—if using a mix of vegetables, check only the heartiest ingredients.

TOSS with your favorite dressing or sauce (see page 302), our seasoning suggestions, or a squeeze of lemon or lime juice and a sprinkling of salt and pepper. Serve warm.

TO STEAM ON THE STOVETOP: Bring 2 cups of water to a boil in a large pot. Place a colander or steamer inside the pot. Add the vegetables, cover, and steam until fork-tender. (Refer to the chart for general time guidelines.) Check the vegetables often by tasting.

TOSS with your favorite dressing or sauce (see page 202), our seasoning suggestions below, or a squeeze cf lemon or lime juice and sprinkling of salt and pepper. Serve warm.

Steaming Vegetables

VEGETABLE	PREP	STEAM TIME	SEASONING SUGGESTIONS
Asparagus	whole	7 to 13 minutes	drizzle of extra-virgin olive oil, squeeze of lemon juice and sprinkle of zest
Beets	1-inch pieces	35 to 50 minutes	squeeze of orange juice and sprinkle of zest and fresh thyme
Broccoli	1-inch florets	5 to 7 minutes	squeeze of lemon juice and sprinkle of zest
Brussels sprouts	whole	8 to 15 minutes	squeeze of lemon juice and sprinkle of zest
Butternut squash	1-inch pieces	7 to 10 minutes	drizzle of ghee, dried thyme
Cabbage	8 wedges	6 to 10 minutes	squeeze of lemon juice, dried chives
Carrots	1 ½-inch pieces	7 to 10 minutes	squeeze of lemon juice, minced fresh parsley and mint
Cauliflower	1-inch florets	5 to 10 minutes	squeeze of lemon juice, dried chives
Fennel	1-inch pieces	8 to 10 minutes	squeeze of orange or lemon juice and sprinkle of zest
Green beans	whole	6 to 10 minutes	splash cf balsamic vinegar
Kale	2-inch pieces	4 to 7 minutes	drizzle cf extra-virgin olive oil, minced garlic
Onion	½ inch slices	8 to 12 minutes	squeeze of lemon juice and sprinkle of zest
Parsnips	1 ½-inch pieces	7 to 10 minutes	sprinkle of dried thyme
Potatoes (all varieties)	1-inch pieces	8 to 12 minutes	drizzle of ghee, sprinkle of fresh rosemary
Radishes	whole	7 to 14 minutes	squeeze of orange juice, fresh parsley
Snap peas/snow peas	whole	5 to 6 minutes	splash of sesame oil, chopped green onions
Spinach	whole leaves	3 to 5 minutes	squeeze of lemon juice and sprinkle of zest
Swiss chard	2-inch pieces	3 to 5 minutes	drizzle of extra-virgin olive oil, minced garlic
Turnips	1-inch pieces	8 to 12 minutes	drizzle of extra-virgin olive oil, dried chives
Zucchini/summer squash	1-inch rounds	5 to 8 minutes	lemon zest, dried chives

Burger "Buns"

No, you're not eating bread (or buns) on the Whole30, but who says your Perfect Burger (page 153) has to be naked? Let's redefine *bun* from "a refined flour-based super-processed, tasteless, flavorless, nutrition-less burger holder" to "a healthy, colorful, nutritious explosion of flavor blanketing your meat."

Way better, right? Enjoy these breadless bun variations, but feel free to create your own buns or wraps, too. You can also use tomato slices, hearty lettuce leaves (like Boston, Bibb, or romaine), or roasted red pepper halves to hold your burger.

Wait—here's a totally mind-blowing thought: Who says the *meat* can't be the bun? Try stacking your fillings between *two* burgers—the mess will be worth the meaty reward.

eggplant buns

SERVES 2 (WITH LEFTOVERS)

PREP TIME: 5 minutes

COOK TIME: 20 minutes

TOTAL TIME: 25 minutes

1 eggplant

3 tablespoons cooking fat

½ teaspoon salt

½ teaspoon black pepper

PREHEAT the oven to 425°F. Line a baking sheet with foil.

SLICE the eggplant evenly into ¾-inch-thick rounds. Arrange in a single layer on the prepared pan. Drizzle half of the cooking fat evenly over the eggplant, then flip each slice and drizzle the remaining fat on the other side. Season with the salt and pepper.

ROAST the eggplant for 20 minutes, until it is browned on the outside and fork-tender. Allow to cool, then stack a burger and fillings between two slices and serve.

STORE extras in foil or in an airtight container in the fridge. They will keep for up to 3 to 5 days, perfect for more burgers, or adding to Kitchen Sink Scrambled Eggs (page 202).

YOU can also grill the eggplant slices, following the instructions for Perfect Grilled Vegetables on page 164.

portabella mushroom buns

SERVES 2

PREP TIME: 5 minutes

COOK TIME: 20 minutes

TOTAL TIME: 25 minutes

---

4 large portabella mushrooms

3 tablespoons cooking fat, melted

½ teaspoon salt

½ teaspoon black pepper

1 clove garlic, minced

You can also grill the mushroom slices, following the instructions for Perfect Grilled Vegetables on page 164.

PREHEAT the oven to 400°F. Line a baking sheet with foil.

RINSE the mushroom tops with cool water or wipe with a wet paper towel to remove any excess dirt. Dry thoroughly. Place the mushrooms upside-down on the prepared baking sheet. Remove the stems by gently breaking them off, and drizzle the cooking fat evenly over the mushrooms. Season with the salt, pepper, and garlic.

ROAST for 10 minutes, then flip and roast for another 10 minutes, until fork-tender. Allow to cool, then stack a burger and fillings between two mushroom caps and serve.

sweet potato buns

SERVES 2 (WITH LEFTOVERS)

PREP TIME: 5 minutes

COOK TIME: 6 to 10 minutes

TOTAL TIME: 11 to 15 minutes

---

2 sweet potatoes

2 tablespoons cooking fat

Salt and black pepper

You can also roast the sweet potato slices, following the instructions for Perfect Roasted Vegetables on page 166.

PEEL the sweet potato and cut into ½-inch-thick rounds. (Choose thick, round sweet potatoes over long, skinny ones.) Heat the cooking fat over medium heat in a large skillet, swirling to coat the bottom of the pan. When the fat is hot, add the largest slices from the middle of the potato, laying them out in a single layer in the pan. (Cook these in batches, if necessary.) Cook until fork-tender and browned, 3 to 5 minutes on each side. Sprinkle with salt and pepper. Let cool, then stack a burger and fillings between two slices of sweet potato and serve.

STORE the extras in foil or an airtight container the fridge. They will keep for up to 3 to 5 days, perfect for more burgers, or adding to tomorrow morning's Frittata (page 206).

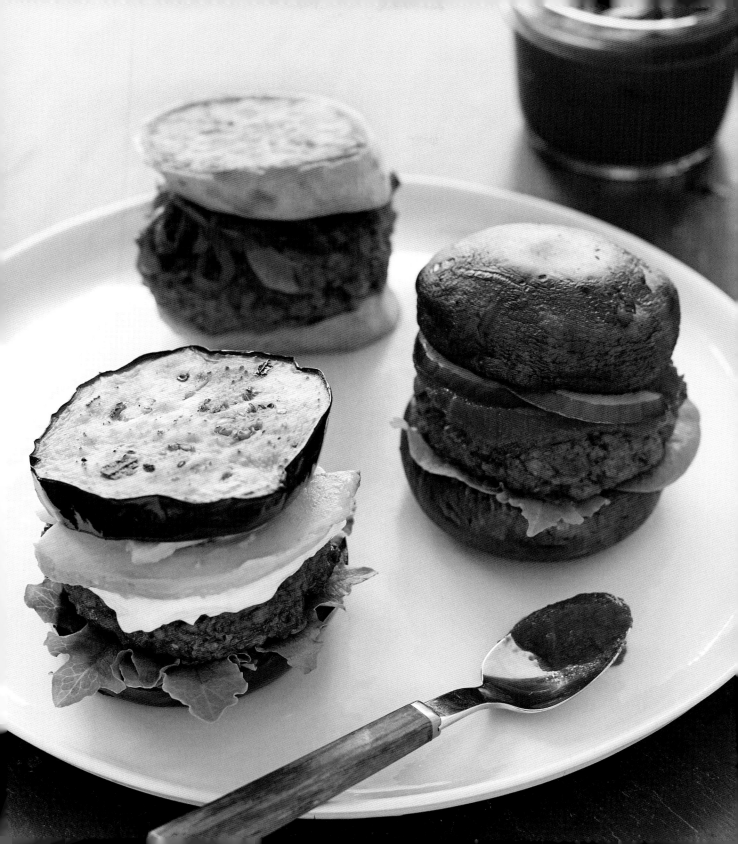

Bone Broth

Bone broth is a Whole30 staple, not just as a cooking ingredient; homemade broth actually functions as a health supplement on the Whole30! It's a source of minerals—like calcium, phosphorus, magnesium, and potassium—in forms that your body can easily absorb. It's also rich in glycine and proline, amino acids not found in significant amounts in muscle meat (the vast majority of the meat we consume). It also contains chondroitin sulfate and glucosamine, the compounds sold as supplements to reduce inflammation, arthritis, and joint pain. Finally, "soup bones" include a form of protein called collagen, abundant in bone, marrow, cartilage, tendons, and ligaments. (The breakdown of collagen in bone broths is what produces gelatin.)

Bone broth aids in healing a leaky gut and regulating digestion, muscle repair, and growth; helps balance your nervous system; and contributes to a strong immune system. (There's a reason your mom always made you chicken soup when you were sick.) The gelatin in broth also reduces joint pain and inflammation, prevents bone loss, and builds healthy skin, hair, and nails.

Unfortunately, broth or "stock" from the grocery store relies on high temperature, fast-cooking techniques, which don't confer the same benefits. In addition, many contain off-plan additives (like MSG) and ingredients (like sugar). If you just need a small amount for a recipe, compliant store-bought stuff will do, but if you're interested in the healing properties of bone broth, you have to make it yourself.

As a supplement, we like to drink a mug of it, just like you would coffee or tea. In fact, a warm cup of broth is a great way to start your morning—try drinking 8 ounces a day, every day. Of course, you can also use it in recipes that call for broth or stock and as a base for your favorite soups.

Source your bones from your local butcher, a local farm (ask around at the farmers' market), a friendly hunter, or your local health food store (if they have a meat department); or order bones online (see page 404). You can also save the bones from a roasted whole chicken, turkey, duck, or goose.

You can use bones from just about any animal—beef, veal, lamb, bison or buffalo, venison, chicken, duck, goose, turkey, or pork. Get a variety of bones—ask for marrow bones, oxtail, and "soup bones." Make sure you include some larger bones like knuckles, or feet (like chicken feet), which will contain more cartilage, and therefore more collagen. You can even mix and match bones in the same batch of broth—some beef, some lamb, some chicken—but know that will change the flavor. (Most folks prefer to stick to one animal source at once.)

If you're making chicken broth, planning ahead will allow you to make three recipes with the same bird. First, purchase a three to four pound chicken and roast it whole using our recipe on page 157. Then, pick the carcass clean and use the meat in a Protein Salad (page 161) or Harvest Chicken Salad (page 232). Finally, use the carcass to make your chicken broth.

Ideally, you're sourcing pastured or grass-fed, organically raised bones. The animals have to be healthy to impart the maximum health benefit. Do your best to seek out pastured chicken or 100-percent grass-fed beef bones from a local source.

We've given you our basic recipes here, but you can add many different herbs, spices, or vegetables to your broth to change the flavor. Consider adding green onion, leek, mushrooms, garlic, red pepper flakes, bay leaves, rosemary, sage, or ginger. Avoid using broccoli, turnip peels, cabbage, Brussels sprouts, green peppers, collard greens, or mustard greens as they will make your broth bitter.

Finally, for an easy addition of small amounts of broth to recipes, store some broth in an ice cube tray in the freezer. One cube is about an ounce (2 tablespoons), so recipes that call for ¼ cup of broth would take 2 cubes, ½ cup would take 4 cubes, etc. You can store larger amounts in glass mason jars, but be sure to let the broth cool down before transferring to glass. Finally, make sure you leave enough space in a glass container for the frozen broth to expand—otherwise, the glass could break.

chicken bone broth

MAKES 1 GALLON

PREP TIME: 15 minutes
COOK TIME: 12 to 24 hours
TOTAL TIME: 12 to 24 hours

Carcass from a 3- to 4-pound roasted chicken

2 carrots, roughly chopped

3 stalks celery, roughly chopped

2 onions, roughly chopped

5 to 6 fresh parsley stems

1 sprig fresh thyme

2 tablespoons apple cider vinegar

10 black peppercorns

1 teaspoon salt

ADD all ingredients to a large stockpot, cover with water, and bring to a boil. Cover and reduce the heat to low. Simmer for 12 to 24 hours without stirring. (You can also do this in a slow cooker. Set the cooker to high until it boils, then turn the temperature down to low and simmer for 12 to 24 hours.)

STRAIN the broth through a fine mesh colander. Discard the solids. Transfer the broth to multiple containers to speed up cooling—don't freeze or refrigerate while hot! Allow the broth sit in the fridge (uncovered) for several hours, until the fat rises to the top and hardens. Scrape off the fat with a spoon and discard.

A properly prepared chicken broth might look a little jiggly when cold. That's just the gelatin from the collagen in the bones. Gently heat the broth and it will return to a liquid state.

REFRIGERATE the broth for up to 3 to 4 days, or freeze for up to 6 months.

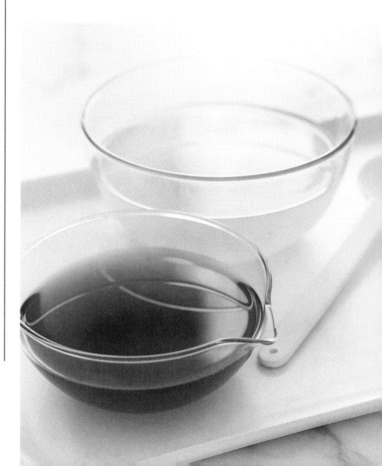

beef bone broth

MAKES 1 GALLON

PREP TIME: 15 minutes

COOK TIME: 12 to 24 hours

TOTAL TIME: 12 to 24 hours

---

3 to 4 pounds beef bones

2 carrots, roughly chopped

3 stalks celery, roughly chopped

2 onions, roughly chopped

5 to 6 parsley stems

1 sprig fresh thyme

2 tablespoons apple cider vinegar

10 black peppercorns

1 teaspoon salt

ADD all ingredients to a large stockpot, cover with water, and bring to a boil. Cover and reduce the heat to low. Simmer for 12 to 24 hours without stirring. (You can also do this in a slow cooker. Set the cooker to high until the broth boils, then turn the temperature down to low and simmer for 12 to 24 hours.)

STRAIN the broth through a fine mesh colander. Discard the solids. Transfer the broth to multiple containers to speed up cooling—don't freeze or refrigerate while hot! Allow the broth to sit in the fridge (uncovered) for several hours, until the fat rises to the top and hardens. Scrape off the fat with a spoon and discard.

A properly prepared beef broth will look solid but jiggly when cold—think "meat Jell-O." That's just the gelatin from the collagen in the bones. Gently heat the broth and it will return to a liquid state.

REFRIGERATE the broth for up to 3 to 4 days, or freeze for up to 6 months.

Vegetable Broth

Follow the recipe for chicken broth (page 177), omitting the chicken carcass and adding any additional vegetables, herbs, and spices you desire. Bring to a boil, then reduce the heat to low and simmer for 1 to 2 hours, without stirring. Strain, cool, and store or freeze.

coconut cream

This is the easiest thing you will do in this entire book, but it's a game-changer for so many recipes. Adding coconut milk to soups or sauces is a great way to add thickness and texture, but sometimes coconut milk can water down a dish (like our Cauliflower Mash on page 270). Here's where coconut cream comes in.

Take a can of full-fat coconut milk and put it in the refrigerator for an hour or two—although we recommend leaving at least one can in the fridge at all times for emergency coconut cream situations. (That is something that can actually happen on the Whole30.)

When you open the can, the cream will have risen to the top and become solid, while the coconut water remains at the bottom of the can. Just scoop out the thick stuff at the top and use it in recipes that call for coconut cream.

You can also find prepared coconut cream or "culinary coconut milk" at some health food stores, but why would you pay extra when the only thing required to make your own is opening your refrigerator?

Perfect Mayo

Homemade mayonnaise is a staple in the Whole30 kitchen. It forms the base for an unlimited number of sauces and dressings; holds together chicken, tuna, salmon, and egg salad; and coats meat and seafood before cooking or grilling.

This is one recipe for which you *don't* want to use extra-virgin olive oil—the flavor is just too strong. Use a light-tasting olive oil, avocado oil, or a high-oleic safflower or sunflower oil instead.

You can use a food processor or blender, or mix using a handheld immersion (stick) blender, but please don't try to whisk your mayonnaise by hand—you'll give yourself tennis elbow *and* have really runny mayo to boot.

Mayonnaise will last in the fridge for about a week after your eggs expire, so check the date on your egg carton, add a week, and write *that* date on your mayonnaise jar.

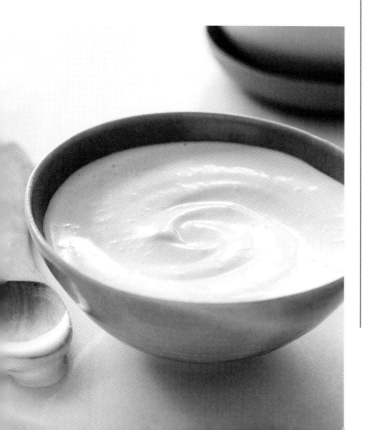

basic mayonnaise

MAKES 1½ CUPS

PREP TIME: 10 minutes

1¼ cups light olive oil

1 large egg

½ teaspoon mustard powder

½ teaspoon salt

Juice of ½ lemon

You can change up our Basic Mayonnaise any number of ways to create a variety of different flavors. For inspiration, see Mayonnaise Variations starting on page 309.

PLACE ¼ cup of the olive oil, the egg, mustard powder, and salt in a blender, food processor, or mixing bowl. Mix thoroughly. While the food processor or blender is running (or while mixing in a bowl with an immersion blender), slowly drizzle in the remaining 1 cup olive oil. After you've added all the oil and the mixture has emulsified, add the lemon juice, blending on low or stirring to incorporate.

⭐ PRO TIP *The key to this emulsion is making sure all ingredients are at room temperature. Leave your egg out on the counter for an hour, or let it sit in a bowl of hot water for 5 minutes before mixing. Keep one lemon on the counter at all times for the express purpose of making mayo—trust us, you'll be making a lot of this. The slower you add your oil, the thicker and creamier your emulsion will be. You can slowly pour oil by hand out of a spouted measuring cup, or use a plastic squeeze bottle to slowly drizzle it into the bowl, food processor, or blender. If you're using an immersion blender, pump the stick up and down a few times toward the end to whip some air into the mixture, making it even fluffier.*

The Perfect Egg-free Mayo

One of the biggest bummers of being allergic or sensitive to eggs is that our Basic Mayonnaise is out. We really didn't want you to miss out on this most versatile condiment, however, so we asked our friend Mickey Trescott, author of *The Autoimmune Paleo Cookbook,* if we could adapt her recipe for egg-free mayo here.

The base of this mayo is coconut butter (also called "coconut manna" or "coconut concentrate"). It's available at most health food stores, or online. While this version of mayo won't taste the same as the creamy concoction you're used to, it still makes a great base for all of the dressings, sauces, and dips on page 302.

This keeps in the fridge for several weeks, but it does harden. Just bring it up to room temperature before using—either leave it out on your counter for an hour or so, or place the container in a bowl of hot water until it softens.

egg-free mayonnaise

MAKES 1¼ CUPS

PREP TIME: 10 minutes

½ cup coconut butter, slightly warmed

½ cup warm water

¼ cup light olive oil

2 cloves garlic, peeled

1 tablespoon lemon juice

¼ teaspoon salt

If you plan on using this egg-free mayo as a base for dressings and sauces, skip the lemon juice. You then have a neutral-flavored base to which you can add any kind of acid (like a citrus juice or vinegar) based on the dressing or sauce you select.

PLACE all of the ingredients in a food processor or blender and blend on high until the mixture thickens, 1 to 2 minutes.

Homemade Coconut Butter

⭐ PRO TIP *If you can't find coconut butter, you can use Mickey's recipe to make your own using coconut flakes and a food processor: Place 4 cups unsweetened coconut flakes in a food processor. Blend on high speed, occasionally stopping to scrape down the sides with a rubber spatula. Process for about a minute at a time, taking breaks so as to not overheat the motor. After 5 or 10 minutes, you should be left with a smooth, creamy liquid. Store in a glass jar at room temperature (no need to refrigerate)—it will keep for up to 6 months.*

Compound Butter

Compound butter is a mixture of butter plus herbs, spices, toasted nuts, or other flavorful ingredients. These tasty butters can be melted on top of meats or vegetables, adding a totally new dimension to your meal. This is also one way to fancy up a simple dinner for company—a slice of compound butter on your Perfect Oven Baked Salmon (page 160) is sure to impress.

compound butter

SERVES 4 TO 8

PREP TIME: 10 minutes

COOL TIME: 2 hours

TOTAL TIME: 2 hours 10 minutes

½ cup (1 stick) unsalted butter, clarified; or ½ cup ghee

¼ cup hazelnuts

1 clove garlic, minced

2 teaspoons fresh thyme leaves

½ teaspoon salt

¼ teaspoon black pepper

⭐ PRO TIP *Some of our favorite compound butter combinations include: ¼ cup sun-dried tomatoes, ¼ cup black olives, pitted, and 2 teaspoons minced fresh rosemary leaves; ¼ cup minced fresh parsley, ¼ cup toasted pine nuts, and 1 tablespoon lemon juice; and 1 minced garlic clove, 2 teaspoons each fresh rosemary, oregano, and chives. Make sure all the ingredients are finely minced.*

PLACE the clarified butter or ghee in a small bowl and leave on the counter until it reaches room temperature.

HEAT a dry pan over medium heat. When the pan is hot, add the hazelnuts and cook, shaking the pan often to prevent burning, until lightly browned, about 5 minutes. Transfer the hazelnuts to a cutting board, allow to cool, then chop.

GENTLY fold the chopped hazelnuts, garlic, thyme leaves, salt, and pepper into the softened butter or ghee. Place a large piece of plastic wrap on a flat surface and place the butter mixture in the center. Form into a rough log, about 1½ inches in diameter. Wrap the plastic wrap tightly around the butter and refrigerate until firm, about 2 hours. You can do this ahead of time if prepping for an event or dinner party—compound butter using fresh ingredients will keep in the fridge for 2 to 3 days.

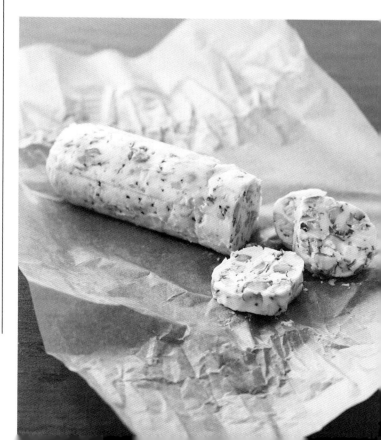

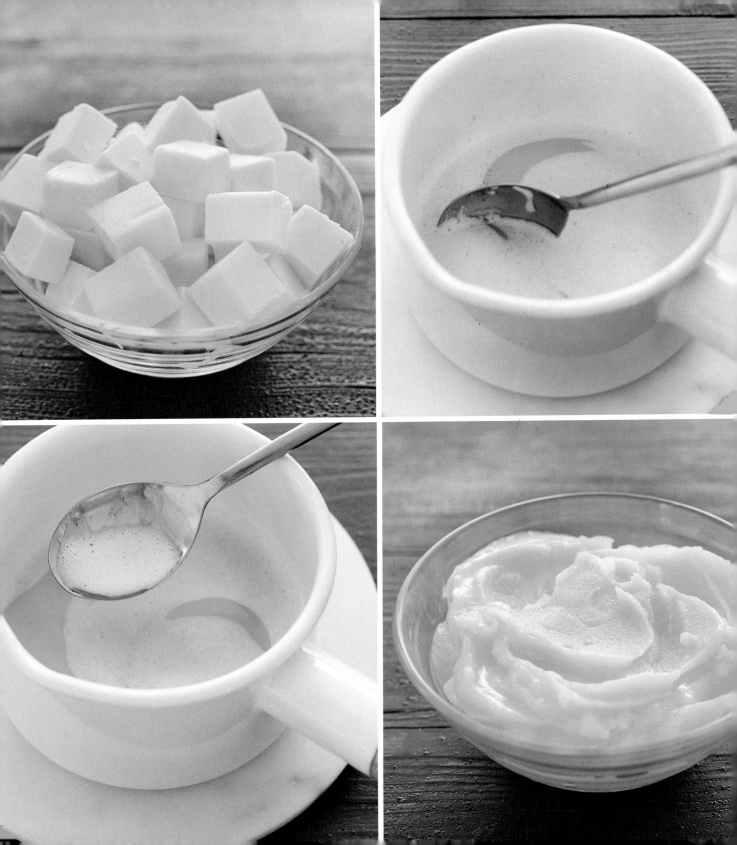

Clarified Butter

Plain old butter isn't allowed on the Whole30 because it contains traces of milk proteins, which may be problematic for sensitive individuals. Clarified butter is the technique of simmering butter slowly at a low temperature to separate the milk solids from the pure butter oil. The end result is a delicious, pure, dairy-free fat, perfect for flavoring dishes or cooking (even on high heat).

You'll also see *ghee* in the recipes—ghee is just a different form of clarified butter. To make ghee, simply simmer the butter longer, until the milk proteins begin to brown, clump, and drift to the bottom of the pan. Ghee has a sweeter, nuttier flavor than clarified butter. (You can also purchase pastured organic ghee online—see page 403 for our favorite brands.)

While it's not part of our official Whole30 rules, we'd always encourage you to look for pastured organic butter when making your own clarified butter or ghee. Common brands available at health food stores nationwide include Strauss, Kerrygold, Kalona Super Natural, and Organic Valley.

clarified butter

MAKES 1½ CUPS

PREP TIME: 5 minutes

COOK TIME: 20 minutes

TOTAL TIME: 25 minutes

---

1 pound (4 sticks) unsalted butter

CUT the butter into 1-inch cubes. Place in a small pot or saucepan over medium-low heat and let melt and come to a simmer without stirring. As the butter simmers, foamy white dairy solids will rise to the surface. With a spoon or ladle, gently skim the dairy solids off the top and discard, leaving just the pure clarified butter in the pan.

ONCE you've removed the majority of the milk solids, strain the butter through cheesecloth into a glass storage jar, discarding the milk solids and cheesecloth when you are done. Allow the butter to cool before storing.

CLARIFIED butter can be stored in the refrigerator for up to 6 months or at room temperature for up to 3 months.

Basic Vinaigrette

Vinaigrette isn't just a mix of oil and vinegar; it's actually a pretty specific equation. Technically, it's an emulsion of one part acid, three parts fat, plus your flavoring. Acids can be any kind of vinegar or citrus juice. Fats are usually some kind of oil, but you can also use a homemade mayonnaise for a creamier dressing. Common emulsifiers include garlic, mustard, and eggs, although you don't have to use an emulsifier—just shake it up and serve!

Vinaigrettes are another Whole30 cooking staple. They're great on salads, sure, but also make for delicious marinades and dressings for meat, seafood and vegetables.

For easy clean up, emulsify vinaigrette the old-fashioned way—by hand! Place all ingredients in a glass container with a lid and shake until well blended, or add to a mixing bowl and whisk until combined. If you'd rather, however, you can use a blender or food processor to do the mixing for you.

basic vinaigrette

MAKES 1 CUP

PREP TIME: 5 minutes

¼ **cup white wine or apple cider vinegar**

¾ **cup extra-virgin olive oil**

¼ **teaspoon salt**

½ **teaspoon black pepper**

Serve your vinaigrette right away, or make ahead of time and store in the refrigerator. If the mixture separates, just whisk or shake before serving. Homemade salad dressings using fresh ingredients (like garlic or herbs) will keep in the refrigerator for up to 2 to 3 days. The olive oil will harden and get cloudy in the cold, so if your dressing has been in the fridge overnight, take it out ahead of time, let it come to room temperature, and shake it up before serving.

PLACE the vinegar in a small bowl. Drizzle in the olive oil while whisking steadily to emulsify. Adjust seasoning with the salt and pepper.

⭐ PRO TIP *You can change up our Basic Vinaigrette any number of ways to create a variety of different flavors. For inspiration, see* *Vinaigrette Variations, page 326.*

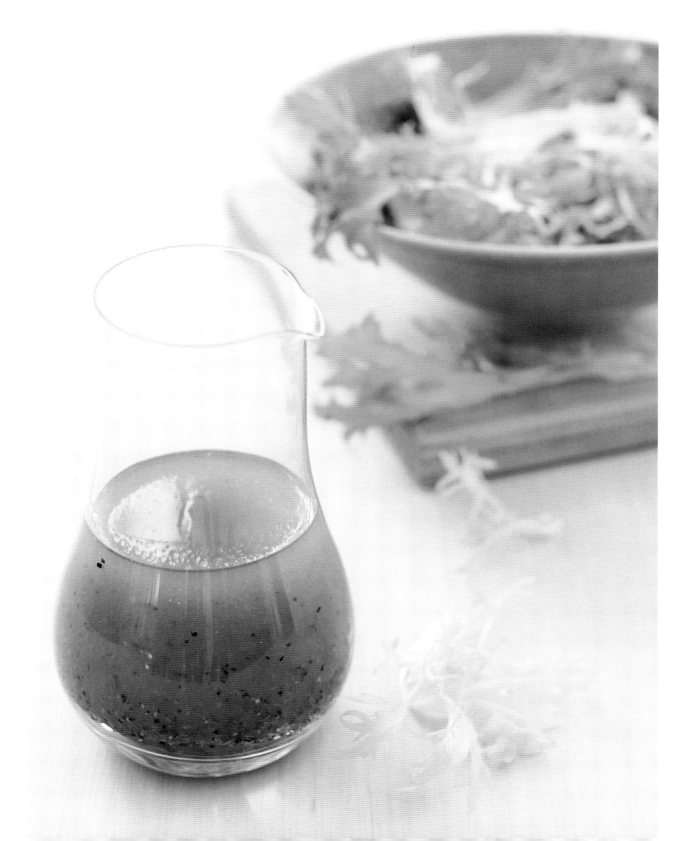

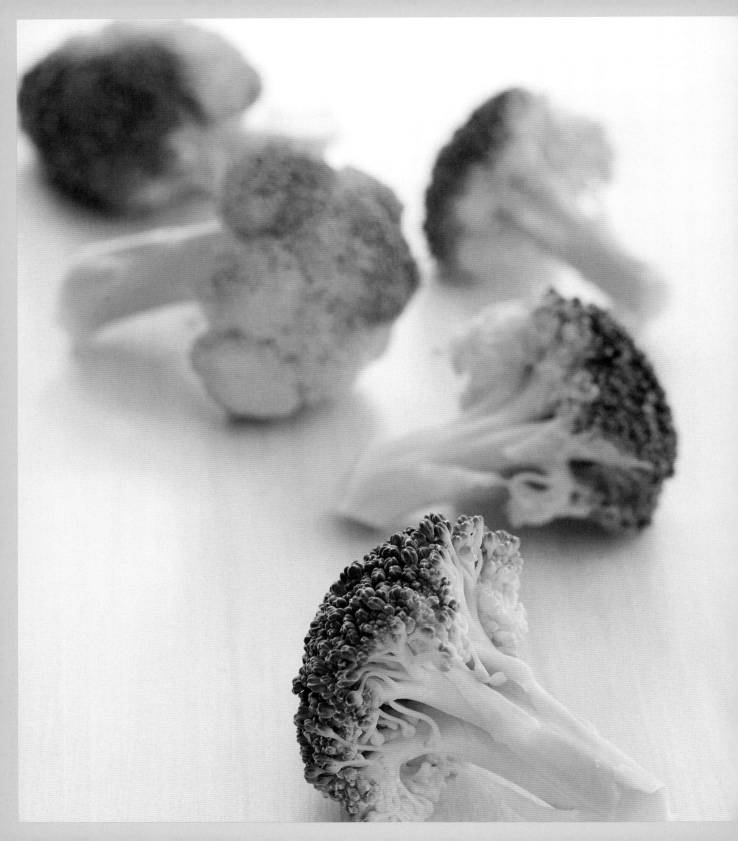

whole30 recipes

Welcome to the heart of The Whole30: our recipes. This section is where you'll put your kitchen skills and the Kitchen Fundamentals you learned in the last section to the test.

Don't be nervous.

This section includes nothing but simple, delicious, nutritious meals made from everyday ingredients. You won't find any specialty food items, hard-to-procure cooking fats or meats, or techniques that call for fancy kitchen tools. We recruited Culinary Institute of America-trained chef Richard Bradford to help us create meals perfect for the beginner chef living in a small town, with access to just one or two regular grocery stores. The recipes in many sections start off simple and get more involved, so you can build confidence in the kitchen as you gain experience with the Whole30.

If you're an experienced chef with a well-stocked Whole30 pantry, you're in for a real treat. These recipes may look basic, but they pack a real flavor punch. Chef Richard has hit the trifecta in that effortless way only a professional chef can pull off—these recipes have simple ingredients and easy preparation techniques, but are incredibly tasty and satisfying. We should know—we've eaten our way through this book more than once.

Not exactly a tough job.

Before you dive in, let's go over some helpful hints for cooking your way through our Whole30 recipes.

First, You Must Read

We know you want to jump right in with both burners, but there is nothing worse than getting halfway through cooking dinner and realizing you're out of a key ingredient. Before you start chopping, dicing, and preheating, take a minute to read through the entire recipe. Like, the whole thing. You'll get a big-picture understanding of what ingredients are involved, whether you have to prep anything in advance (like a sauce or marinade), the tools you'll need, and what the dish should look like when it's done.

Mise-en-place

Remember how we said planning and preparing are everything with the Whole30? Cooking is no exception! *Mise-en-place* is a French term for "putting in place," and it basically means that before you start cooking, all of your ingredients are prepped and your tools are in order. Let's walk through your mise-en-place for the Classic Chili on page 342 First, read through the entire recipe. We'll wait.

Now it's time to prepare the ingredients. First, lay everything but the meat out on a clean section of kitchen counter: the onion, three cloves of garlic, all the spice containers, two peppers, three tomatoes, and your container of beef broth. We'd also pull out a large pot, a small bowl, two medium bowls, a slotted spoon, measuring cups and spoons, a chef's knife, and a cutting board.

Finely chop the onion first, then mince the garlic and put them into the same small bowl. Next, measure out all of your spices and add them to the bowl with the onion and garlic. (As the instructions say these all go into the pot at the same time, why dirty more than one bowl?)

Next, chop the peppers and tomatoes, and place them into a different medium-sized bowl. Measure out your broth and add it to the peppers and tomatoes. (Again, they all go into the pot at the same time.) Place the bowls with prepared ingredients and the empty bowl by the stove, add your large pot to the stovetop, and remove the ground meat from the fridge. For bonus points, take two minutes to put all your spice containers back, and wash your knife, measuring cups, and cutting board.

Now you may cook.

Start at the top of the instructions and prepare your ground meat. Transfer it into the empty bowl sitting by your stove. Add the onion, garlic, and spice mixture from the small bowl to the pot and cook as instructed. Add the peppers, tomatoes, and broth from the other bowl to the pot, return the ground meat in the third bowl to the pot, and finish cooking.

By the way, the only clean up left to do while the table is being set and the chili served is three bowls and a slotted spoon.

This mise-en-place stuff works all right.

Get Your Pan Hot

You'll see our recipe instructions often say, "when the pan is hot . . ." or "once the cooking fat is hot . . ." This is a really important step, so don't rush the process! Adding cold protein to a cold (or warming) pan means it'll likely stick to the bottom, creating a cooking and dishwashing mess. Plus, this techinque causes your ingredients to release moisture as they heat up, leaving you with dry meat or fish. If you're trying to get a good sear on your steak, chicken breast, or fish fillet, that pan or cooking fat needs to be hot to seal in the moisture and lightly brown the surface.

The same goes for sautéing vegetables—a pre-heated pan means faster cooking times, more evenly cooked veggies, and tasty browned bits at the bottom of your stainless steel or cast-iron pan. Yum.

Cooking Times Vary

We've tested all of these recipes in the real world more than once, making sure our cooking times were accurate. Sometimes, we included a range, because things like root vegetables, steaks, or roasts may take longer or shorter to cook based on their size and thickness. However, there are other factors that may impact cooking times, so don't be surprised if you need to add a little more or a little less time to our general recommendations.

First, ovens sometimes run "hot" or "cold." For example, the Hartwigs' oven runs a little cold, so they have to turn the temperature to 365°F for recipes calling for 350°F heat. (You'd naturally figure this out after a few weeks of baking or roasting, or you can use a thermometer to verify the actual temperature versus the temperature on the display.) If your oven runs slightly hot or cold, you may need to adjust your temperature or cooking times to accommodate.

In addition, where you live may impact how long it takes you to steam broccoli.

Seriously.

Altitude has quite an impact on certain cooking methods. As elevation rises, foods you boil, steam, or simmer (like vegetables, roasts, and stews) require a longer cooking time. Our times were based on cooking at sea level, which means mountain men and women may need to adjust. Our Braised Beef Brisket (page 214) may take an hour longer to cook in Salt Lake City than it does in Miami, and residents of Denver may need to add an extra two to three minutes to our Perfect Boiled Egg recipe (page 149). Luckily, oven temperatures are not affected by altitude, so 350°F is always 350°F.

Unless your oven runs hot or cold, of course.

What we're trying to say here is that practice *in your own kitchen* makes perfect. Follow the recipes to the letter if you're unfamiliar with cooking, and adjust them if your environment calls for longer or shorter cooking times. Or, modify our instructions on the fly if you know it takes longer than seven minutes for your broccoli to steam. Make notes in the margins of your favorite recipes, taking note of adjusted cooking times or temperatures, and don't stress if your first few steaks come out more well-done than you'd like.

As with the Whole30, this whole "cooking real food" stuff gets easier with time and experience. On that note . . .

Serves Two(ish)

Most recipes in this book say they serve two people, sometimes with leftovers.

Immediately, you should see the trouble with this.

Which two people?

Our recipes include "average" portion sizes for meat, seafood, eggs, and vegetables per our Meal Template (page 194), but the members of your household may require less food or more food per meal—in fact, you may know this already based on the cooking you did pre-Whole30. If you look at our Perfect Grilled Steak (page 154) and think, "Five ounces, are you kidding me?" just buy bigger cuts of steak and adjust your cooking times if necessary. (Bigger steaks may not take longer, but thicker steaks will.)

You can also adjust this on the fly if you find you're consistently hungry between meals. Buy more protein, the most satiating of all the macronutrients, and make slightly bigger meals until you find the sweet spot. (In fact, even if you're not super hungry, you may want to cook extra meat just so you'll have leftovers!)

You can also adjust for satiety by adding more fat to your meals. Use a little more cooking fat or add some fat, depending on the recipe. Sprinkle more nuts or seeds, add a half an avocado on the side, or toss some olives into your salad. The combination of extra protein and extra fat is especially good at tiding you over from meal to meal. Feel free to add more veggies, too, although they're not very calorie dense and won't help much with satiety.

Unless you're loading your sweet potato with extra ghee, which would totally work.

Now, let's talk about some quick tips for cooking your way through the book.

QUICK TIP: Cooking fat

⭐ You'll notice some of our recipes call for a specific kind of fat, but many just say, "cooking fat." Here's the deal: When the kind of fat you use is important for the flavor or texture of the dish, we'll give you specific options. In our Cauliflower Mash (page 270), we call for clarified butter or ghee because adding extra-virgin olive oil to your mash just wouldn't work.

If you're using fat for cooking, however, just use whatever you have on hand, or whatever you think will taste best for the dish. The list of healthy cooking fats is extensive, so feel free to use coconut oil, clarified butter, ghee, extra-virgin olive oil, palm oil, tallow, lard, bacon fat, or duck fat if we just call for a general "cooking fat" in the recipe.

QUICK TIP: Use a meat thermometer

⭐ On page 140, we recommended some kitchen tools and gadgets that will make cooking real food that much faster, easier, and more fun. One of the most valuable gadgets for the budding chef is a meat thermometer. There are all kinds of tricks for evaluating whether your meat and poultry are done cooking, like pressing on the flesh or using a kitchen timer. But tactile cues take time to learn, and your kitchen timer is probably the least accurate way to measure doneness, as cooking times will vary based on a variety of factors.

A meat thermometer, on the other hand, tells you exactly when to pull your meat or seafood off the heat at just the right time—as long as you use it properly. First, insert the thermometer at the thickest part of the meat, away from any bones. If you're cooking a whole turkey or chicken, place the thermometer in the inner thigh area (near the breast), but don't push it against the bone. If it's a thin cut of meat (like a burger), you can even insert the thermometer sideways!

However, thermometers aren't great for all protein sources, like ribs or flaky fish, so you'll also want to practice your visual skills for evaluating meat and seafood doneness.

Translation: cut into the meat and take a peek.

We know, your food won't look quite as pretty if there's a big slice up the middle, but in the beginning, this is another fantastic way to evaluate whether your meat is actually ready. You'll be able to gauge the perfect pinkness of a medium-rare burger, the glistening flake of a ready salmon fillet, and just the right shade of whiteness in the center of a chicken breast. Just remember that your meat, seafood, and eggs will continue to cook for a few minutes after you pull them off the heat, so grab that burger off the grill while it's just this side of "too red"; by the time you let it rest, it'll be perfect.

QUICK TIP: Make sure all ingredients are Whole30-compliant

⭐ There are places in the book where we use ingredients like mustard, chicken broth, or hot sauce. Though we don't specify this in the recipe itself, here is your friendly reminder to make sure all packaged foods used in your meals still fit the Whole30 guidelines. Read your labels! Make sure your hot sauce doesn't include added sugar, your mustard doesn't use wine or sulfites, and your chicken broth doesn't include cornstarch or rice bran.

We give you some tips for finding Whole30-compliant condiments in the "Can I Have?" section starting on page 60, but finding compliant broth may be more challenging. Luckily, it's super easy to make yourself—just follow our instructions on page 176.

QUICK TIP: Create an "emergency meal plan"

⭐ *There will be nights when you get home from work or school tired and cranky, and the idea of making dinner will seem overwhelming. You will want to call for pizza. You will want to eat popcorn and wine for dinner. You will be tempted to give up.*

You are not going out like that.

After flipping through this book, come up with three emergency meals you could prep in under 15 minutes, using ingredients you always have on hand. Something like Perfect Scrambled Eggs (page 150), hot sauce, avocado, and whatever leftover veggies you have on hand. Or maybe the No-Fuss Salmon Cakes from page 346—you'll always have canned salmon and sweet potato in your pantry, and if you're out of green onion, it's not a big deal. Maybe it's the Protein Salad (page 161) always waiting in your fridge, with a side of Roasted Sweet Potato (page 296). Or maybe it's a frozen shrimp and frozen vegetable stir-fry drizzled with our Asian Vinaigrette (page 330).

Now, write these meals down and stick the list on your refrigerator. Doesn't that feel better already? The brain loves a plan. You feel stress when you're faced with a situation that feels threatening and unfamiliar, with no plan to move through it. Writing down your emergency meals and knowing you'll always have Good

Food on hand is your plan. And now your brain can relax, and you don't have to worry about bailing halfway through your Whole30 because you had a really bad day.

You're welcome.

QUICK TIP: Feel free to have some fun

⭐ *No, really. Cooking is fun! The kitchen is where you feel accomplished, get creative, be proud of the fact that you took these ingredients and made this meal and then got to eat it. Use our recipes as a jumping-off point, but if you notice that you like a lot more spice than we usually call for, feel like extra veggies make things more interesting, or want to road test your own creation based on what you've learned in our Kitchen Fundamentals section, go for it!*

You might mess some meals up. (We sure have. Rarely was anything inedible, though.) Your meals may turn out ugly, but taste delicious—still winning in our book. Your kitchen may look like a bomb went off after making something relatively simple. Don't stress, because it gets easier.

Remember, any new skill requires practice and dedication. You've got the dedication part down, because for the next 30 days, you've committed to eating real food three times a day. Now, just practice! Use the tips throughout this book (especially the clean-up section on page 333) to help you streamline the process, stick to the Kitchen Fundamentals section to build confidence, and recruit the help of family or friends to help make the chopping and washing go by faster.

Okay, we've talked enough here.
Time to eat!

shopping list for omnivores

Protein

SEAFOOD
- BEST: wild-caught and sustainably fished
- BETTER: wild-caught and/or sustainable
- GOOD: farm-raised

RUMINANTS (beef, buffalo, lamb, elk, venison, etc.)
- BEST: 100 percent grass-fed and organic
- BETTER: grass-fed and/or organic
- GOOD: lean, fat trimmed/drained

EGGS
- BEST: pastured and organic
- BETTER: organic (omega-3 enriched optional)
- GOOD: store-bought

POULTRY (chicken, turkey, duck, pheasant, etc.)
- BEST: pastured and organic
- BETTER: organic
- GOOD: store-bought, skin removed

NON-RUMINANTS (pork, wild boar, rabbit, etc.)
- BEST: pastured and organic
- BETTER: organic
- GOOD: lean, fat trimmed/drained

PROCESSED MEATS (bacon, sausage, deli meat, etc.)
- BEST: 100 percent grass-fed/pastured and organic
- BETTER: organic
- AVOID: those with added sugar, MSG, sulfites, or carrageenan

Vegetables
- Acorn Squash
- Anise/Fennel Root
- Artichoke
- Arugula
- Asparagus
- Beets
- Bell Peppers
- Bok Choy
- Broccoli/Broccolini
- Broccoli Rabe
- Brussels Sprouts
- Buttercup Squash
- Butternut Squash
- Cabbage
- Carrots
- Cauliflower
- Celery
- Collard
- Cucumber
- Delicata Squash
- Eggplant
- Garlic
- Green Beans
- Greens (beet, mustard, turnip)
- Jalapeño
- Jicama
- Kale
- Kohlrabi
- Leeks
- Lettuce (all)
- Mushrooms (all)
- Okra
- Onions/Shallots
- Parsnips
- Potatoes (all)
- Pumpkin
- Radish
- Rutabaga
- Rhubarb
- Snow/Sugar Snap Peas
- Spaghetti Squash
- Spinach
- Sprouts
- Summer Squash
- Sweet Potato/Yams
- Swiss Chard
- Tomato
- Turnip
- Watercress
- Zucchini

Fruit
- Apples (all varieties)
- Apricots
- Bananas
- Blackberries
- Blueberries
- Cherries
- Dates
- Exotic Fruit (star fruit, quince)
- Figs
- Grapefruit
- Grapes (green and red)
- Kiwi
- Lemon
- Lime
- Mango
- Melon
- Nectarines
- Oranges
- Papaya
- Peaches

- Pears (all varieties)
- Pineapple
- Plum
- Pomegranate
- Raspberries
- Strawberries
- Tangerines
- Watermelon
- LIMIT: Dried Fruit

Fats

- BEST: COOKING FATS
  - Animal Fats
  - Clarified Butter
  - Coconut Oil
  - Extra-Virgin Olive Oil
  - Ghee
- BEST: EATING FATS
  - Avocado
  - Cashews
  - Coconut Butter
  - Coconut Meat/Flakes
  - Coconut Milk (canned)
  - Hazelnuts/Filberts
  - Macadamia Nuts
  - Macadamia Butter
  - Olives (all)
- OCCASIONAL: NUTS & SEEDS
  - Almonds
  - Almond Butter
  - Brazil Nuts
  - Pecans
  - Pistachio
- LIMIT: NUTS & SEEDS
  - Flax Seeds
  - Pine Nuts
  - Pumpkin Seeds/Pepitas
  - Sesame Seeds
  - Sunflower Seeds
  - Sunflower Seed Butter
  - Walnuts

Fresh herbs and spices

- Basil
- Bay Leaves
- Chives
- Cilantro
- Dill
- Ginger Root
- Lemongrass
- Oregano
- Parsley
- Rosemary
- Thyme

Dried herbs and spices

- Allspice
- Black Pepper
- Black Peppercorns
- Cayenne Pepper
- Chili Powder
- Chipotle Powder
- Cinnamon
- Cumin
- Curry Powder (red and yellow)
- Dill
- Garlic Powder
- Ground Cloves
- Ground Ginger
- Mustard Powder
- Nutmeg
- Onion Powder
- Oregano
- Paprika
- Red Pepper Flakes
- Sage
- Salt
- Thyme
- Wasabi Powder

Pantry items

- Apple Cider Vinegar
- Arrowroot Powder*
- Balsamic Vinegar
- Beef Broth
- Canned Salmon
- Canned Tuna
- Capers
- Chicken Broth
- Dill Pickles
- Dried Cranberries (sweetened with apple juice)
- Hot Sauce
- Red Wine Vinegar
- Rice Vinegar
- Roasted Red Peppers
- Sesame Oil
- Sun-Dried Tomatoes
- Tomato Paste
- Tomatoes (crushed and diced)
- Vegetable Broth
- White Vinegar

Beverages

- Apple Cider
- Club Soda
- Coconut Water
- Coffee
- Fruit Juice (orange, apple, pomegranate)
- Kombucha
- Mineral Water
- Naturally Flavored Water
- Seltzer Water
- Sparkling Water
- Tea (all varieties)
- Vegetable Juice

Optional

- Almond Flour
- Canned Vegetables (sweet potato, butternut squash, pumpkin)
- Cocoa (100 percent cacao)
- Coconut Aminos
- Coconut Flour
- Fish Sauce
- Mustard

Download this list at:
www.whole30.com/pdf-downloads

*Used only in Holiday Dinner on page 380.

making healthy meals easy

PRACTICE GOOD MEALTIME HAB-ITS. Eat meals at the table in a relaxed fashion. Do not allow distractions like TV, phone, or email while you are eating. Chew slowly and thoroughly, don't gulp. Take the time to enjoy the delicious, healthy food you have prepared!

Meals

Eat three meals a day, starting with a good breakfast. Base each meal around 1 to 2 palm-sized protein sources. Fill the rest of your plate with vegetables. Occasionally add a serving of fruit. Add fat in the following recommended amounts per meal:

- **ALL OILS AND COOKING FATS** (olive oil, animal fats, etc.): 1 to 2 thumb-sized portions

- **ALL BUTTERS** (ghee, coconut butter, nut butters, etc.): 1 to 2 thumb-sized portions

- **COCONUT** (shredded or flaked): 1 to 2 open (heaping) handfuls

- **OLIVES**: 1 to 2 open (heaping) handfuls

- **NUTS AND SEEDS:** Up to one closed handful

- **AVOCADO:** ½ to 1 avocado

- **COCONUT MILK:** Between ¼ and ½ of one (14-ounce) can

Make each meal large enough to satisfy you until the next meal—don't snack, if you can help it. Stop eating a few hours before bed.

Pre-workout

Eat 15 to 75 minutes pre-workout, as a signal to prepare your body for activity. If you train first thing in the morning, something is better than nothing. Choose foods that are easily digestible and palatable. This is the most variable factor in our template, so experiment with different foods, quantities, and timing.

Include a small amount of protein (half a meal size or smaller), and (optionally) a small amount of fat (half a meal size or smaller). Do not add fruit or carb-dense vegetables to your pre-workout snack.

Post-workout

Eat immediately following exercise (15 to 30 minutes). Eat a meal-sized easily digestible protein, plus the appropriate amount of carb-dense vegetables based on the Carb Curve in *It Starts With Food*. Do not use fruit as your primary post-workout carb, and add little to no fat. Examples of carb-dense vegetables appropriate for post-workout include sweet potatoes/yams, taro/poi, butternut squash, acorn squash, pumpkin, or beets.

Note, your PWO meal is a special bonus meal—not meant to replace breakfast, lunch, or dinner. Think of it as a necessary source of additional calories and nutrients, designed to help you recover faster and more efficiently from high intensity exercise.

good food on the road

Protein

- Deli meat
- Canned tuna, salmon, or chicken
- Hard-boiled eggs
- Smoked salmon (wild-caught)
- Shrimp (buy pre-cooked, or cook and peel them yourself)
- Your grocery store's brand of pre-cooked "simple" chicken breast or salmon
- Jerky (beef, salmon, etc.) like Primal Pacs, Chomps, or Wild Zora

Vegetables

- Carrots, celery, cucumber, sugar snap peas, snow peas, bell peppers
- Jicama (peel and slice into chunky sticks)
- Kale chips (make your own!)
- Toasted nori sheets like SeaSnax
- Fresh salsa
- Canned sweet potato, pumpkin, or butternut squash
- Baby food! (Sweet potato, butternut squash, or other vegetable varieties)

Fruit

- Whatever is fresh, local, in-season, and not too expensive
- Unsweetened applesauce
- Baby food (fruit varieties)
- Dried fruits (perfect for hiking)

Healthy fats

- Canned olives
- EVOO (extra virgin olive oil)
- Avocado or fresh guacamole
- Coconut milk
- Coconut meat or flakes
- Coconut butter
- Nuts, seeds, and nut butters

Kitchen tools

- Sharp paring knife (not in your carry-on!)
- Flexible cutting board
- Can opener, portable silverware, and (optionally) dishes and bowls
- One glass or porcelain container, for microwaving on the go

Bonus tips

PLANNING AND PREPARATION ARE KEY!

See page 402 for where to stock up on the Whole30 Approved brands mentioned above, and turn back to page 93 for more helpful Whole30 travel tips.

PROTEIN is the toughest on-the-go food. Plan ahead and stock up to cook chicken or salmon the night before, boil a dozen eggs, or purchase some compliant jerky ahead of time.

SMOKED SALMON is often overlooked, but the wild-caught stuff is a great source of omega-3 fatty acids and protein. Slice, roll around chunks of honeydew melon or kiwi, secure with a toothpick, and go.

FRUIT is way too easy to overdo when traveling, so swap some out for veggies. The flexible cutting board, sharp knife, and plastic silverware help you branch out from just carrots and celery.

FRESH SALSA and **GUACAMOLE** are lifesavers. Roll deli turkey around pepper slices and lettuce, secure with a toothpick, and dip in salsa and guacamole.

NUTS are also easy to overeat on when traveling. Try olives instead. They're portable, don't need refrigeration, and are the perfect plane food (if you drain the can before going through security).

ALL-IN-ONE "EMERGENCY" BARS (like Epic Bars) are a good source of protein, carbs, and fat on the go, but don't overdo them! Real food should always come first.

7-Day Meal Plan

	MONDAY	TUESDAY	WEDNESDAY	THURSDAY	FRIDAY	SATURDAY	SUNDAY
1	Spinach Frittata (page 206), side of fruit, avocado	Leftover ground beef & spaghetti squash topped with a Perfect Fried Egg (page 149)	Leftover chicken and roasted potatoes, drizzle of Pesto (page 315)	Perfect Scrambled Eggs (page 150) with berries, side of Perfect Steamed Spinach (page 171) with ghee	Leftover salmon, Butternut Squash Soup (page 266)	Kitchen Sink Scrambled Eggs (page 202, using leftover pork and greens), side of applesauce	Leftover carnitas topped with a Perfect Fried Egg (page 149), pan-fried plantains
2	Protein Salad (page 161, using our "traditional approach") on a bed of baby spinach, Ranch Dressing (page 316), side of fruit	Protein Salad in hollow bell pepper, sliced carrots, celery, and apple, with Ranch Dressing (page 316) for dipping	Mexican Tuna (page 238) in romaine leaves, leftover slaw, side of fruit	Leftover brisket and butternut squash, drizzle of pesto, side of fruit	Greek Salad (page 278) with Perfect Boiled Eggs (page 149), side of fruit	No-Fuss Salmon Cakes (page 346), leftover butternut squash soup, Green Beans with Onions, Mushrooms, and Peppers (page 280)	Leftover salmon cakes, Cold Thai Salad (page 274) with Sunshine Sauce (page 320)
3	Perfect Ground Meat (page 152) with Italian Seasoning, Tomato Sauce (page 324), Roasted Spaghetti Squash (page 294)	Perfect Seared Chicken Breast (page 157), Roasted Red Pepper Mayonnaise (page 312), Perfect Roasted Potatoes (page 166), Green Cabbage Slaw (page 282)	Slow Cooker Beef Brisket (page 214), with the butternut squash "Make it a Meal" variation, garden salad with dressing from Greek Salad (page 278)	Perfect Oven-Baked Salmon (page 160) with Broccoli, Mushrooms, and Yellow Squash with Red Pepper Sauce (page 264)	Pork Chops with Spiced Applesauce (page 258)	Roasted Sweet Potato (page 296) stuffed with Pulled Pork Carnitas (page 254), drizzle of Avocado Mayonnaise (page 310)	Chicken Sausage, Pepper, Onion, Kale Frittata (page 206), drizzle avocado mayo, fruit salad, Cauliflower Mash (page 270)

We'll address this up front—no, we are not giving you a 30-day meal plan. It's not because we're lazy, and it's not because we couldn't randomly slap 90 recipes into a calendar and call it your "meal plan." We're not, and we could have, and we are deliberately choosing not to.

The Whole30 is built on a foundation of tough love. All of the resources we give you in this book and on our website are the "love" part. We've done our best to give you all the information, guidance, support, and encouragement you'll need to succeed.

But here's the "tough" part:

You have to meet us halfway.

You're all grown-ups, and you are all perfectly capable of deciding what to eat a week from next Wednesday. Not only that, you *should* be in charge of exactly what you eat and when. Your Whole30 success, and your ability to take these new, healthy habits you create on the program with you for the rest of your life, depends on your ability to figure out how to make this work in your own life. If you blindly eat exactly what we tell you to eat for the next 30 days, how will you learn to meal plan, food prep, handle "food emergencies," and learn new cooking techniques? (Trick question—you won't.)

We've got a teach-you-how-to-fish kind of mindset, but we're not going to throw you out into the river with nothing but a rod and a lure. We'll give you a meal plan to get you through your first week—that's 21 opportunities for you to meal prep, cook, and figure out how to make this "cooking real food" thing work in your own life. We've included a good variety of protein options, vegetables, and added fats, flexibility with your fruit, and a number of simple cooking techniques to get you comfortable in the kitchen. We're using Whole30 kitchen fundamentals and recipes for your first five days, then allowing you to freestyle a bit on the weekend.

And in a minute, we're going to tell you exactly how we'd prep for your week, day by day.

Like we said, we would never just leave you out in the middle of the river.

Your Whole30 Week One Meal Plan

We designed this meal plan to stretch your grocery store budget, minimize the time you spend in the kitchen, and convince your taste buds that this Whole30 thing is tasty and satisfying. Meal prep is done throughout the week, but you'll have a little bit of a heavier load on Sundays, when most people take an hour or two to get ready for the week.

Many lunches and breakfasts involve leftovers. If you're cooking for one, you can just follow our recipes exactly as outlined, as they all serve two. If you're cooking for two (or more), make sure you double or adjust our ingredient quantities so you've got dinner and enough left over for the next day.

As we'll explain in the Recipes section, make sure you read through this entire plan before you head to the grocery store. It's important that you know what meals you'll be eating again the next day, which nights require the most prep time, and which mornings you'll be cooking breakfast versus just reheating breakfast.

Finally, we haven't built in any snacks, but especially in the first week, you'll want to make sure you have some extra food on hand should you find yourself hungry between meals. (It's common for your appetite to take a week or two to regulate—if you need a snack during this transition, no big deal.) Hard-boil a dozen eggs, stock up on some Whole30 Approved on-the-go foods (page 195), and make sure you always have some "emergency food" in your car, your gym bag, your purse, and your desk at work, just in case.

As we may have mentioned a few times already, when it comes to the Whole30, planning and preparation are key.

Sunday

You're in meal-prep mode! First, take an egg out of the fridge and put it in a glass of hot water, as you'll need it for your mayonnaise soon. Then, start your tomato sauce and roast your spaghetti squash—both take an hour of pretty hands-off time. While those are cooking, take 5 minutes to prepare a batch of Basic Mayonnaise (page 179). Use that to make a batch of Ranch Dressing, and to add to your Protein Salad. Finally, start making your Frittata about 5 minutes before your spaghetti squash timer goes off. When you pull the squash out of the oven, turn the heat to broil, pop in your frittata, and let it finish cooking. Finally, pack up a portion of protein salad, some baby spinach, and a small container of Ranch Dressing for tomorrow's lunch.

Whew. That wasn't so bad, was it? You'll be happy you took the time tomorrow!

Monday

Reheat your frittata for breakfast and walk out your front door with lunch in hand. When you get home for dinner, all you have to do is brown the ground beef and reheat the tomato sauce and spaghetti squash—dinner in under 15 minutes on a Monday night is way worth some extra prep on a lazy Sunday. After dinner, get used to setting aside a half hour or so to prep for the next day. Make it part of your nightly routine, before you sit down to watch a movie, read a book, or play a game.

Monday night, your job is to pack the rest of the protein salad, a hollowed-out pepper, and some carrot, celery, and apple slices with the rest of the ranch dressing for lunch. You'll also want to make the Roasted Red Pepper Sauce (page 316) and use some of it to prepare tomorrow night's mayo variation.

Bonus: Make the cabbage slaw for tomorrow night's dinner—it tastes better if the flavors meld in the fridge overnight.

Tuesday

Once again, breakfast is leftovers, and lunch is packed. When it's time for dinner, make the chicken, and roast your potatoes. A few potato tips: first, make extra! You'll eat the leftovers later. Because the chicken and potatoes both use the oven, start your spuds roasting at 425°F about 20 minutes before you start the chicken, then turn temp down to 350°F and finish baking them together.

Tuesday night, your post-dinner prep includes making a batch of Pesto (page 315), preparing your Mexican Tuna Boats (page 238), and peeling and chopping your butternut squash for the morning. Look—no cooking required! Pack up your lunch (the tuna, a few romaine leaves, your side of fruit, and any leftover slaw) and stash the squash in the fridge overnight.

Wednesday

Get up 15 minutes earlier so you can brown the brisket and get the slow cooker set up for dinner. (You can handle that, as breakfast is leftovers and lunch is packed). Wednesday at dinnertime, make a garden salad (pick any ingredients you want—lettuce, cucumber, peppers, onions, tomatoes, mushrooms, shredded carrots, olives, etc.) and prepare the dressing for the Greek Salad (page 278)—in fact, double the dressing, because you'll use it again on Friday. You'll be sitting down to a hot slow-cooked meal and a fresh, crisp salad in under 15 minutes.

Wednesday night, you're off! No food prep for tomorrow, just pack up your leftovers, some pesto, and a side of fruit for Thursday's lunch.

Thursday

Thursday morning, you actually do have to make breakfast, but don't worry—it'll only take about 10 minutes. As always, lunch is packed, giving you something delicious to look forward to at noon.

(Are your co-workers noticing your amazing meals yet?) At dinner, cook the salmon and vegetable side, topping your veggies with the leftover roasted red pepper sauce.

Thursday night, make your Butternut Squash Soup (page 266) and Greek Salad (page 278), hard-boil half a dozen eggs, and pack up your lunch. (Don't forget the leftover Greek dressing you made yesterday!)

Friday

Breakfast is leftovers and the soup you made last night, lunch is packed, and it's Friday! Friday night after work, make your Pork Chops with Spiced Applesauce. (Oh, but double the applesauce recipe—everything from the onion to the nutmeg—as you'll be eating more of that for breakfast tomorrow.)

Now, take the rest of the night off. It's the weekend!

Saturday

Your breakfast is pork chop leftovers and freshly wilted greens scrambled into some eggs, topped with leftover applesauce. You'll either start your slow-cooker Pulled Pork Carnitas (page 254) now, or wait and cook it in the oven mid-afternoon—your choice.

At lunchtime, make your No-Fuss Salmon Cakes (page 346) and Green Beans with Onions, Mushrooms, and Peppers (page 280), and reheat the rest of the butternut squash soup. Sometime during the day, make a batch of basic mayo and use some of it to prepare your Avocado Mayonnaise (page 310) for dinner.

Start your sweet potatoes roasting an hour before dinnertime, and pull them out when the carnitas are done. Saturday night, you can either make your Sunshine Sauce (page 320), or take the night off.

Sunday

Your Sunday breakfast is fun and easy—plantains add a sweet and festive side to your carnitas and eggs. (Look for them in your local Mexican market. Buy them very ripe and soft, not green. Slice them in ¼-inch rounds, melt some ghee in a skillet, and fry them on medium heat in batches, letting them brown on one side before flipping them once.)

Lunch is leftover salmon cakes, but first, prepare your Cold Thai Salad (page 274) and (if you skipped it last night) Sunshine Sauce. (Note: if you can't find sunflower seed butter, prep our Asian Vinaigrette on page 330 or the Cilantro-Lime Mayonnaise on page 310 instead).

Dinner is "brinner" (breakfast for dinner), taking our Spinach Frittata (page 206) recipe and adding your own variations. If you can't find compliant chicken sausage, substitute a half-portion of cooked Perfect Ground Meat (page 152), or prepare a double-batch of our Perfect Sausage (page 162), use two patties in your frittata, and save the rest for Monday's breakfast, lunch, or dinner. You'll also make a Cauliflower Mash (page 270)—we'd recommend doubling the recipe. (We see a delicious breakfast of frittata and cauliflower mash in your Monday future.)

Congratulations! You made it through your first week of the Whole30 eating a wide variety of nutrient-dense foods, cooking simple but delicious meals, and not feeling chained to your cutting boards or dishwasher. We're confident you can take it from here. Now let's get to the recipes!

Download our shopping list template at: www.whole30.com/pdf-download to make shopping for this 7-day meal plan easier.

EGGS

EGGS ARE ONE OF THE MOST VERSATILE AND COST-EFFECTIVE PROTEIN SOURCES ON THE WHOLE30, which can be a really good thing for your budget, but a not-so-good thing for your taste buds. It's easy to get burned out on eggs for breakfast, so maybe it's time we redefine "breakfast."

What do you think of when the word "breakfast" comes to mind? Typically, foods like cereal, muffins, bagels, and eggs. This can be a real problem on the Whole30, since three of those four traditional breakfast foods are off-limits on the program. (Make that four out of four for people with a specific sensitivity or allergy to eggs.) So let's start thinking of breakfast in different terms, and change the name to plain old "Meal 1." That brings about an entirely new perspective, doesn't it? It's no longer a traditional meal consumed in the morning—now it's just another meal in your three-meals-a-day template. Isn't that freeing?

We've given you some really versatile egg dishes in this book, both in Whole30 Cooking Fundamentals (starting on page 149) and in the recipes to come. These pages showcase a variety of cooking techniques to produce eggs five different ways (hard-boiled, scrambled, fried, poached, and frittata-fied), a proven way to stave off egg boredom.

But now, let's address the question we know you'll have at some point during your Whole30: "Do you have any egg-free breakfast ideas?" The answer is yes, we do. *Thousands.* Anything you could possibly eat on the Whole30 is just as good for Meal 1 as it is for Meal 3. Any recipe in this book, for instance. But some people can't imagine eating a dry-rubbed steak or short ribs first thing in the morning.

Those people are lacking imagination, and that makes us sad.

So let's talk about what you could eat for breakfast if you're not eating eggs. First, think of poultry. Chicken and turkey are easy to prepare, cook, or reheat, which makes it practical to prepare at 6 a.m. before you're fully caffeinated. Any one of our poultry recipes (starting on page 224) would be fantastic as an alternative to eggs in the morning—in fact, Melissa's Chicken Hash was invented for that specific purpose.

Salmon is another obvious choice—most of you have eaten smoked salmon for breakfast in the past, even if it was draped across a bagel and smeared with cream cheese. You can roast it, poach it, or buy it smoked add it into our hearty Greek Salad (page 278).

Wait, salad?

Yes! Don't overlook an early-morning salad. They're light, delicious, and make you feel like you started your day off with extra nutrition from those leafy greens. Channel your inner Scandinavia and enjoy some cold cuts (like salami, roast beef, or prosciutto), pickled vegetables, and a fresh garden salad first thing in the morning, or top your favorite salad fixings with grilled chicken, salmon, or even ground beef. Prep your ingredients and cook your protein the night before, and you've got a hearty, satisfying Meal 1 in under five minutes. (Don't tell us you don't have five minutes to prep in the morning—it takes longer than that to toast a frozen waffle.)

Here are some additional egg-free breakfast ideas from this book:

- Leftovers from last night—just eat the same meal all over again!

- Perfect Burger (page 153), topped with caramelized onions with a side of steamed spinach

- Perfect Oven-Baked Salmon (page 160), topped with compound butter (page 181), your favorite vegetable side, and fruit salad

- Protein Salad (page 161) served over salad greens

- Sausage and Sweet Potato Home Fries (page 208—skip the fried eggs)

- Leftover Brisket (page 214) with Butternut Squash Soup (page 266)

- Stuffed Peppers (page 222)

- Chicken Meatballs (page 226) and Gazpacho (page 276)

- Melissa's Chicken Hash (page 228)

- Harvest Chicken Salad (page 232)

- Halibut with Citrus Ginger Glaze (page 240) and Cauliflower Mash (page 270)

- Poached Salmon with Cucumber Dill Sauce (page 246) over fresh baby spinach

- Leftover Carnitas (page 254) "stuffed" inside a baked sweet potato

- Leftover Pork Ribs with BBQ Sauce (page 256) with sautéed peppers and onions

- Pork Chop and Applesauce (page 258) with a side of Sweet Potato Soup (page 300)

- Banger Sausage and Sweet Potato Mash (page 249—you won't even notice the egg in the sausage patties, or just skip adding it altogether if you're allergic)

Of course, if you really want to, you can still put an egg on any of these dishes. In fact, we've determined you can actually put a fried egg on anything. Trust us. It's science.

One last thing, because we know you're going to ask—yes, we want you to eat the whole egg. That's because half the protein and many of the vitamins, minerals, and phytonutrients are found in the yolk. And no, we're not worried about your cholesterol levels. The Whole30 is designed to minimize *systemic inflammation*, which is a way bigger driver of high cholesterol than your diet—even if you're regularly eating eggs and red meat. In fact, many doctors love our program because it offers a natural way to lower your "bad" cholesterol and triglycerides while boosting your "good" cholesterol.

Plus, in addition to the protein and micronutrients, all the fat in an egg is found in the yolk. Ready for some more science? Fat is what makes food taste good.

Really, this is all excellent news. Egg whites are so 1992.

kitchen sink scrambled eggs

SERVES 2

PREP TIME: 10 minutes
COOK TIME: 10 minutes
TOTAL TIME: 20 minutes

---

2 tablespoon cooking fat

½ onion, finely chopped

½ bell pepper, any color, cut into strips

1 cup sliced button, cremini, or portabella mushrooms

1 cup chopped greens (kale, spinach, chard, or mustard greens)

6 large eggs, beaten

1 avocado, split lengthwise, pitted, peeled, and diced

¼ teaspoon salt

¼ teaspoon black pepper

The whole point of the "kitchen sink" is to include any combination of cooked meat, seafood, vegetables, and fruit you like. (Yes, fruit! Eggs and fruit are a surprisingly delicious combination.) Use up stuff that's about to go bad, finish up those leftover vegetables from dinner last night, or shop deliberately and create something new.

Try sautéed peaches, spinach, and basil; smoked salmon, leeks, arugula, fennel, and dill; butternut squash, apples, and pecans; chicken sausage, roasted red peppers, and Kalamata olives; or roasted sweet potatoes, blueberries, and kale.

HEAT a large skillet over medium-low heat. Add the cooking fat and swirl to coat the bottom of the pan. When the fat is hot, add the onion, bell pepper, and mushrooms and cook, stirring, until the onions are translucent, 4 to 5 minutes.

STIR in the greens and cook until they begin to wilt (the time will vary depending on the type of green). Add the eggs and cook, stirring frequently and scraping the bottom and sides of the pan to prevent sticking, until the eggs are scrambled, fluffy, and still look wet but not runny, 5 to 7 minutes.

REMOVE the pan from the heat, top with the diced avocado, season with the salt and pepper, and serve.

⭐ SCRAMBLES *are less pressure than omelets and frittatas, as you don't have to try to hold them together. Remember to whisk or beat the eggs until they are completely blended, stir often while cooking, and don't be tempted to rush the process by cooking eggs over high heat, or you'll risk turning your scramble into rubber.*

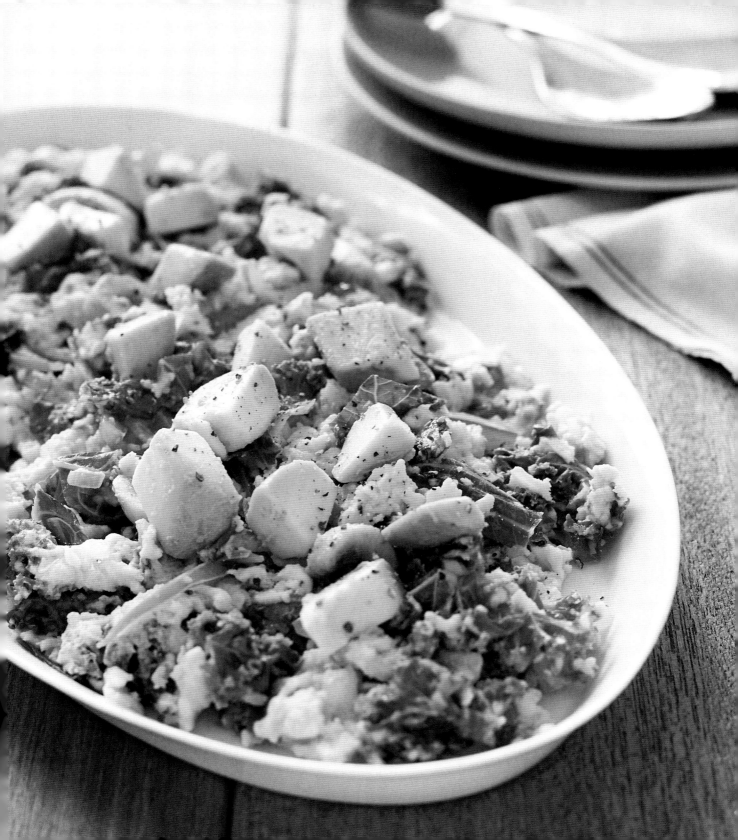

southwest scrambled eggs

SERVES 2

PREP TIME: 15 minutes
COOK TIME: 5 to 7 minutes
TOTAL TIME: 20 to 22 minutes

---

1 avocado, split lengthwise, pitted, and peeled

2 tablespoons cooking fat

6 large eggs, beaten

1 teaspoon salt

½ teaspoon black pepper

1 cup Salsa (page 319)

Crunched for time? Make your salsa up to two days ahead of time, or buy salsa from your grocery or health food store. Just read the label carefully—many salsas add sugar. (We have no idea why.) These eggs would also be delicious with a side of Guacamole (page 308) instead of the avocado.

SET the avocado halves flat side down on a cutting board and cut into thin slices.

HEAT the cooking fat in a large skillet over medium heat. In a mixing bowl, whisk the eggs with the salt and pepper. When the oil is hot, add the eggs and cook, stirring and scraping the bottom and sides of the pan to prevent burning, until the eggs are scrambled, fluffy, and still look wet but not runny, 5 to 7 minutes.

DIVIDE the eggs between 2 plates, top with the avocado, and spoon the salsa evenly over both portions.

MAKE IT A MEAL: Serve with steamed spinach and pan-fried plantains; or last night's leftover veggies and a side of berries.

⭐ PREPPING AVOCADOS *To easily remove an avocado pit, halve the avocado by carefully running a knife lengthwise along the seed, then quickly (and cautiously) tap a knife into the pit. Once it sticks, twist the knife slightly until the pit loosens from the avocado flesh and pull it out. Use a large spoon to separate the avocado from the peel.*

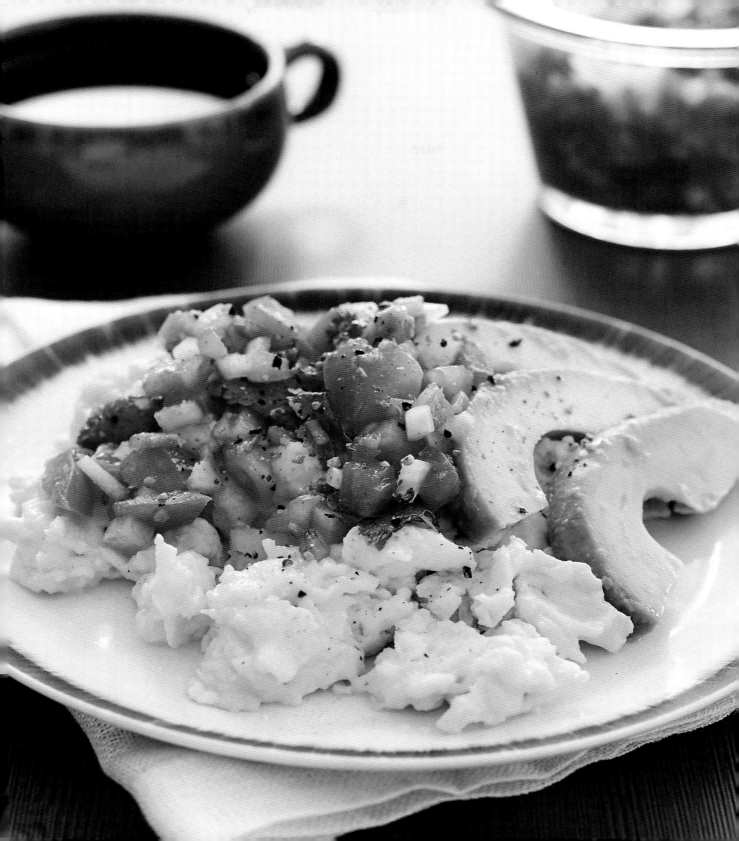

spinach frittata

SERVES 2

PREP TIME: 10 minutes

COOK TIME: 10 to 15 minutes

TOTAL TIME: 20 to 25 minutes

---

6 large eggs, beaten

¼ teaspoon salt

¼ teaspoon black pepper

2 tablespoons cooking fat

½ onion, diced

1 cup diced seeded tomato (plus a few slices for topping the frittata)

1 bag (about 9 ounces) baby spinach, roughly chopped

Grated zest and juice of ¼ lemon

Mix and match vegetables and meat to vary the flavors of your frittatas. Try making it Mexican (spiced cooked ground beef, thinly sliced jalapeños, diced tomato, and cilantro), Italian (cooked sausage, red peppers, onions, and basil), Greek (cooked chicken, sun-dried tomatoes, black olives, and artichoke hearts), or use any leftover meat and vegetables you happen to have in your fridge for a kitchen sink frittata.

SET the oven to broil (or preheat to 500°F).

IN a mixing bowl, whisk the eggs with the salt and pepper.

HEAT a large oven-safe skillet over medium heat. Add the cooking fat to the pan and swirl to coat the bottom. When the fat is hot, add the onion and tomato and cook, stirring, until softened, 2 to 3 minutes. Add the spinach and let it wilt for 30 seconds. Add the eggs and fold them into the vegetables with a rubber spatula. Cook, without stirring to let the eggs set on the bottom and sides of the pan, until the eggs are firm and still appear wet, 3 to 4 minutes. Lay a few tomato slices on top. Drizzle the lemon juice and sprinkle the lemon zest over the top.

TRANSFER the pan with the eggs to the oven and broil 4 to 6 inches from the heat (or bake in the preheated oven) for 3 to 5 minutes, until the top is golden brown. Cut into slices and serve hot out of the pan.

⭐ COOKING VARIATIONS *If you don't have an oven-safe skillet, you can cook the frittata in a regular pan on the stovetop, then transfer the frittata to a Pyrex dish to broil. Preheat the oven to 350°F, and grease the bottom and sides of your baking dish with coconut oil or ghee. Cook the vegetables in a large frying pan on the stovetop as directed. Then, add the cooked vegetables to the bowl with the eggs, and transfer the mixture to the baking dish. Bake for 25 to 30 minutes, until the frittata is set in the center and slightly golden on top. Drizzle the lemon juice and sprinkle the zest over the top just before serving. Your frittata will reheat beautifully the next day. Or enjoy it cold! A slice is a really easy and delicious on-the-go breakfast or lunch.*

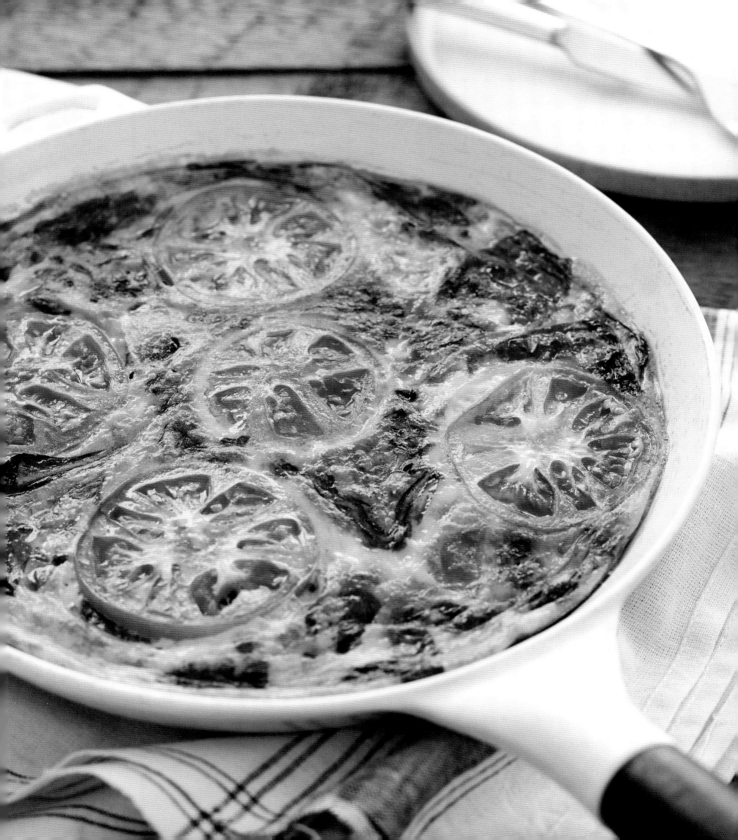

diner breakfast: eggs, sausage, and home fries

SERVES 2

PREP TIME: 5 to 10 minutes
COOK TIME: 15 to 20 minutes
TOTAL TIME: 20 to 30 minutes

3 tablespoons cooking fat

¼ cup finely diced white onion

½ pound ground meat (pork, chicken, turkey)

¼ teaspoon dried sage

¼ teaspoon salt

⅛ teaspoon black pepper

⅛ teaspoon garlic powder

1 sweet potato, peeled and cut into large dice

½ bell pepper, (any color), seeded, ribs removed, and diced

4 large eggs, cracked into a bowl

This all-in-one breakfast would be delicious with some Hollandaise (page 314), Ranch Dressing (page 316), Chimichurri (page 306), or Buffalo Sauce (page 304) drizzled over the top.

PREHEAT the oven to 350°F. Line a baking sheet with parchment paper.

TO make the sausage, heat 1 tablespoon of the cooking fat in a large heavy skillet over medium-high heat. When the fat is hot, add the onion and cook, stirring, for until softened, about 2 minutes.

TRANSFER the onion to a mixing bowl and add the ground meat, sage, salt, pepper, and garlic powder. Form the mixture into 4 equal patties and set the sausage aside.

TO make the home fries, return the same skillet to the stove and heat over medium-high heat. Melt 1 tablespoon of the cooking fat and swirl to coat the bottom of the pan. When the fat is hot, add the sweet potato and cook, stirring occasionally so all sides make contact with the hot pan, for 4 minutes. Add the bell pepper and cook, stirring, until softened, 2 to 3 minutes. Spread the home fries mixture evenly onto the prepared baking sheet. Bake for 5 minutes.

MEANWHILE, to cook the sausage, return the same skillet to the stove and heat over medium heat. Add the sausage patties and cook until browned, about 2 minutes on each side.

ADD the sausage to the home fries on the baking sheet. Return to the oven and bake for 5 to 7 minutes, until the sausage is no longer pink in the middle and the home fries are fork-tender.

MEANWHILE, to cook the eggs, add the remaining 1 tablespoon cooking fat to the same skillet and melt over medium heat. Slide all 4 eggs gently into the pan and let them cook slowly, yolk-side up, until the yolks are cooked but still bright in color, 5 to 8 minutes.

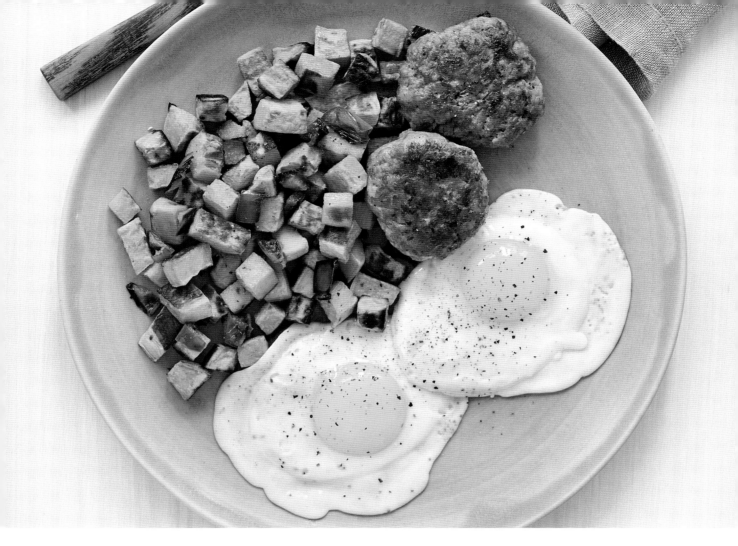

ARRANGE the sausage patties and home fries on 2 plates. With a spatula, carefully remove the eggs from the pan and either lay them over the home fries or place on the side.

⭐ CRACKING EGGS *Having trouble cracking your eggs without breaking the yolk? The key is a brief, sharp tap (not a hard rap) on a sharp surface. The side of your pan or mixing bowl might be too blunt to do the trick, so try a sharp tap with a butter knife, or use a pan or bowl with a more defined edge. And if the yolks do break, no big deal! Just drop them into the pan as-is, and let the yolk cook without mixing or stirring for that fried egg taste.*

seared salmon benedict

SERVES 2

PREP TIME: 15 minutes
COOK TIME: 10 minutes
TOTAL TIME: 25 minutes

---

2 salmon fillets (5 ounces each), skin removed

1 teaspoon salt

½ teaspoon black pepper

3 tablespoons cooking fat

2 large eggs, poached (see page 150)

½ cup Hollandaise (page 314)

1 pinch cayenne pepper

It's important that the fat be very hot to properly sear fish. To test, toss in a few grains of sea salt, or a small piece of your ingredients (like a bit of garlic or a small square of onion). If it sizzles, your pan is ready! You can also stick the end of a chopstick or a wooden spoon into the oil. If bubbles form around the wood, you've reached the right temperature.

PREHEAT the oven to 350°F.

SEASON both sides of salmon evenly with the salt and pepper. In a large oven-safe skillet, heat the cooking fat over medium-high heat, swirling to coat the bottom of the pan. When the fat is hot, add the salmon fillets skinned-side down. Sear the salmon until you see the edges start to pull away from the pan, 3 to 4 minutes. Slide a metal spatula under each fillet and turn. (If they are ready, they will come off with little effort, so don't rush this step! If the fillets don't readily release, allow another minute before turning them over.)

TRANSFER the pan to the oven and bake for 5 to 7 minutes, until white "curd" protein starts to show on the sides of the salmon. Check often, as thinner salmon will cook faster. Transfer the cooked salmon to a plate.

PLACE the poached eggs over the salmon fillets and drizzle evenly with the hollandaise. Top with a dash or two of cayenne pepper and black pepper.

⭐ SKINNING SALMON *To remove the skin from salmon, place the fillet skin-side down on a flat surface. Pressing gently on the top of the fillet to hold it in place, slide a sharp knife between the skin and the flesh closest to your body. While holding on to the flap of skin you just created, slide the knife away from you, separating the skin from the flesh. Discard the skin. Most fish markets and health food stores will skin your fish for you, so feel free to ask your fishmonger for this service before he wraps up your purchase.*

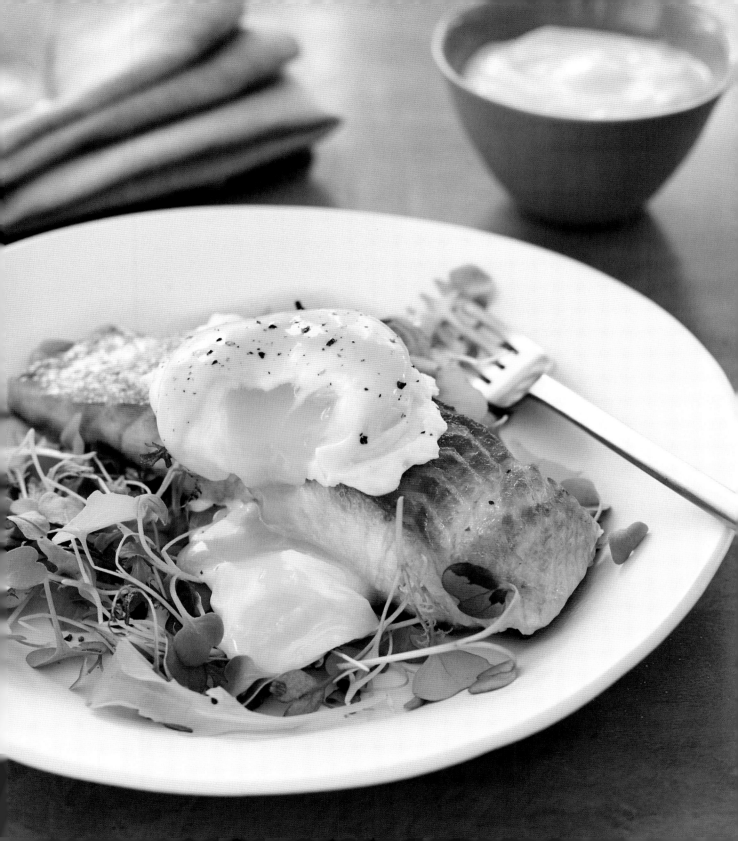

RED MEAT

WE'RE TELLING YOU UP FRONT, some of our beef recipes involve marinating your meat for up to eight hours. Why the warning? A few reasons—which apply to every recipe in the book that requires a marinade, brine, or rub.

First, you'll be tempted to skip this step. Please don't. If you do, you'll be missing out on (a) infusing your meat with a glorious array of flavors, (b) transforming tougher cuts to tender, melt-in-your-mouth goodness, and (c) feeling like an accomplished adult who does grown-up things like returning library books on time and marinating steak.

Second, discovering this can be maddening when you're flipping through a cookbook an hour before dinner. "This looks delicious . . . I have all these ingredients . . . Oh, come on! I have to marinate this?! I'm hungry *now*."

Don't be mad. Remember, you *want* to do this additional step with some of these recipes—but if your meat needs a few hours of soak time, you can't leave your preparations until the last minute. Plus, it's really not that hard to work this into your busy schedule. If we were you, here's how we'd do it:

In your Sunday meal planning session, you decide to make the Steak Salad on page 220 for dinner on Monday. But wait—this dish requires a marinated steak, so you're already thinking ahead!

Sunday night after dinner, you take fifteen minutes to make the Cilantro-Lime Mayonnaise and prepare your marinade, and toss them in the fridge in preparation for the next day.

Come Monday morning, you take two minutes to transfer your steaks and the marinade to a gallon-size resealable plastic bag, squeeze out the air, and put it back in the fridge. You spend the next eight hours working hard at the office while your steak is working hard getting tender and flavorful. (Don't worry if there's more than eight hours between when you leave the house and when you return—an hour or two either way doesn't matter with red meat.)

Now Monday night when you return home, all you have to do is chop a few veggies, cook the steak, and dress the salad—dinner in under 20 minutes. See, wasn't that easy?

If you *really* wanted to plan ahead, you could even reserve a small amount of the marinade in a separate container when you make it, drizzling the fresh stuff over your cooked meat just before serving to add even more flavor. (Please don't reuse your marinade after it's been in contact with raw meat. Ew.)

We're careful to note long cooking times (like the Braised Beef Brisket on page 214) or marinate times in each recipe, so if you just pay attention during your meal planning sessions, you'll never have to get mad at your cookbook—or eat tough, dry, flavorless meat—ever again.

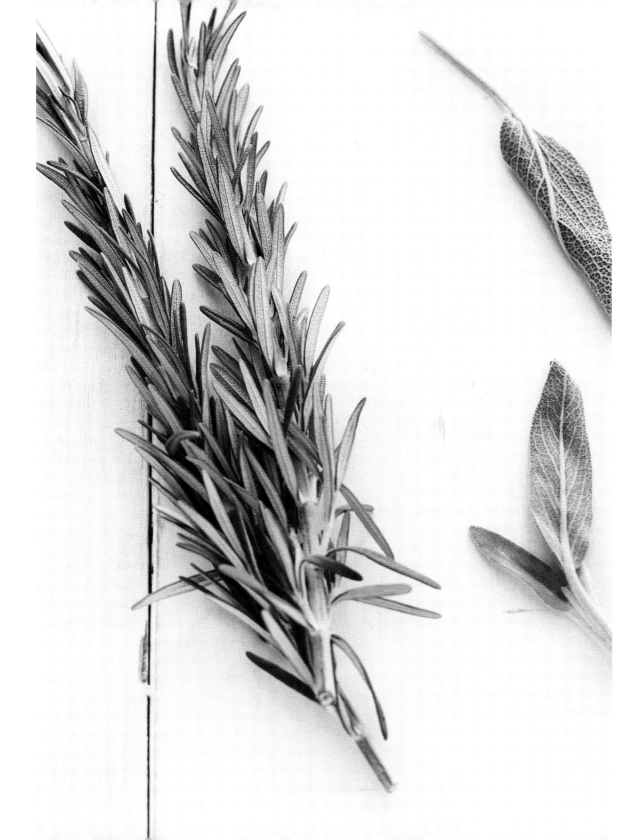

braised beef brisket

SERVES 2

PREP TIME: 15 minutes
COOK TIME: 4 hours
TOTAL TIME: 4 hours 15 minutes

1 tablespoon salt

1 teaspoon black pepper

1½ pounds beef brisket, trimmed

3 tablespoons cooking fat

½ medium onion, peeled and quartered

4 cloves garlic, peeled

2 sprigs fresh thyme

5 cups Beef Bone Broth (page 178) or water

You could skip the first step, but we don't recommend it: Browning the brisket creates a crust-like texture on the outside and a deep, rich flavor inside. Trust us, it's worth the extra effort (and if you use the same pan for stovetop and oven, it doesn't create any more dishes to wash).

⭐ FOR THE SLOW COOKER *This is the perfect dish to prep in the morning— you'll have dinner waiting for you as soon as you walk in the door from work. Add all ingredients to the slow cooker, covering with broth or water just to the top of the meat (it should not require the full 5 cups). Cover and cook over low heat for 8 to 9 hours. If you have the time, follow the recipe instructions and brown the brisket on the stovetop first for extra flavor.*

PREHEAT the oven to 350°F.

MIX the salt and pepper in a small bowl and use to season the brisket evenly on both sides.

IN a Dutch oven or deep flameproof roasting pan, melt the cooking fat over medium-high heat, coating the bottom of the pan. When the fat is hot, add the brisket and sear until golden brown, about 2 minutes on each side. Remove the brisket from the pan.

REDUCE the heat to medium under the same pan and add the onion. Cook, scraping the bottom of the pot with a wooden spoon to prevent burning, until the onion is softened, 2 to 3 minutes. Add the garlic and cook until aromatic, about 1 minute. Add the thyme, broth or water, and brisket, increase the heat to medium-high, and bring to a boil.

COVER the pot, transfer to the oven, and bake, turning the meat after each hour, for 3½ to 4 hours, until the brisket is fork tender.

TRANSFER the brisket to a bowl and shred or slice thin, discarding the excess fat. Discard the thyme stems.

LADLE the cooking liquid, onions, and garlic from the pan into a food processor or blender. Blend the sauce completely. Place the pan back on the stovetop, return the sauce to the pan, and bring to a simmer over medium-high heat. Simmer until the sauce coats the back of a wooden spoon, about 5 minutes.

SERVE the brisket warm with the sauce.

MAKE IT A MEAL: Make this an easy dinner by adding 2 quartered peeled sweet potatoes, 1 diced peeled large butternut squash, and/or 4 to 6 roughly chopped carrots to the pan and cooking with the brisket.

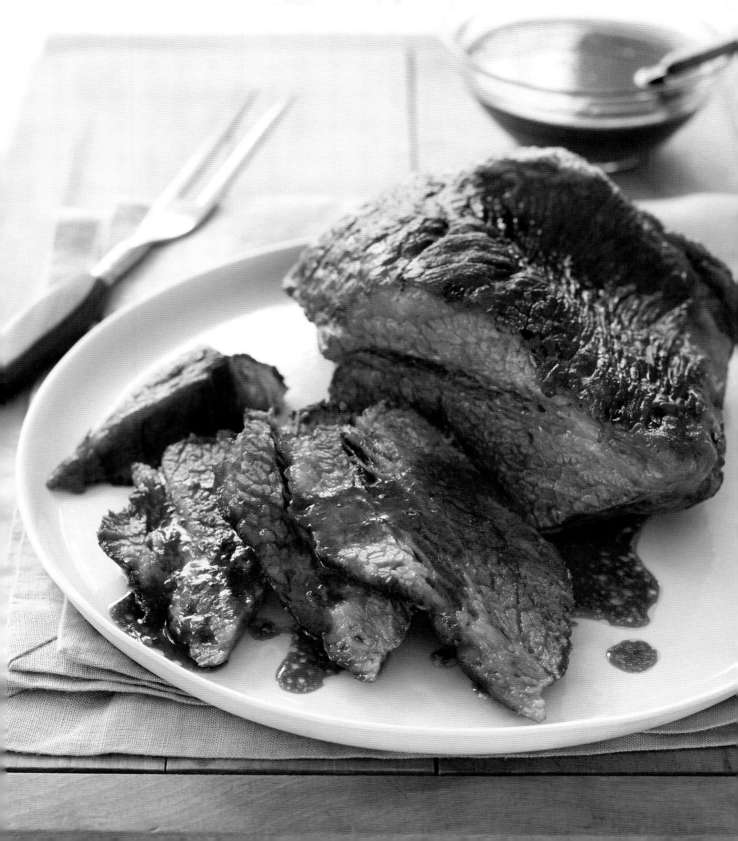

grilled steak with garlic-shallot puree and avocado

SERVES 2

PREP TIME: 15 minutes

COOK TIME: 25 minutes

TOTAL TIME: 40 minutes

---

2 steaks (5 ounces each) for grilling
(sirloin, strip, rib eye, tenderloin)

1 teaspoon salt

1 teaspoon black pepper

2 cloves garlic, peeled

1 shallot, peeled

2 tablespoons extra-virgin olive oil

1 avocado, split lengthwise, pitted,
and peeled

Roasting the shallot and garlic imparts a
rich, deep flavor, but you could cut about
20 minutes off your cooking time by
sautéing instead of roasting: First mince
the shallot and garlic. Heat a large
skillet over medium-high heat. Add
1 tablespoon cooking fat and swirl to
coat the bottom of the pan. Add the
shallot and cook until translucent (2 to
3 minutes), then add the garlic and
cook until aromatic (about 1 minute).
Puree in the blender as directed.

REMOVE the steaks from the refrigerator 30 minutes
before cooking. Preheat a grill to high heat (500°F) and the
oven to 350°F. Line a baking sheet with foil.

MIX the salt and pepper in a small bowl and use two-thirds
of the mixture to season the steaks.

TOSS the garlic and shallot in 1 tablespoon of the olive oil
and arrange on the prepared baking sheet. Season evenly
with the remaining salt and pepper. Roast in the oven for
25 minutes, until the cloves are soft throughout. Transfer
the garlic and shallots to a food processor, add the remaining 1 tablespoon olive oil, and puree. Transfer the puree to
a dish, cover with foil to keep warm, and set aside.

LAY the steaks on the hot grill and sear for 2 to 3 minutes.
The steaks should pull off easily when they are seared. Turn
the steaks over and sear the other side—the second side
doesn't take as long, 1 to 2 minutes, or to desired doneness (see chart on page 154). Let the steaks rest for 5 to 10
minutes.

MEANWHILE, sear the avocado halves pitted side down
on the grill until lightly browned, 3 to 4 minutes.

ARRANGE the avocado and steaks on plates and top the
steaks with the warm garlic and shallot puree.

MAKE IT A MEAL: This flavorful steak goes great with
the Roasted Beet, Orange, and Avocado Salad (page 290)
or Green Beans with Sautéed Onion, Mushrooms, and
Peppers (page 280).

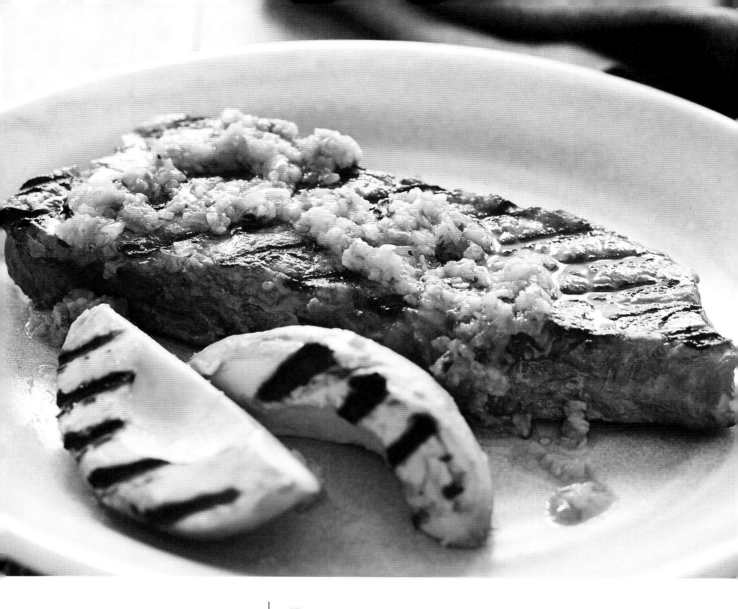

⭐ GRILLING STEAK *Grilling room-temperature steak keeps the outside from overcooking while waiting for the cold inside to reach the right temperature. And don't just tuck right into that gorgeous steak when you pull it off the grill—let it rest! If you cut into your steak fresh off the grill (or out of the pan), all those juices (and flavor) will spill out onto your plate, making your meat both drier and less tasty. Letting it rest allows the steak to cool slightly, causing the muscle fibers to relax and retain all those delicious juices in the meat.*

chimichurri beef kabobs

SERVES 2

PREP TIME: 20 minutes

MARINATE TIME: 1 to 8 hours

COOK TIME: 15 minutes

TOTAL TIME: 35 minutes plus marinating

---

1 pound lean steak (sirloin, strip, flank), cut into 1-inch dice

1½ cups Chimichurri (page 306)

1 red, yellow, or orange bell pepper, seeded, ribs removed, and cut into 1½-inch squares

1 onion, cut into 6 wedges

1 zucchini, cut into 1½-inch-thick rounds

If you don't have a grill, you have two other options for the kabobs. First, buy a grill plate for your stove and follow the same directions—it's just like a barbecue, minus the mosquitoes. Or, you can broil, and then bake the skewers: Preheat the oven to Broil (or 500°F) and place the skewers on a foil-lined baking sheet. Broil the kabobs for 3 minutes, then flip the skewers and broil for another 3 minutes. Reduce the oven temperature to 350°F and brush the skewers with the remaining chimichurri. Bake to desired doneness, 12 to 15 minutes.

IF using wooden skewers, soak them in water for 30 minutes to 1 hour to prevent them from burning.

PLACE the steak in a resealable plastic bag or nonreactive bowl with a lid. Cover the steak with enough chimichurri (about 1 cup) to coat thoroughly. Seal the bag or cover the bowl and marinate the steak in the refrigerator for 1 to 8 hours; more is better, especially for tougher cuts. (Feel free to leave your steak marinating overnight.)

REMOVE the steak from the refrigerator 30 minutes before cooking. Preheat the grill to high heat (500°F).

REMOVE the steak from the marinade; discard the marinade. Prepare the kabobs by threading the steak, bell pepper, onion, and zucchini onto soaked wooden skewers or metal skewers, alternating meat and vegetables. You should be able to make about 6 skewers.

GRILL the kabobs directly over high heat for 2 minutes on each side. Reduce the heat to medium (or move the kabobs to indirect heat). Grill to desired doneness, 12 to 15 minutes, and serve with the remaining chimichuri. (The easiest way to check is to remove one of the kebabs from the heat and cut into the meat, checking for color.)

MAKE IT A MEAL: This summertime BBQ favorite goes great with Watermelon Salad (page 359) and the Green Cabbage Slaw (page 282).

⭐ MARINATING *Don't marinate in a bowl made of copper, cast iron, aluminum, or easily stained plastic. When you add high-acid foods like citrus juice or tomato sauce to these kinds of bowls, they can react with the metal and impart a metallic taste to your foods. Instead, use a nonreactive bowl like glass or stainless steel. Always marinate in the fridge to avoid bacteria growth, and make sure to discard any remaining marinade, since it's been in contact with raw meat.*

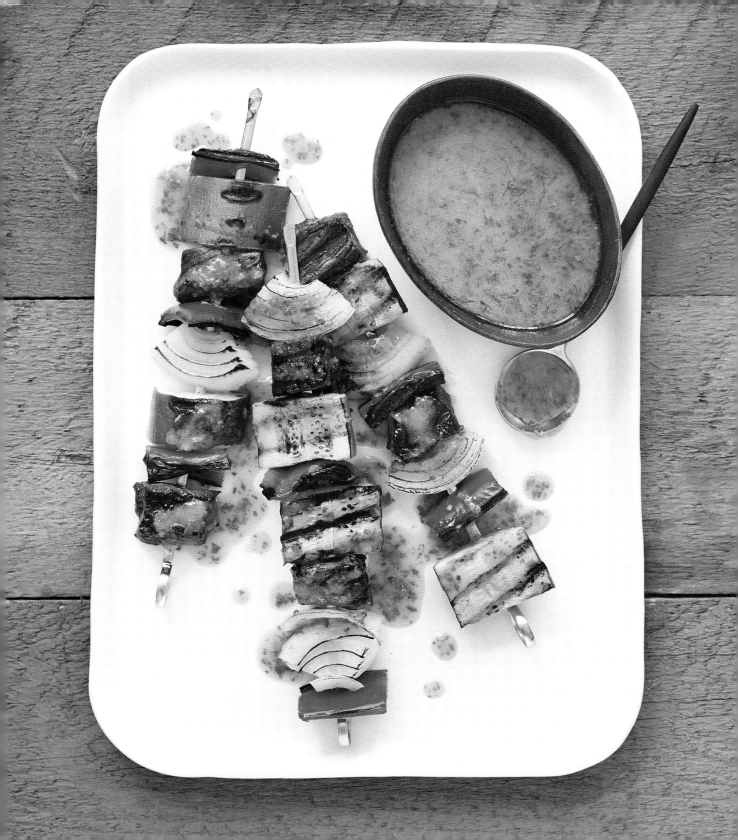

steak salad with cilantro-lime mayo

SERVES 2

PREP TIME: 20 minutes

MARINATE TIME: 1 to 8 hours

COOK TIME: 20 minutes

TOTAL TIME: 40 minutes plus marinating

½ cup extra-virgin olive oil

4 limes, juiced

¼ cup finely diced onion

2 cloves garlic, minced

2 tablespoons roughly chopped fresh cilantro

1 teaspoon mustard powder

1 pound beef (flank steak, sirloin, or strip steak)

4 cups salad greens

1 avocado, split lengthwise, pitted, peeled, and cut into large dice

½ cup halved cherry tomatoes

1 red, yellow, or orange bell pepper, seeded, ribs removed, and cut into large dice

½ cup Cilantro-Lime Mayonnaise (page 310)

You can easily swap out the steak for chicken, shrimp, salmon, or cod. Chicken can marinate for the same amount of time, but seafood should only "soak" for 20 minutes—any longer and the acid from the lime juice will start to turn the fish to mush. For a vegetarian version, use hard-boiled eggs in place of meat.

TO make the marinade, in a food processor, combine the olive oil, lime juice, onion, garlic, cilantro, and mustard powder and blend on low speed. Place the beef in a resealable plastic bag or a nonreactive bowl with a lid and add the marinade. Seal the bag or cover the bowl and marinate in the refrigerator for 1 to 8 hours; more is better, especially for tougher cuts of meat. (Feel free to leave your steak marinating overnight, or start your dinner prep in the morning before work.)

REMOVE the steak from the refrigerator 30 minutes before cooking. Preheat the oven to 350°F. Heat a grill to high heat (500°F) or heat a heavy skillet over high heat on the stovetop. Line a baking sheet with foil.

REMOVE the beef from the marinade; discard the marinade. On the grill or in the skillet on the stovetop, sear the beef over high heat until a light crust is formed, 2 to 3 minutes each side. Transfer the beef to the prepared baking sheet. Roast the beef in the oven for 8 to 15 minutes (depending on thickness) to desired doneness. (See page 154 for temperature guidelines.) Let the steak rest for 5 to 10 minutes, then thinly slice.

WHILE the beef rests, toss the salad greens with the avocado, tomato, and bell pepper in a large bowl, then divide between 2 plates.

PLACE slices of steak on top of the greens. Add 1 tablespoon water (or more) to the cilantro-lime mayo and mix thoroughly, until it's the consistency of salad dressing. Drizzle the dressing over the steak and salad and serve.

⭐ SALAD GREENS *You may want to choose a heartier green for this dish to stand up to the warm steak and bold dressing. Try romaine, endive, or arugula, or make a bed of baby spinach or ribbon-cut kale in colder months. If you're serving your leftovers cold, a butter head lettuce variety (butter, Boston, or Bibb) would be delicious.*

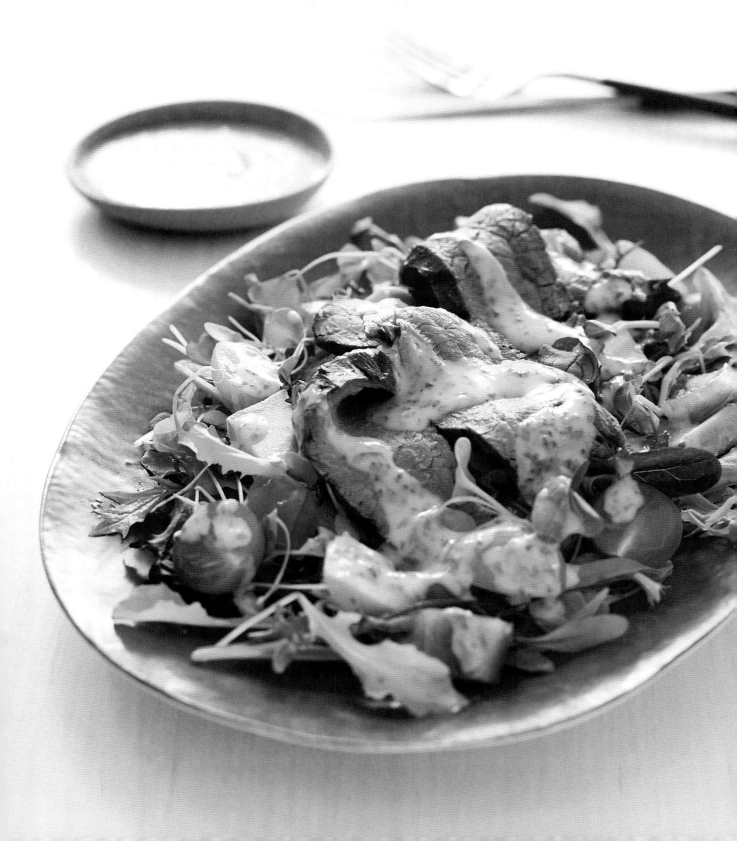

stuffed peppers

SERVES 2

PREP TIME: 20 minutes

COOKING TIME: 30 minutes

TOTAL TIME: 50 minutes

---

4 red, yellow, or orange bell peppers (preferably round in shape)

3 tablespoons cooking fat

¼ cup finely chopped onion

2 cloves garlic, minced (or 1 teaspoon garlic powder)

4 kale leaves, stems removed, leaves finely chopped

1 pound ground meat (beef, lamb, bison)

2 tablespoons tomato paste

¼ teaspoon cumin

¼ teaspoon chili powder

½ teaspoon salt

¼ teaspoon black pepper

1 cup finely chopped peeled winter squash (butternut, acorn, etc.)

This dish just begs you to use up all of the leftover vegetables you have in your fridge. Add some chopped mushrooms, spinach, cauliflower, or broccoli in place of or in addition to the kale. The more vegetables you add to the mix, the more peppers you'll need to hold all that stuffing, so buy one or two extra just in case—or enjoy any filling that doesn't fit in the peppers on top of a salad or in a bowl drizzled with some Pesto (page 315) or Ranch Dressing (page 316) for lunch the next day.

PREHEAT the oven to 350°F. Line a deep baking dish with parchment paper.

WITH a paring knife, slice around the top of each bell pepper and gently pull up on the stem. Discard the seeded core. Place the peppers in the prepared dish. Bake for 10 minutes, until softened. Set aside.

MEANWHILE, melt the cooking fat in a large skillet over medium heat and swirl to coat the bottom. When the fat is hot, add the onion and cook, stirring with a wooden spoon, until translucent, 2 to 3 minutes. Add the garlic and continue to cook until aromatic, about 1 minute. Add the kale and cook for 1 minute, stirring. Add the ground meat and cook, breaking up the meat with a spatula or wooden spoon and stirring it into the vegetables, for 2 to 3 minutes. Stir in the tomato paste, cumin, chili powder, salt, and pepper. Cook until the meat is mostly browned, 7 to 9 minutes. Stir in the squash and cook until the squash is slightly softened, 2 to 3 minutes.

DIVIDE the meat and squash mixture evenly among the softened bell peppers. Return to the oven and bake for 10 minutes, until the peppers look wrinkly and the beef is slightly browned on top.

⭐ STABILIZING PEPPERS *If your peppers won't stay upright in the pan, gently slice across the bottom to create a flat surface. Only skim the bottom of the pepper with your knife, however—you don't want to cut too much away and create a hole for the meat and juices to leak through.*

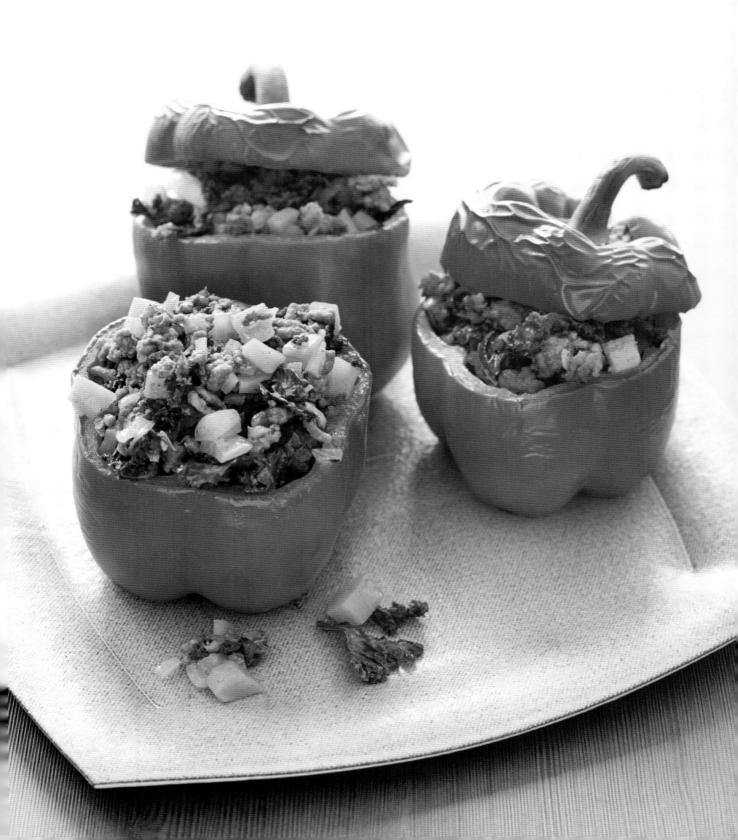

POULTRY

LET'S PLAY A GAME: we'll say the word "chicken" and you'll say the first word that comes into your head. Ready? Chicken.

Did you just say "dry," "boring," "rubbery," or "meh"? Yeah, that's what we thought. Chicken (and turkey, and poultry in general) gets kind of a bum rap as being the vanilla of the meat world, and you're probably not super excited about the idea of eating even more chicken. But we've got one piece of advice that is going to change your chicken-views forever. Ready for it?

Stop overcooking your birds.

Seriously, people. You *think* you don't like chicken, but the truth is, you're just cooking it to death, which leaves it dry, rubbery, and flavorless. We know you're worried about undercooked meat, and we're not suggesting anyone eat their chicken rare. But there are a few things you can do to ensure your chicken is properly cooked and juicy, tender, and flavorful.

First, you must pound. Buy a meat tenderizer (page 145) and pound your chicken breasts so they're uniform in thickness. This prevents the thinner ends from drying out while you're waiting for the thicker part to cook through. This step takes approximately 60 seconds, and is actually an effective stress-reliever.

Next, get a good sear. We describe this technique in several recipes, but the idea is simple. Get your pan and cooking oil hot, place the chicken breast in the pan, and leave it alone for a few minutes. Don't poke it, stir it, or move it. Just let it sit, allowing the outside to crust up to a nice golden brown. (This takes 3 to 4 minutes.) You'll know it's done when it lifts easily from the pan, and doesn't stick. Optionally, you can flip it and sear the other side too, or just continue on with your cooking technique. This traps the juices inside the chicken (where they belong), instead of letting them escape into the pan.

Finally, don't guess using visual cues—use a meat thermometer (page 143) to tell you when your chicken is done. According to the experts, a chicken is properly (safely) cooked when it reaches 165°F. But remember, meat keeps cooking even after you pull it off the heat. If you wait until your bird is 165°F (or 170°F, for good measure) *before* you remove it from the pan, it'll keep cooking on your plate, leaving you with dry, tough chicken.

Stick your thermometer in the thickest part of the bird, without touching any bones. If you're making boneless chicken breasts (pounded evenly, right?) you'll have to get creative and stick the thermometer in sideways. Keep an eye on the temperature as you approach the recommended cooking times, and pull your bird off the heat when it's 160°F. Let it "rest" (sit on the kitchen counter on a dish or serving tray) for 5 minutes, or until the thermometer reads 165°F.

Perfection! A delicious, evenly cooked, juicy, tender, flavorful bird. *Now* you like chicken.

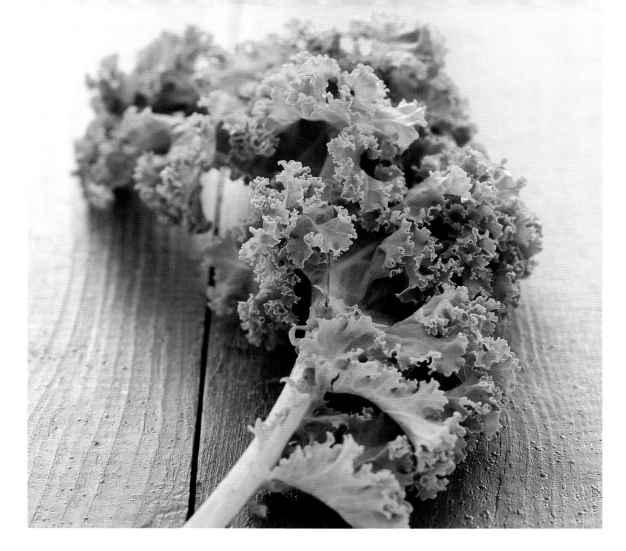

BONUS TIP: Marinating or brining your bird before cooking it can impart even more delicious flavor. We've given you some marinades in the Dressings and Sauces section starting on page 306, but here's a simple brining technique you can employ on any kind of poultry, whether it's the whole bird, breast, or thigh:

Mix ¼ cup of salt into 4 cups of lukewarm water until the salt is fully dissolved, then place in a plastic resealable bag or bowl with your poultry. (Make sure the poultry is fully covered—double the brine if necessary.) Place in the fridge for 30 minutes to 1 hour. Remove the chicken from the brine, rinse it, then pat it dry. Proceed to the Perfect Seared Chicken Breast recipe on page 157 and prepare to have your socks knocked off.

You can even mix various herbs and spices (like minced garlic or ginger, sprigs of rosemary, thyme, sage, slices of citrus, or bay leaves) into your brine to impart even more flavor.

Now you *love* chicken. Happy day.

chicken meatballs

SERVES 2

PREP TIME: 20 minutes
COOK TIME: 15 minutes
TOTAL TIME: 35 minutes

1 pound ground chicken thigh

1 large egg, beaten

¼ onion, finely chopped

2 cloves garlic, minced

2 teaspoons minced fresh oregano, (or 1 teaspoon dried oregano)

1 teaspoon salt

½ teaspoon black pepper

2 tablespoons cooking fat, plus more if needed

While it's not necessary, if you stock grain-free flours in your pantry, you could add ¼ cup of almond flour or 2 tablespoons of coconut flour to your meat mixture to make your meatballs more dense in texture. Change the flavor of this dish by swapping out the oregano for fresh rosemary, sage, or thyme. Or add 2 tablespoons of your favorite hot sauce to the mixture and serve with our Ranch Dressing (page 316). These also reheat like a dream, so double the batch and enjoy for a few extra meals.

PREHEAT the oven to 350°F. Line a baking sheet with parchment paper.

THOROUGHLY mix the chicken, egg, onion, garlic, oregano, salt, and pepper in a large bowl. Roll into 15 to 20 meatballs, each about the size of a golf ball.

MELT the cooking fat in a large skillet over medium-high heat. When the fat is hot, add the meatballs (depending on the size of your pan, you may have to do this in batches). Cook for about 30 seconds per side, turning to prevent burning, until browned all over, about 5 minutes. Reduce the heat and add more cooking fat if the pan begins to smoke.

TRANSFER the meatballs to the prepared baking sheet. Transfer to the oven to finish cooking for 8 to 10 minutes, until the internal temperature reaches 160°F. Let the meatballs rest for 5 minutes and serve.

MAKE IT A MEAL: Pair these meatballs with Roasted Red Pepper Sauce (page 316), Tomato Sauce (page 324), or Pesto (page 315), and serve over Roasted Spaghetti Squash (page 294) or on top of our Ratatouille (page 288).

⭐ VEGETABLE "SPAGHETTI" *Meatballs are just begging to be placed over a pile of noodles. Did you know you can make "noodles" out of many vegetables if you have the right tools? A julienne peeler is great for softer vegetables like cucumber or zucchini (see our Romesco Garlic Shrimp with Zucchini Noodles on page 244), but it can be a little time-consuming to prepare large batches. A spiral slicer can turn nearly anything—potatoes, carrots, parsnips, even apples—into thin, spaghetti-like strings, and the process is so fun your kids (or partner) will actually want to participate. Just whip up a batch of your favorite "noodles," leave raw or steam until they're al dente (check often by tasting, as you don't want soggy noodles), and serve.*

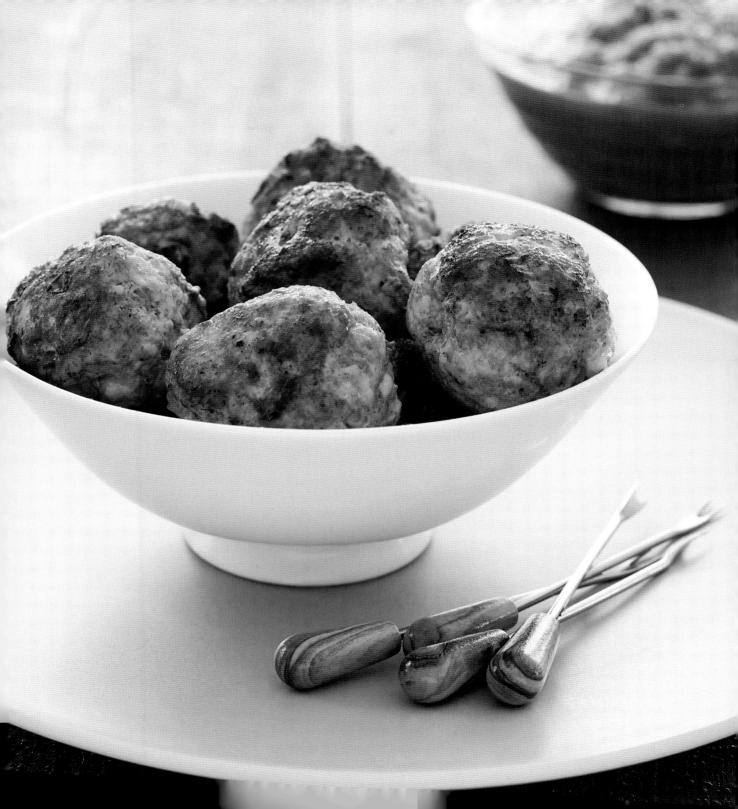

melissa's chicken hash

SERVES 2

PREP TIME: 15 minutes
COOK TIME: 5 to 10 minutes
TOTAL TIME: 20 to 25 minutes

---

2 tablespoons cooking fat

1 pound boneless, skinless chicken thighs, cut into 1-inch dice

½ teaspoon salt

½ teaspoon black pepper

¼ cup chopped walnuts

1 sweet potato, peeled and grated

1 Granny Smith apple, cored, peeled, and diced

½ teaspoon red pepper flakes

¼ cup apple cider

2 generous handfuls arugula or baby spinach

Splash of apple cider vinegar

Melissa Hartwig created this recipe out of egg-boredom one morning, and found that chicken and apple is a surprisingly delicious combination. One night over dinner, she shared her favorite egg-free breakfast idea with Chef Richard, who envisioned adding texture and punch in the form of walnuts and apple cider vinegar. Now, it's one of Pre-Made Paleo's best-selling meals (see page 403 for details), and remains one of Melissa's favorite no-egg breakfasts.

IN a large skillet, heat the cooking fat over medium-high heat, swirling to coat the bottom of the pan. When the fat is hot, add the chicken, being sure not to crowd the pieces. Season the chicken with the salt and pepper. Cook until browned, 2 to 3 minutes. Turn the chicken to brown the other sides, add the walnuts, and cook until the chicken is browned and the walnuts are toasted, 2 to 3 minutes. (Shake the pan occasionally so the walnuts don't burn.) Add the sweet potato, apple, and red pepper flakes and cook, stirring often, until the chicken is fully cooked, 3 to 4 minutes.

ADD the apple cider and mix all the ingredients together, scraping the bottom of the pan with a wooden spoon to bring up any tasty bits. Add the arugula and cook for another 30 seconds, gently stirring to the wilt leaves. Drizzle with the splash of apple cider vinegar and serve immediately.

⭐ LEFTOVERS *You can also spiral slice your sweet potato instead of grating it to save some time. Use your spiral slicer to create thin noodles, then chop them into 1-inch pieces and cook as directed. This dish is just as delicious eaten cold, like a fancy chicken salad. Spoon leftovers on a bed of fresh greens, drizzle with a little olive oil and apple cider vinegar, and garnish with some diced avocado.*

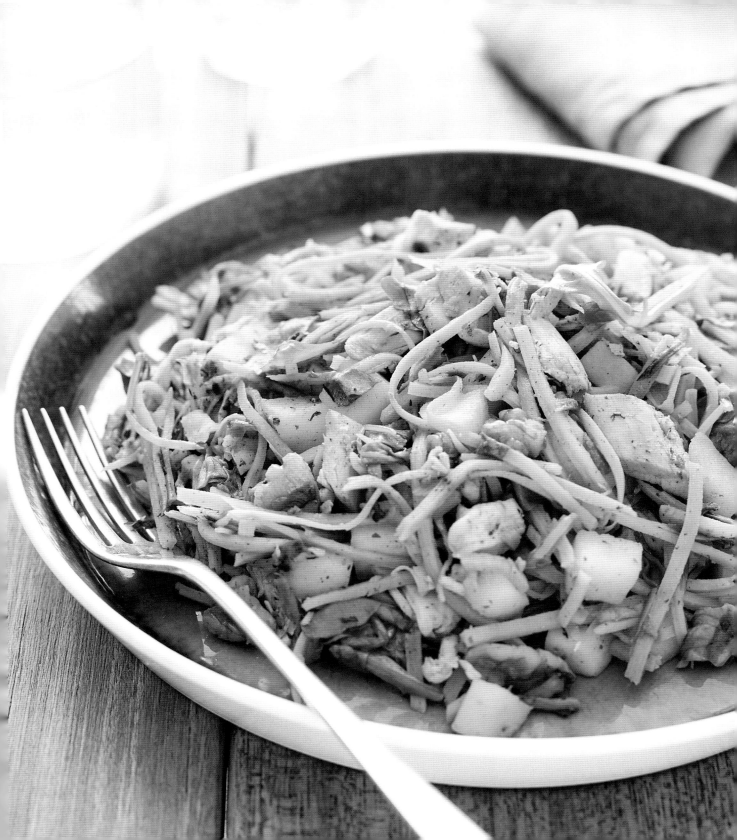

grilled coconut-curry chicken

SERVES 2

PREP TIME: 15 minutes
COOK TIME: 15 minutes
TOTAL TIME: 30 minutes

---

3 tablespoons cooking fat

½ onion, finely diced

2 cloves garlic, minced

1 tablespoon yellow curry powder

1 cup canned crushed tomatoes

½ cup coconut cream (see page 178)

1 teaspoon salt

½ teaspoon black pepper

1½ pounds bone-in, skin-on, split chicken breasts (2 pieces)

1 lime, quartered

Don't pour all the curry sauce over the chicken; once the mixture has come into contact with the raw meat, you have to throw it out. Instead, place your chicken in a shallow bowl, and pour a little of the sauce over the chicken. Brush or rub it evenly over the meat, then flip and repeat on the other side. Save the extra sauce to drizzle over the top of this dish before serving, or use it to top tomorrow night's chicken, shrimp, or vegetables.

TO make the curry sauce, melt the cooking fat in a saucepan over medium heat and swirl to coat the bottom of the pan. When the fat is hot, add the onion and cook, stirring, until translucent, 2 to 3 minutes. Add the garlic and stir until it becomes aromatic, about 30 seconds. Add the curry powder and stir for 15 to 20 seconds, taking care that the garlic and curry powder don't burn. Add the tomatoes and simmer until thickened, about 5 minutes. Transfer the contents of the pan to a food processor or blender and puree until smooth. Pour into a mixing bowl and let cool. Mix in the coconut cream, salt, and pepper.

PLACE the chicken in a shallow bowl. Pour some of the sauce over the chicken and brush it on each side.

PREHEAT a grill to high heat (500°F).

REMOVE the chicken from the curry sauce and discard the extra sauce. Add the chicken, breast-side down, to the grill and sear until golden brown, about 2 minutes. (When the meat is properly seared it will pull off the grates very easily, so don't rush this step.) Turn the chicken over so the bone side is down and place over indirect heat. Cover with the grill lid and continue to cook until the internal temperature of the chicken is 160°F, or the breast meat springs back when pressed with a finger. This will take 10 to 15 minutes, depending on thickness.

LET the chicken rest for 5 minutes. Serve with a squeeze of lime juice and the reserved curry sauce.

MAKE IT A MEAL: This recipe goes great with Cauliflower Rice (page 272) and Sautéed Kale with Almonds (page 298), or grilled peppers, onions, and pineapple (see page 164).

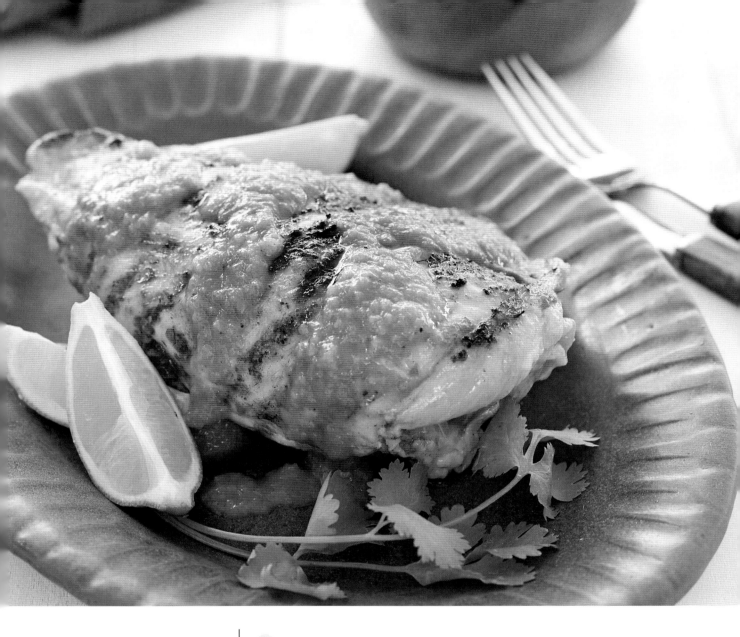

⭐ BAKED COCONUT-CURRY **CHICKEN** *If you don't have a grill, you can bake the chicken in the oven. Turn the oven to Broil (or 500°F), and place the raw chicken in a baking dish. Sear the chicken in the oven for 5 minutes. Reduce the oven temperature to 350°F. Brush the chicken with the curry sauce and finish cooking in the oven for 10 to 15 minutes (depending on thickness), until the internal temperature reaches 160°F.*

harvest grilled chicken salad

SERVES 2

PREP TIME: 20 minutes
COOK TIME: 10 minutes
TOTAL TIME: 30 minutes

½ **teaspoon salt**

½ **teaspoon black pepper**

½ **teaspoon ground cumin**

½ **teaspoon chili powder**

½ **teaspoon garlic powder**

½ **teaspoon onion powder**

1 **pound boneless, skinless chicken breasts**

4 **cups lettuce leaves (torn into 1-inch pieces)**

½ **Granny Smith apple, cored and sliced or diced**

½ **cucumber, sliced or diced**

¼ **cup dried cranberries (sweetened with apple juice)**

Raspberry Walnut Vinaigrette (page 328)

If you can't find cranberries sweetened with apple juice, substitute raisins or currants. For the perfect office lunch, just layer the salad in a large mason jar and throw on the lid. Layer the ingredients in this order for maximum awesomeness and minimum sogginess: dressing, chicken (make sure it's cool), vegetables and fruit, and as much lettuce as you can fit on top. When you're ready to eat, just shake and serve!

PREHEAT a grill to medium-high heat (375° to 450°F).

IN a small bowl, mix together the salt, pepper, cumin, chili powder, garlic powder, and onion powder. Season the chicken evenly with the mixture. Grill the chicken, turning once, until the internal temperature reaches 160°F or until the flesh springs back when pressed, 3 to 4 minutes per side. Let the chicken rest for 5 minutes before slicing into thin strips.

IN a large salad bowl, combine the lettuce, apple, cucumber, and cranberries. Top with the sliced chicken. Toss all of the ingredients lightly with the vinaigrette just before serving.

⭐ CHICKEN SUBSTITUTIONS *Don't want to fire up the grill? Follow our Perfect Seared Chicken Breast technique on page 157. No time to cook? Purchase a compliant rotisserie chicken (and use the carcass to make the Bone Broth from page 177), add a scoop of the Protein Salad (page 161) sitting in your fridge, or substitute canned chicken, tuna, salmon, or hard-boiled eggs.*

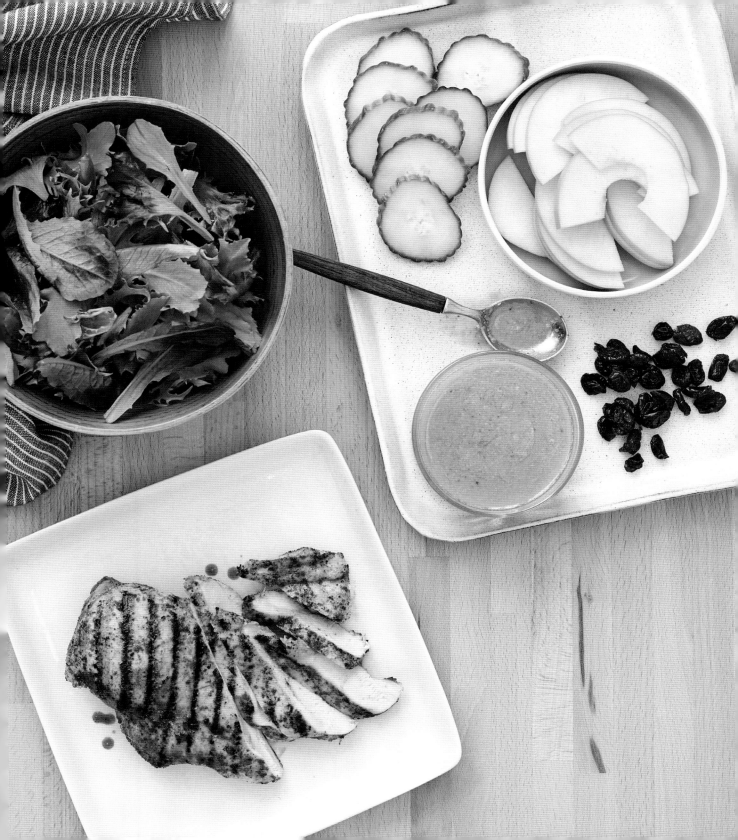

thai cucumber cups

SERVES 2

PREP TIME: 20 minutes
COOK TIME: 15 minutes
TOTAL TIME: 35 minutes

---

2 cloves garlic, minced

1 tablespoon minced fresh ginger

½ jalapeño, seeded and minced

Grated zest and juice of 2 limes

½ cup + 2 tablespoons extra-virgin olive oil

¼ teaspoon salt

¼ teaspoon black pepper

½ cup cashews

1 cup roughly chopped button, cremini, or portabella mushrooms

¼ cup finely diced red, yellow, or orange bell pepper

2 tablespoons thinly sliced green onion

1 pound ground turkey

4 cucumbers, hollowed into cups (see below)

2 tablespoons chopped fresh cilantro

The cucumber cups make this dish the perfect appetizer, pot-luck contribution, or baby shower dish, but they may be too time-consuming for a mid-day lunch. The turkey, vegetable, and dressing mixture is just as tasty over a bed of crisp greens, wrapped in a romaine lettuce leaf, scooped into a bell pepper, or spooned on top of any of our breadless bun options on page 173–174. It's also delicious reheated in the morning (and topped with a fried egg or two).

TO prepare the dressing, whisk together the garlic, ginger, jalapeño, and lime zest and juice in a medium non-reactive mixing bowl. Whisking, drizzle in ½ cup of the olive oil. Whisk in the salt and pepper. Set aside.

IN a large skillet over medium-high heat, add 1 tablespoon of the olive oil and swirl to coat the bottom of the pan. When the fat is hot, add the cashews and toast, shaking the pan to keep them from burning, until lightly browned, 2 to 3 minutes. Transfer to a cutting board, roughly chop, and let cool.

IN the same skillet over medium-high heat, heat the remaining tablespoon of olive oil. Add the mushrooms and cook, stirring, for 3 minutes. Add the bell pepper, green onion, and turkey. Cook, breaking up the turkey with a spatula or wooden spoon and mixing it into the vegetables, until the turkey is thoroughly browned, 7 to 10 minutes.

REMOVE the pan from the heat, add most of the dressing, and mix well. Sprinkle the chopped cashews into the turkey mixture.

SPOON the turkey mixture into the cucumber cups and top with the chopped cilantro and a drizzle of the remaining dressing.

⭐ CUCUMBER CUPS *To make the cucumber cups, cut each cucumber into 3 logs (approximately 2 inches long). Scoop out the inner flesh using a small spoon or small melon baller, but don't scoop out all the way through to the bottom, as the cups need to hold the meat mixture. Lightly salt the cucumber rounds and place on paper towels to drain.*

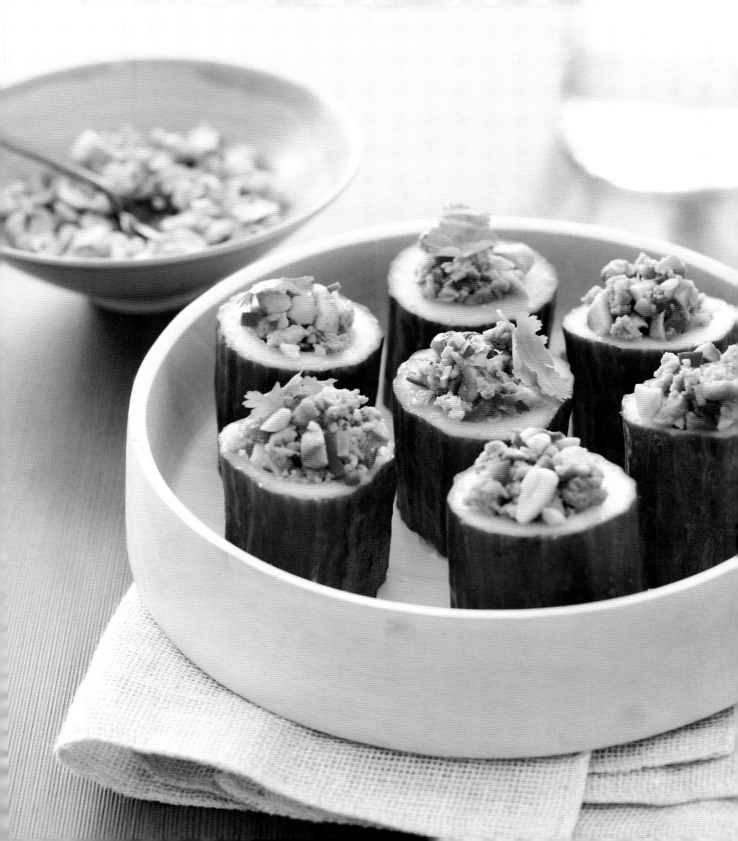

SEAFOOD

WHILE THE WHOLE30 WASN'T DESIGNED SPECIFICALLY FOR VEGETARIANS, we do have a loyal following who prefer leaving red meat and poultry off their plate. The good news is that seafood, especially the wild-caught varieties, is packed with nutrition (including anti-inflammatory omega-3 fats found in cold-water fatty fish like salmon) *and* protein. We've had many a pescetarian complete the Whole30 using only a variety of seafood and eggs as their protein source, with great success. (See page 120 for our Whole30 recommendations for vegetarians and vegans.)

Fish and shellfish are sometimes intimidating for new cooks. You wonder how you'll know if the fish is fresh, whether frozen fish really tastes as good, and how to cook it.

The good news is that fish is actually easy *and* fast to cook (the recipes we give you here generally require less than 20 minutes of active cooking time), and it's really easy to swap out one kind of fish for another in these recipes. Plus, frozen fish and shellfish are a cost-effective way to source healthy protein. And don't overlook the little guys! While we haven't included any specific recipes here, small fish like sardines, herring, mackerel, and anchovies are loaded with healthy fats and are low in toxins.

You can categorize fish into three simple categories, based on texture: firm, moderate, and flaky. Use these classifications to help you find the best substitutions if the fish we call for isn't available (or is too expensive).

FIRM: catfish, grouper, halibut, sea bass, snapper, mahi-mahi, salmon, swordfish, tuna

MODERATE: rockfish, shrimp, tilapia, walleye, orange roughy, ocean perch, trout, mackerel

FLAKY: cod, flounder, haddock, pollock, scallops, lingcod, whitefish

When buying fresh fish, the best rule of thumb is actually a rule of nose. Smell your fresh fish—it should remind you of seawater, or cucumber. (Strange, but true.) If it gives off a strong odor, that means it's past its prime, so pass on it. The flesh should look shiny and clean, with no dull or discolored patches. If you're allowed, press the flesh with your finger. It should spring back quickly—if the dent remains, you know the fish isn't super fresh. Make sure you either cook or freeze fresh fish within two days of purchase.

High quality frozen fish will have basically no odor at all, but if there are ice crystals on the fish itself, that means it's lost some moisture, and likely won't taste as good. Never thaw frozen fish on the counter—either thaw it overnight in

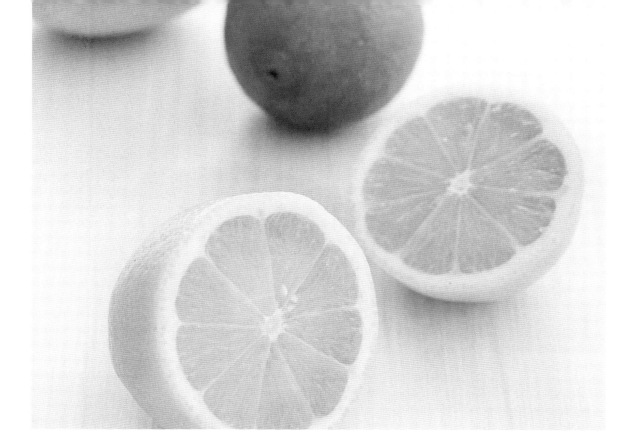

the refrigerator (plan on about 24 hours for one pound), or thaw it faster by placing it in a bowl under running cold water. And once it's thawed, cook it right away—don't delay more than a day, and don't ever re-freeze.

Scallops are sold either fresh and shucked, or frozen and vacuum-sealed. Both are delicious, fast-cooking options. You can also buy shrimp fresh, frozen, or pre-cooked; the latter are a great option to add to a salad or leftover veggies for a quick and easy lunch or dinner.

Don't try to defrost scallops or shrimp under running water, however—they're pretty sensitive, and the water can ruin the texture. Use your refrigerator or thaw them under cold water while

they're still inside the bag, and pat them dry before cooking.

You'll want to check your fish often during cooking. That's because unlike beef, seafood becomes tougher the longer you cook it. Plan to stick close to your oven or pan during these recipes, to make sure your shrimp don't have the consistency of a bicycle tire. But if you're in the kitchen checking on your fish anyway, why not whip up a batch of Basic Mayonnaise (page 179)? In fact, your Whole30 rule of thumb should be this: If I'm in the kitchen waiting for something to cook, I'm thinking ahead and doing some food prep.

No need to thank us for this tip—you'll thank yourself later.

mexican tuna boats

SERVES 2

PREP TIME: 10 minutes

1 avocado, pitted and peeled

2 cans (5 ounces each) tuna, drained

3 green onions, thinly sliced

Juice of 1½ limes

½ jalapeño, minced

1 tablespoon minced fresh cilantro

½ teaspoon chili powder

½ teaspoon salt

⅛ teaspoon black pepper

1 head endive, separated into leaves

This dish makes for the perfect lunch—just pack up your tuna in a glass container and wrap your leaves in a slightly damp paper towel inside a resealable bag to keep them crisp. Or, stuff the tuna salad inside a romaine lettuce leaf, hollowed-out bell pepper, tomato, or the cucumber cups from page 234. This dish would also work with canned chicken or salmon and would taste amazing with a drizzle of cool Ranch Dressing (page 316) or Avocado Mayonnaise (page 310).

IN a medium sized bowl, mash the avocado with a fork, leaving it slightly chunky. Add the tuna to the bowl, flaking it apart with a fork, and mix to combine with the avocado. Add the onions, juice of 1 lime, jalapeño, cilantro, chili powder, salt, and pepper and mix well.

SPOON the tuna mixture into the endive leaves. Sprinkle a dusting of chili powder. Squeeze the juice from the remaining ½ lime over the top and serve.

MAKE IT A MEAL: While there are some greens in this dish, you're lacking serious veggie power. Try serving the lettuce wraps with Roasted Sweet Potatoes (page 296), Gazpacho (page 276), or raw carrots, bell pepper strips, and celery with Avocado Mayonnaise (page 310) for dipping.

⭐ VEGETABLE CHOPPER *You could trim a few minutes off your prep time with a chopper, which makes fine dicing your jalapeño a snap. You can get one for around $20, and while it's not a must-have kitchen tool, it will make things like our Salsa (page 319) and Gazpacho (page 276) 74 percent faster to prepare.*

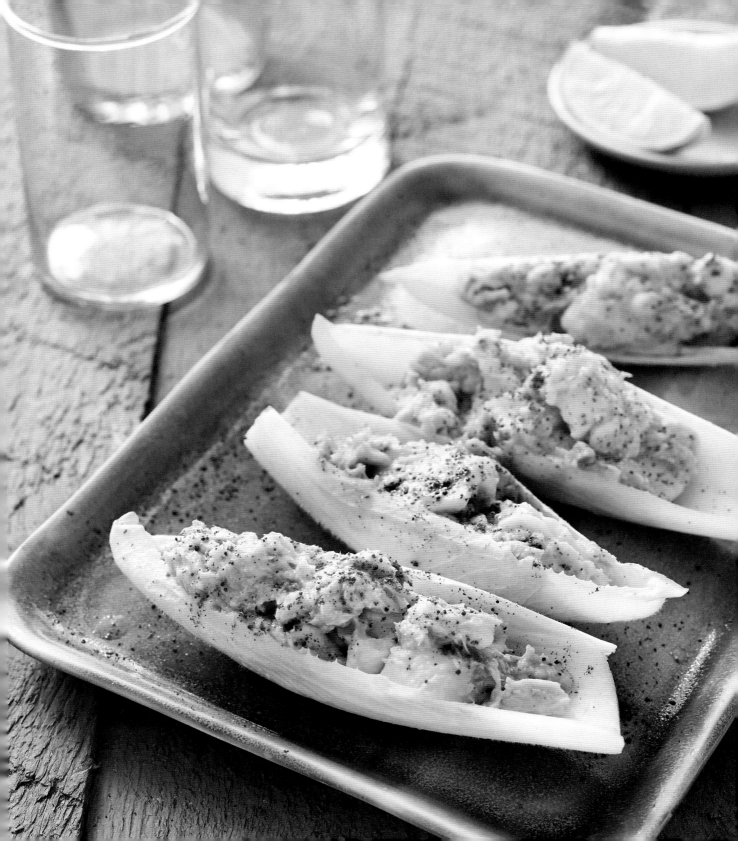

halibut with citrus-ginger glaze

SERVES 2

PREP TIME: 10 minutes

COOK TIME: 20 minutes

TOTAL TIME: 35 minutes

FOR THE GLAZE

½ cup apple cider

Grated zest and juice of 2 lemons

Juice of 1 orange

½ tablespoon grated fresh ginger
(or ½ teaspoon ground ginger)

FOR THE FISH

3 tablespoons cooking fat

2 halibut fillets (5 ounces each)

1 teaspoon salt

½ teaspoon black pepper

Halibut is delicious, but it can also be expensive. You can substitute a variety of white fish here—try cod, turbot, dogfish, haddock, or striped bass. If you don't want to juice the orange by hand, substitute ¼ cup store-bought orange juice.

PREHEAT the oven to 400°F.

FOR THE GLAZE: Cook the apple cider in a small saucepan over medium-high heat until reduced to about 1 tablespoon, 4 to 6 minutes. Add the lemon juice, orange juice, and ginger and cook until reduced by half, 3 to 5 minutes. Remove the pan from the heat and add the lemon zest. Set aside.

FOR THE FISH: Heat 2 tablespoons of the cooking fat in a large skillet over high heat, swirling to coat the bottom of the pan. While the fat is heating, season the halibut with the salt and pepper. When the fat is hot, place the fish top-side-down in the pan and sear for 2 to 3 minutes. While the fish is searing, melt the remaining 1 tablespoon cooking fat (if necessary), line a baking sheet with parchment paper, and brush half of the fat on the paper.

REMOVE the halibut from the pan and transfer seared-side-up to the greased, lined baking sheet. Brush the remaining cooking fat over the top of the halibut. Bake in the oven for 10 to 12 minutes, until the flesh is just barely firm and flakes easily with a fork. Transfer the fish to a serving dish or individual plates and spoon the glaze over the top just before serving.

⭐ HALIBUT *Halibut and other white fish are a little tricky to cook; there is very little oil in halibut, so it dries out fast. Check this dish in the oven every few minutes as it gets close to the end of cooking. If you're worried about overcooking, pull it out just before it looks done (when the flesh almost flakes with a fork) and let it rest on the pan for a minute, as it will keep cooking once you take it out of the oven. You can also use a meat thermometer—pull it out of the oven when the center of the fish is between 130° and 135°F.*

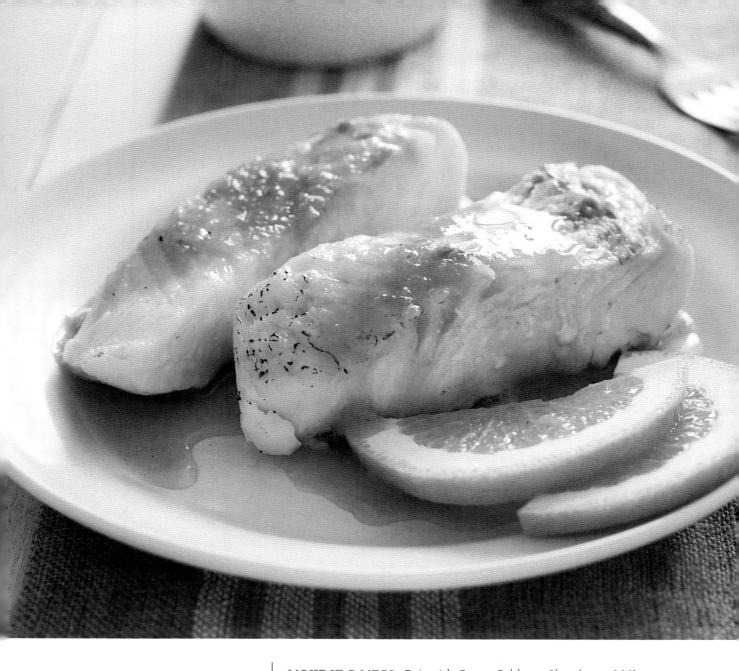

MAKE IT A MEAL: Pair with Green Cabbage Slaw (page 282) and Cauliflower Rice (page 272) for an Asian-inspired feast. Or serve with our Roasted Beet, Orange, and Avocado Salad (page 290) for a fresh, simple meal.

cod with mushroom and red pepper relish

SERVES 2

PREP TIME: 10 minutes

COOKING TIME: 15 minutes

TOTAL TIME: 25 minutes

---

1 pound cod

½ teaspoon salt

¼ teaspoon black pepper

2 tablespoons cooking fat

¼ onion, finely chopped

2 teaspoons grated fresh ginger (or ½ teaspoon ground ginger)

2 cloves garlic, minced

1 pint (2 cups) button, cremini, or portabella mushrooms, sliced

1 cup roasted red peppers, chopped

This dish isn't in our Fancypants Meal section, but it's beautiful enough to wow guests. Plus, our pairing suggestion of roasted squash can cook at 350°F, so your oven can easily pull double duty. The squash will take about an hour to roast at this temperature (assuming a large dice), so put it in the oven about 45 minutes before you start cooking the fish. Or, start your cauliflower steaming just before you start prepping the fish—it should be done and ready to blend in the food processor as the fish is coming out of the oven. Make your dressing ahead of time and throw together a salad while the fish cooks and you've got a company-worthy meal.

PREHEAT the oven to 350°F. Line a baking pan or glass baking dish with parchment paper.

CUT the fish into portions and gently pat dry with a paper towel. Season evenly with ¼ teaspoon of the salt and ⅛ teaspoon of the pepper and place in the baking pan. Bake for 12 to 15 minutes, until the flesh in the center of the fish no longer appears wet or spongy in texture when you pierce it with a fork. It's done when it just barely starts to flake when pulled apart.

WHILE the fish is cooking, add the cooking fat to a large skillet over medium heat. When the fat is hot, add the onion and cook, stirring, until the onion is translucent, 2 to 3 minutes. Add the ginger and stir for 30 seconds. Add the garlic and stir until aromatic, about 1 minute. Add the mushrooms and continue to cook, stirring, for 1 to 2 minutes. The mushrooms will release moisture, bringing the flavors together, and then become more dry in appearance. Add the roasted red peppers and the remaining ¼ teaspoon salt and ⅛ teaspoon pepper and stir for 2 minutes, allowing the peppers to warm. Remove the pan from the heat and hold covered to keep warm.

REMOVE the fish from the oven, spoon the mushroom and pepper mixture generously over the top of the fish, and serve immediately

MAKE IT A MEAL: This dish goes beautifully with a simple green salad dressed with our Balsamic Vinaigrette (page 328) and either roasted butternut squash (see page 166–167) or a simple Cauliflower Mash (page 270).

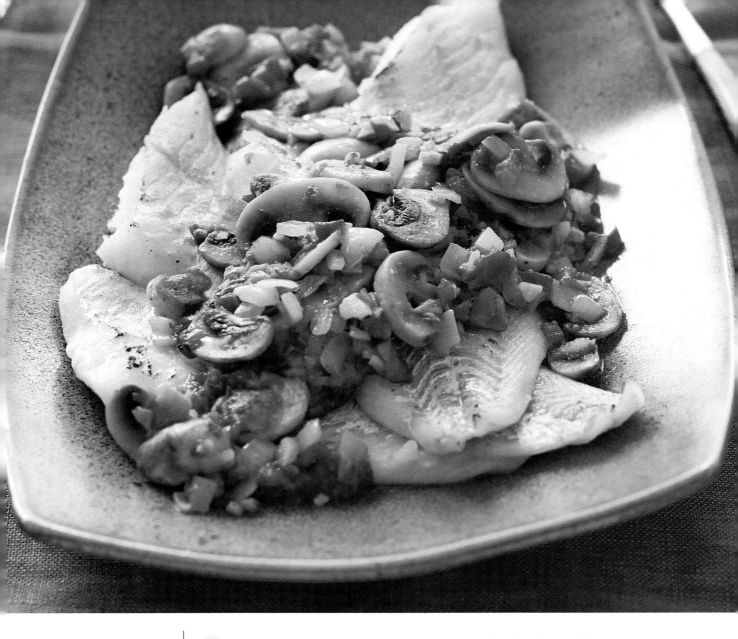

⭐ DRIED MUSHROOMS *Using a mix of more exotic dried mushrooms like shiitakes, porcini, morels, or chanterelles in this dish will boost the flavor and texture of your relish, and make the finished look even more impressive to company. You'll want to use about 3 ounces of dried mushrooms for this dish—feel free to mix and match varieties. Soak them in warm water for 30 minutes first, to rehydrate them and rinse off any dirt or grit. Then, slice them (or dice them, depending on their shape and size) and prepare your "relish" as directed.*

romesco garlic shrimp with zucchini noodles

SERVES 2

PREP TIME: 45 minutes

COOK TIME: 10 minutes

TOTAL TIME: 55 minutes

---

4 medium zucchini (about 4 cups of "noodles")

2 tablespoons cooking fat

¼ onion, finely chopped

2 cloves garlic, minced

1 pound large shrimp, peeled and deveined

1 teaspoon salt

½ teaspoon black pepper

2 teaspoons chopped fresh parsley leaves

Romesco Sauce (page 318)

You can save yourself 25 minutes of prep time and make your Romesco Sauce up to two days in advance. This dish is just as delicious served cold, substituting Pesto (page 315) for the Romesco Sauce, and cold cucumber noodles instead of steamed zoodles. You can also cheat and buy cooked shrimp—just skip the ¼ cup water and covered cooking at the end of the third step.

PEEL the zucchini with a regular peeler. Then, using a julienne peeler, make long slices along one side of each zucchini until you get down to the seeded core. Rotate the zucchini and continue to peel until you've done all four sides. (If you have a spiral slicer, you can use that instead of a julienne peeler.) Discard the core, and set the noodles aside.

ADD 2 cups of water to a large pot over medium-high heat and bring to a boil while you begin cooking the shrimp.

MELT the cooking fat in a large skillet over medium heat, swirling to coat the bottom of the pan. When the fat is hot, add the onion and cook, stirring, until translucent, about 2 minutes. Stir in the garlic and cook until aromatic, about 1 minute. Add the shrimp, toss to coat with the onion and garlic, and cook stirring, for 2 minutes. Add ¼ cup water to the skillet and cover with a lid. Cook until the shrimp form the shape of a "C," 4 to 6 minutes. Transfer to a serving bowl (draining any remaining water), and season with the salt and pepper.

AFTER you add the water and cover the shrimp, place a colander or steamer inside the large pot of boiling water. Add the zucchini noodles, cover, and steam until the zucchini is al dente in texture, 2 to 3 minutes. Drain the "zoodles" and transfer to a serving dish or individual plates.

SPRINKLE the shrimp with the parsley, toss, and spoon over the zoodles. Spoon the Romesco Sauce over the shrimp and zucchini and serve.

⭐ SHRIMP *Shrimp are quite easy to prepare, but they get tougher the longer you cook them. Perfectly cooked shrimp will be pink in color, and shaped like a "C"—if they are curled up tightly into an "O" shape, they're overcooked. If you're using frozen shrimp, make sure they are completely thawed before you start cooking.*

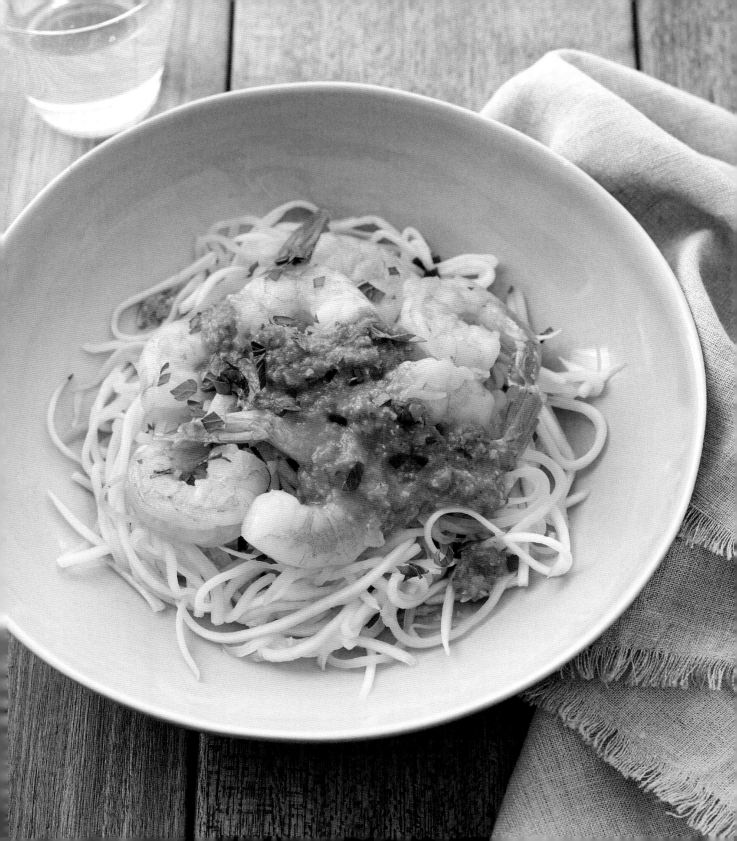

poached salmon with cucumber dill sauce

SERVES 2

PREP TIME: 25 minutes
COOK TIME: 20 minutes
TOTAL TIME: 45 minutes

½ cup rice vinegar

Juice from 3 lemons, divided

1 bay leaf

6 black peppercorns

2 salmon fillets (5 ounces each)

½ cup Basic Mayonnaise (page 179)

¼ cup coconut cream (see page 178)

½ cucumber, peeled and diced

½ shallot, minced

2 sprigs fresh dill, leaves only, chopped

1 teaspoon salt

½ teaspoon black pepper

½ lemon, thinly sliced

Poaching fish helps keep it moist while adding and infusing flavor, but if you're short on time (or ingredients), you can use our Perfect Oven-Baked Salmon technique on page 160. Make a double batch of this Cucumber Dill Sauce, as it's delicious mixed into a Protein Salad (page 161).

PREHEAT the oven to 400°F.

TO make the poaching liquid, combine 2 cups of water with the rice vinegar, the juice of 2 lemons, the bay leaf, and peppercorns in a small saucepan. Bring to a boil over high heat, then remove from the heat.

PLACE the salmon fillets skin-side down in a casserole dish (choose a dish that is deeper than the thickness of the salmon). Pour the poaching liquid over the salmon. Transfer to the oven to poach until it's slightly translucent when you cut into the center, around 15 to 20 minutes, depending on the thickness of the fillets.

WHILE the salmon is poaching, mix the juice of the remaining lemon, the mayonnaise, coconut cream, cucumber, shallot, dill, salt, and pepper in a small bowl.

DISCARD any poaching liquid left in the casserole, along with the bay leaf and peppercorns. Place the salmon on a serving dish or individual plates. Spoon the sauce over the salmon and garnish with the lemon slices.

⭐ PERFECT POACHED SALMON *Overcooked salmon loses its moisture and tenderness, so check often as you're nearing the end of your cooking time. It's better to remove the salmon from the oven slightly underdone, as it will continue to cook even on a serving plate. Poke a butter knife into the salmon at the thickest part and gently pull it apart. The flesh should be easily parted, and look mostly opaque (not red and raw at the top). You should see some white at the edges from the fat, and the flesh should feel firm. Don't cook it until the flesh easily flakes, though—that's a sign of overcooking. Poaching is a very forgiving technique, even if you leave it in the poaching liquid a little too long, your fish will still be moist and tender.*

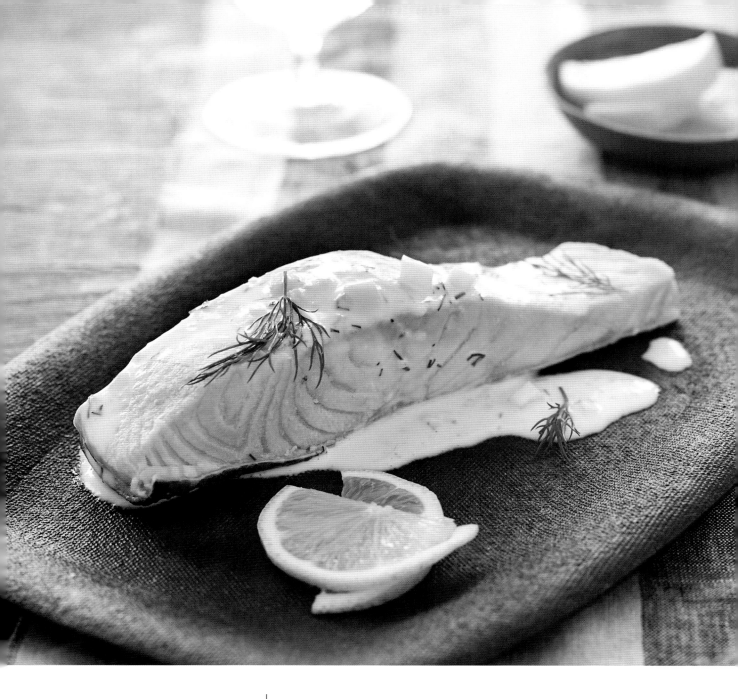

MAKE IT A MEAL: This dish is perfect for Sunday brunch, or any old Meal 1. Serve with our Butternut Squash Soup (page 266) or Grilled Asparagus with Lemon Zest (page 284).

PORK

BACON. THERE. WE SAID IT. We *know* you were thinking it, because in our larger Paleo community, pork is often considered synonymous with bacon. In fact, in our bounce-back from the low-fat craze, people are more than a little bacon-crazy.

Except you won't find any bacon in this section of our recipe book. In fact, you won't find bacon in here at all, except for an explanation of our favorite bacon cooking technique on page 162. We suspect this makes you sad, and maybe even a little angry. But we're not here to be popular—we're here to give you our best recommendations for being healthy while eating real food. And while bacon *is* real food, it's not even close to the most nutritious part of the pig, and it's all too easy to overindulge, leading to the eviction of other nutrients off your plate.

First, it's *really* hard to find Whole30-compliant bacon. We've given you our favorite brands on page 404, but if you're in small-town America shopping at your local grocery store, you're simply not going to find bacon that wasn't cured with sugar (and likely contains lots of other nasty ingredients). We didn't want to give you recipes that three-quarters of you wouldn't be able to make as directed, so this book is basically a bacon-free zone.

In addition, news flash: pork is more than just bacon, sausage, and pork chops. There are a number of cost-effective, delicious cuts that are often overlooked, and including them as part of your meal rotation means you're getting a variety of nutrients and flavors without breaking the bank. Many of these cuts are perfect for slow-cooking (like our Carnitas on page 254) making for easy dinners with way less clean up.

Okay, you're starting to like us again.

Finally, there are some Whole30 Approved foods that are so close to the sweet, fatty, salty stuff you used to eat that they can become problematic too, promoting unintended over-consumption. Nut butters, dried fruit, and bacon are three common examples—all foods that can promote less-than-desired health effects when overeaten, and all too easy to overeat.

So for those of you who can find Whole30-compliant bacon, let's keep it in its place. Use it as a condiment, sprinkled over salads, soups, or stews, or as the occasional protein side at one of your meals. Feel free to keep it in the general rotation, but don't rely on it too much, because to be honest, it's not really a very good source of protein. (In fact, a slice of bacon contains just as much fat as protein.)

And if you can't find approved bacon, don't worry—there are more than enough delicious cuts of pork in this section to make you forget all about the crispy, salty, fatty belly you're craving for the next 30 days. That last thing probably isn't true, but you'll survive.

banger sausage patties with sweet potato mash and caramelized onions

SERVES 2

PREP TIME: 25 minutes
COOK TIME: 25 minutes
TOTAL TIME: 50 minutes

FOR THE SAUSAGE

1 pound ground pork

¼ teaspoon ground sage

¼ teaspoon garlic powder

¼ teaspoon dried thyme

¼ teaspoon onion powder

⅛ teaspoon cayenne pepper

⅛ teaspoon nutmeg

1 teaspoon salt

⅛ teaspoon black pepper

Grated zest of 1 lemon

2 medium sweet potatoes, peeled and cut into large dice

4 tablespoon ghee or clarified butter

½ cup full-fat coconut milk

1 onion, thinly sliced

¼ teaspoon salt

¼ teaspoon black pepper

PREHEAT the oven to 350°F. Bring 4 cups of water to a boil in a medium pot over medium-high heat. Line a baking sheet with parchment paper.

PREPARE THE SAUSAGE: In a large mixing bowl, mix all the sausage ingredients. Form into 8 equal patties. Place on a plate and chill in the freezer for 10 to 15 minutes while starting the sweet potato mash.

COOK the sweet potatoes in the boiling water until fork tender, 10 to 15 minutes. Drain and return the potatoes to the pot. Add 1 tablespoon of the ghee and coconut milk. Using a potato masher, immersion blender, or large kitchen fork, mash and mix the sweet potatoes with the ghee and the coconut milk. Cover the pot to keep warm and set aside.

REMOVE the sausage from the freezer and place on the parchment paper–lined baking sheet. Bake the sausage patties in the oven for 12 to 15 minutes, until the internal temperature reaches 145°F, and no pink remains in the middle of the patty.

MEANWHILE, heat the remaining 3 tablespoons of ghee in a large skillet over medium heat, swirling to coat the bottom of the pan. When the ghee is hot, add the onion and cook for 15 minutes, turning them periodically as they begin to brown and caramelize. (Do not rush this step—the browner the color, the more concentrated the flavor will be.)

TRANSFER the mashed sweet potatoes to a bowl or serving dish and top with the caramelized onions. Season with salt and pepper and stir to combine. Serve with the sausage patties.

Don't be intimidated by the long list of spices in this fancier sausage mixture—measuring and mixing is actually really quick. To make it easier on future you, quadruple the spice mixture (the ingredients from sage to pepper), use one-fourth of it (2 heaping teaspoons) in this batch, and store the rest in an airtight container in your pantry for the next time you want to make the sausage.

MAKE IT A MEAL: Double the sweet potato mash recipe and you've got an easy side dish for tomorrow night's dinner—serve with Braised Beef Brisket (page 214), Walnut-Crusted Pork Tenderloin (page 252), or Halibut with Citrus-Ginger Glaze (page 240).

⭐ CARAMELIZING ONIONS *Caramelizing the onion adds so much flavor to this dish, but it takes care and patience. First, don't slice the onions too thin or they'll dry out too much while cooking. Aim for slices about ⅛ inch thick. Make sure you use a large enough pan—crowd your onions and they'll steam instead of caramelize. Finally, don't rush the process! Onions should be soft in texture and a rich brown color before you pull them off the stove.*

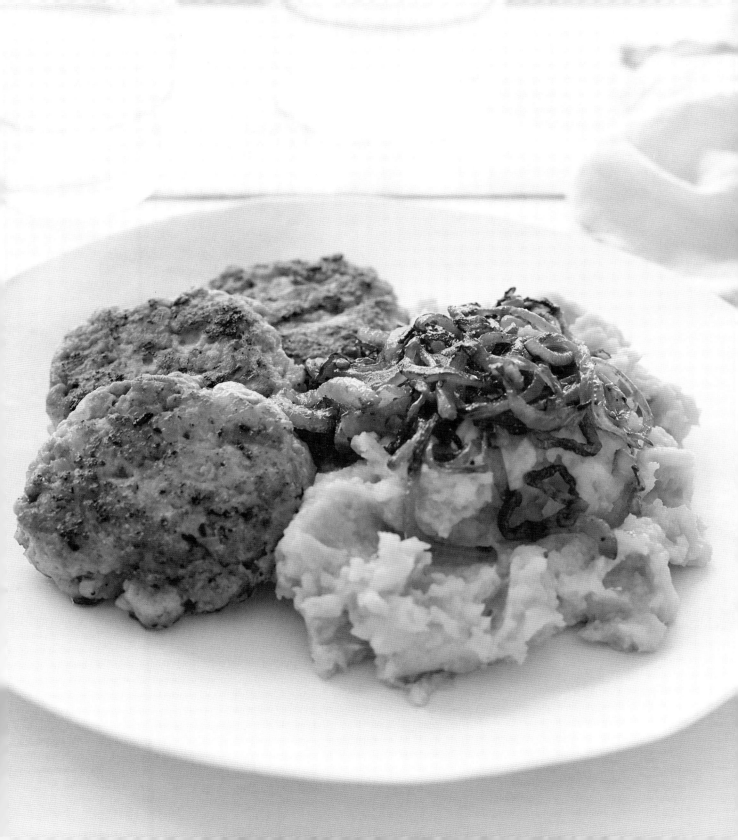

walnut-crusted pork tenderloin

PREP TIME: 20 minutes

COOK TIME: 30 minutes

TOTAL TIME: 50 minutes

---

1 pound pork tenderloin

2 tablespoons mustard powder

1 tablespoon paprika

1 tablespoon onion powder

1 tablespoon garlic powder

1½ teaspoons salt

1½ teaspoons black pepper

½ cup chopped walnuts

3 cups salad greens

½ cup Balsamic Vinaigrette (page 328)

Pork tenderloin is one of the leanest and most tender cuts of pork, but it's also easy to overcook and dry out. It's best to rely on your meat thermometer and not the clock for this cut—so watch your temperatures carefully. This recipe would work just as well with pork chops; the cooking time in the oven would be about the same.

REMOVE the pork from the refrigerator approximately 30 minutes before cooking.

PREHEAT the oven to 375°F.

IF necessary, trim the pork tenderloin, removing the tough outer skin. (This is generally not necessary on boneless cuts of pork loin, but see the tip below for details.) Pat the tenderloin dry with a paper towel. Mix the mustard powder, paprika, onion powder, garlic powder, salt, and pepper in a small bowl. Rub the pork evenly with the spice mixture.

IN a food processor or by hand, pulse or chop the walnuts until finely chopped. Coat the pork evenly with three quarters of the chopped walnuts. Place the tenderloin in a baking pan and roast for 25 to 30 minutes, until the internal temperature reaches 145°F. Let the pork rest for 10 minutes.

SLICE the tenderloin into ½-inch-thick medallions. Place the salad greens on plates, top with the pork slices, sprinkle the remaining chopped walnuts, and drizzle with the Balsamic Vinaigrette.

⭐ REMOVING PORK LOIN'S TOUGH OUTER MEMBRANE *Most boneless cuts of tenderloin won't have much "silver skin" (the tough membrane covering the top of a pork loin). However, if yours does, you'll want to remove it before cooking—otherwise it dries out in the oven and turns quite tough. With a sharp paring or boning knife, pinch the meat to pull the membrane away from the muscle. Remove the outer skin by sliding the knife blade just beneath the membrane and slowly cut along the muscle (with the grain of the meat) in smooth sawing motions. You can also ask your butcher to do this for you before he or she wraps up your purchase.*

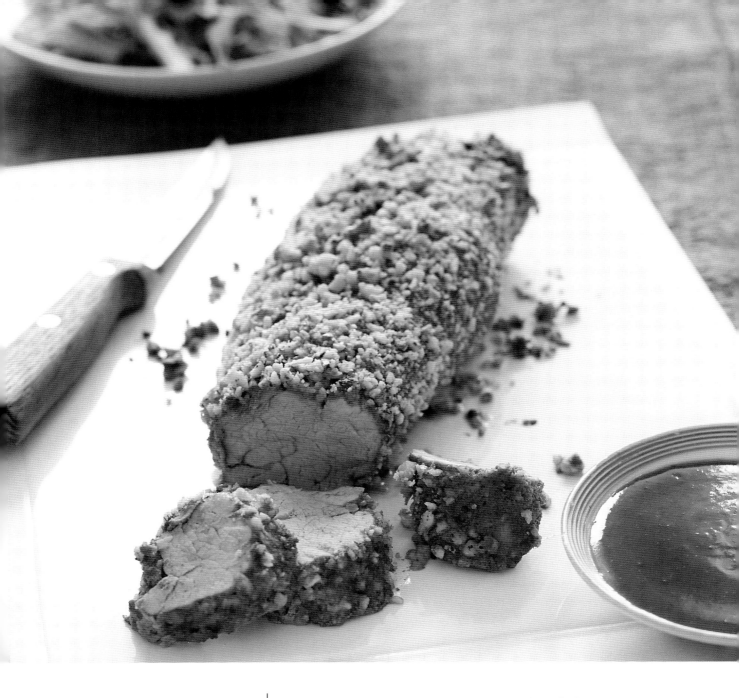

MAKE IT A MEAL: This dish goes great with Grilled Asparagus with Lemon Zest (page 284), Sweet Potato Soup (page 300), or Oven-Roasted Butternut Squash and Brussels Sprouts (page 286).

pulled pork carnitas

SERVES 2

PREP TIME: 15 minutes

COOK TIME: 2 hours 45 minutes

TOTAL TIME: 3 hours

1½ tablespoons salt

1 teaspoon black pepper

2 pounds pork butt, cut into 4-inch cubes

2 tablespoons cooking fat

½ medium onion, roughly chopped

3 cloves garlic, minced

½ teaspoon chili powder

¼ teaspoon ground cinnamon

¼ cup sliced (½-inch pieces) green onions

Juice of ½ lime

Make your evening easier by letting your slow cooker do the cooking. Before you leave for the day, complete the recipe through the fourth step (just before transferring the pot to the oven). At that point, just put everything in the slow cooker. Set the cooker on low and let it cook all day (8 to 10 hours). When you get home, not only will your house smell amazing, but you'll have the ultimate ready-to-eat, pull-apart pork!

PREHEAT the oven to 350°F.

MIX 1 tablespoon of the salt and all of the pepper in a bowl. Use to season the pork butt evenly.

IN a heavy pot or Dutch oven over medium heat, melt the cooking fat, swirling to coat the bottom of the pan. When the fat is hot, add the pork (be sure not to overcrowd) and brown all sides, 3 to 4 minutes per side. Remove the pork from the pot and set aside.

IN the same pot, reduce the heat to medium-low, add the onion, and cook, stirring, until translucent, 4 to 5 minutes. Add the garlic and cook, stirring vigorously to prevent burning, until aromatic, about 1 minute. Add 1 cup of water, the chili powder, and cinnamon. Increase the heat to medium high, return the pork to the pot, and bring to a boil.

COVER the pot with a lid or tightly wrapped foil. Transfer to the oven and bake for 2 ½ hours, turning the meat after each hour. The pork should be fork-tender when done.

TRANSFER the pork to a bowl and shred with a fork or two, discarding any excess fat. Incorporate the cooking liquid from the pot, then add the green onions and lime juice. Season with the remaining ½ tablespoon salt.

MAKE IT A MEAL: Turn your carnitas into a taco salad by serving over crisp greens along with Salsa (page 319) and Guacamole (page 308); serve with Green Cabbage Slaw (page 282) drizzled with Ranch Dressing (page 316).

⭐ CUTS FOR PULLED PORK *Pork butt is the most common cut used for pulled pork because it is marbled with flavor-enhancing fat. It's also known as Boston butt, Boston shoulder, and pork shoulder roast. If you get a cut with the bone, throw it in the pot with the meat and let the nutrients and fat from the bone infuse your carnitas.*

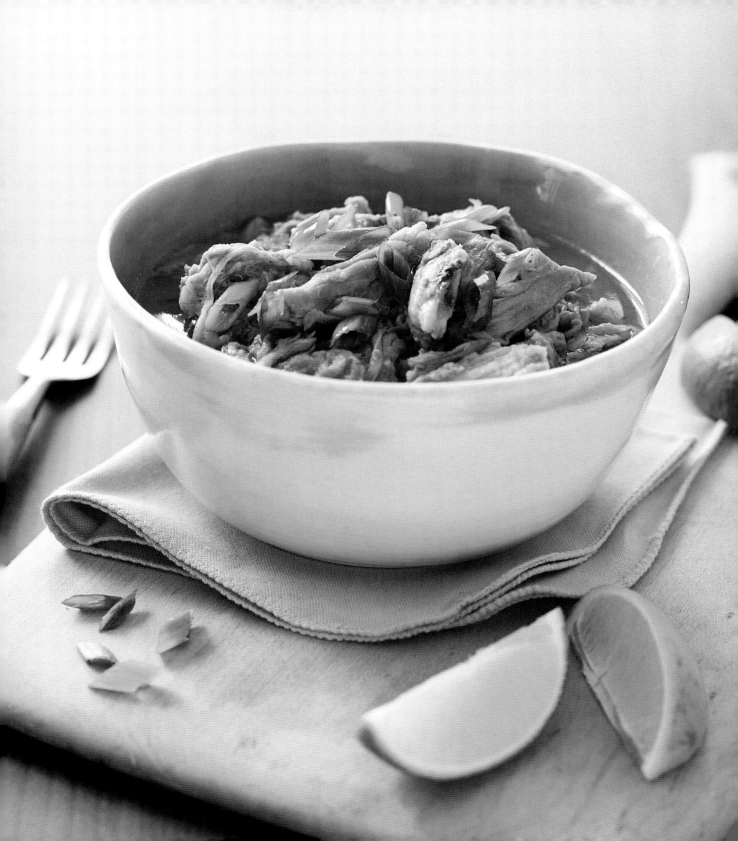

baby back ribs with tangy bbq sauce

SERVES 2

PREP TIME: 20 minutes

MARINATE TIME: 3 to 24 hours

COOK TIME: 1 hour 15 minutes

TOTAL TIME: 1 hour 35 minutes plus marinating time

FOR THE RUB

2 tablespoons dried oregano

1 teaspoon mustard powder

1 teaspoon onion powder

1 teaspoon garlic powder

1 tablespoon paprika

½ teaspoon cumin

1 teaspoon salt

1 teaspoon black pepper

2 pounds baby back ribs

1 cup chicken broth (page 177) or water

2 cups Tangy BBQ Sauce (page 322)

Cut your prep in half by making the BBQ Sauce up to two days ahead of time. Feel like skipping this step? Tessemae's makes a Whole30-compliant BBQ sauce. See page 403 for where to buy.

MAKE THE RUB: Mix the oregano, mustard powder, onion powder, garlic powder, paprika, cumin, salt, and pepper in a small bowl. Set the ribs flesh-side up on a large piece of foil and coat evenly with the rub. Marinate in the refrigerator for 3 to 24 hours (the longer the better).

PREHEAT the oven to 300°F.

PLACE the ribs in a casserole or glass baking dish. Pour the chicken broth or water into the dish and cover with foil. Bake for 1 hour, or until the meat pulls back from the rib bones.

PREHEAT a grill to medium heat (350°F). Place the ribs directly over the heat and grill until nicely charred, 6 to 8 minutes on each side. If you don't have a grill, increase the oven temperature to 475°F and cook the ribs for 10 minutes on each side.

REMOVE the ribs from the grill or oven and immediately baste generously with the BBQ sauce. Serve with the remaining sauce.

MAKE IT A MEAL: This recipe goes great with a serving of Butternut Squash with Kale and Swiss Chard (page 268), Green Cabbage Slaw (page 282), or Roasted Sweet Potatoes (page 296).

⭐ **WHEN ARE THE RIBS DONE?** *While you should cook ribs to 180° to 190°F, a meat thermometer is not much help here: It is very hard to get an accurate reading because the bones get in the way of measuring the temperature. A few ways to test whether your ribs are done: Pick up the slab with a pair of tongs and bounce them slightly. If they are ready, the slab will bow and be close to breaking. You can also poke a toothpick into the meat between the bones. When it slides in with little or no resistance (like with baked goods) your ribs are ready.*

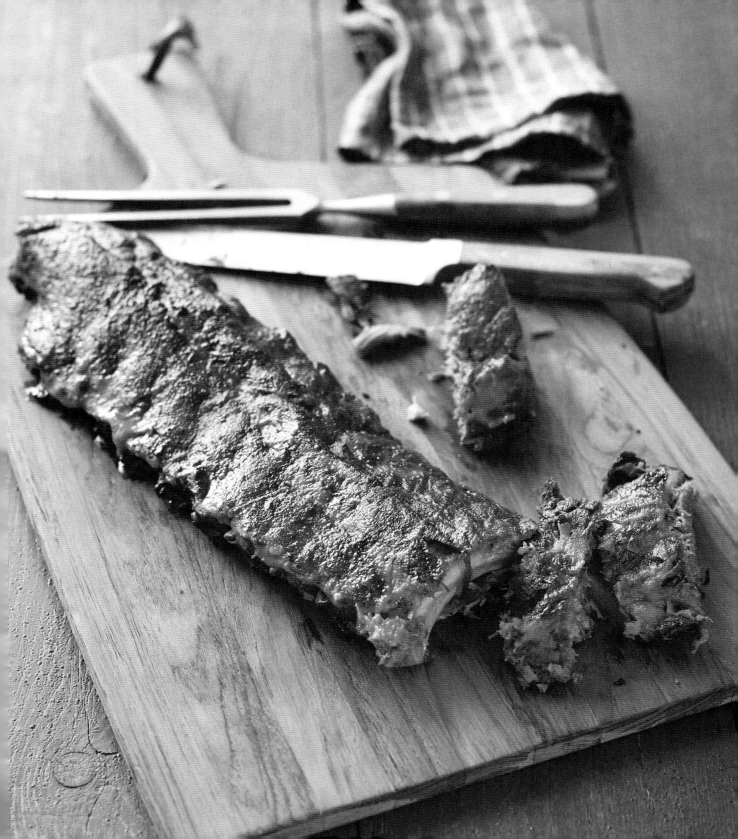

pork chops with spiced applesauce

SERVES 2

PREP TIME: 5 minutes
COOK TIME: 20 minutes
TOTAL TIME: 25 minutes

1 teaspoon salt

1 teaspoon black pepper

2 bone-in pork chops (about 1 pound total)

3 tablespoons cooking fat

1 onion, sliced

2 apples, peeled, cored and diced

½ cup apple cider

½ teaspoon ground ginger

½ teaspoon allspice

1 pinch nutmeg

2 generous handfuls frisée

Don't have access to frisée? You can use arugula, baby kale, or baby spinach. This dish can also make a delicious reappearance at breakfast—fry an egg or two and place over the top of the leftover pork, using the applesauce and freshly wilted greens as your side.

PREHEAT the oven to 350°F.

MIX the salt and pepper in a small bowl and use to season both sides of the pork chops.

MELT 2 tablespoons of the cooking fat in a large skillet over medium-high heat. When the fat is hot, add the pork chops and sear until you see a golden brown crust, 2 to 3 minutes. Turn and sear the other side for 2 minutes.

TRANSFER the pork chops to a baking dish and roast in the oven until the internal temperature reaches 140°F, 10 to 15 minutes, depending on thickness.

WHILE the pork is roasting, combine the remaining 1 tablespoon fat and the onion in the same skillet. Cook over medium heat until the onion is translucent, 2 to 3 minutes. Add the apple, apple cider, ginger, allspice, and nutmeg. Cook (while scraping all the tasty bits off the bottom with a wooden spoon), until the apples soften, about 5 minutes.

TRANSFER the applesauce to a food processor or blender and blend until smooth.

PLACE the frisée on plates. Top with the pork and serve with the applesauce.

⭐ BACON FAT *If you're lucky enough to have access to Whole30-compliant bacon, save the fat the next time you cook a batch. You can use it in heartier recipes like this one. See page 404 for a list of Whole30 Approved bacon brands (like the sugar-free pork bacon from U.S. Wellness Meats) and sources.*

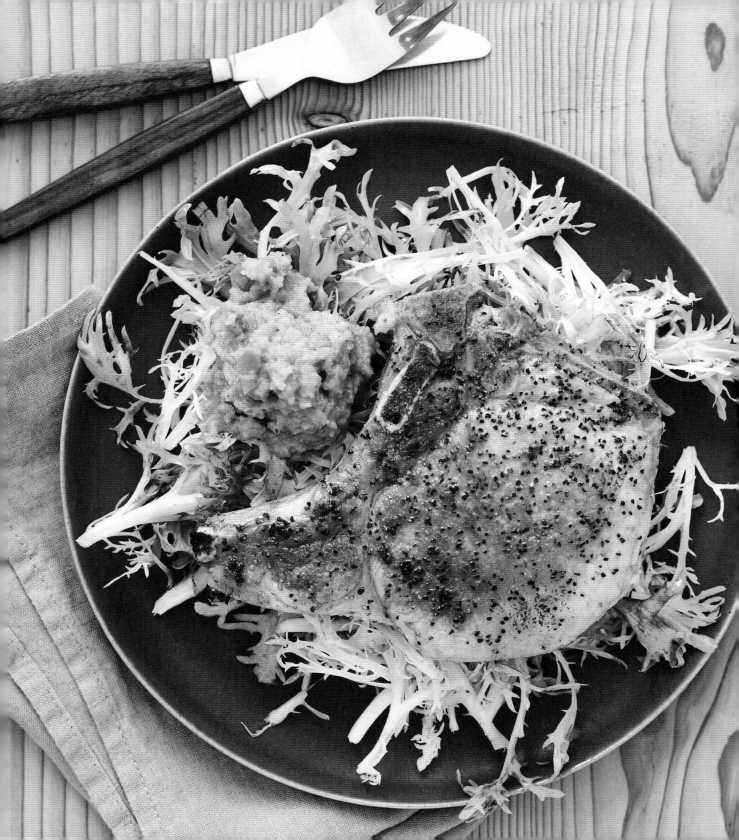

SIDE DISHES

CONTRARY TO WHAT THE MAINSTREAM MEDIA OCCASIONALLY PRESENTS, our healthy eating plan isn't carnivorous. If you follow our Meal Template (page 194), you'll be eating only a moderate amount of protein with each meal. In fact, if you do the math—and we did—the lower end of our protein recommendations are *exactly* in line with the United States Recommended Daily Allowance (US RDA). And we balance the animals we eat with a copious amount of plants—both vegetables and fruit. In fact, after serving yourself some protein, we suggest you fill the *rest of your plate* with vegetables at each meal.

So we're not really sure why some people think the Whole30 is nothing but meat. We suspect an "all you can meat" diet just sounds sexier to the television advertising folks. Extreme is sexy. Moderate is not sexy. But moderate is *healthy*, and we're all about healthy.

Plus, we think healthy is pretty darn sexy.

First, we don't care if you buy fresh or frozen, or eat them cooked or raw. We just want you to eat your veggies, so to borrow a line from the musical group Journey, any way you want it . . . Yes, you'll lose a small amount of nutrients if you buy them frozen, but who's to say you're not losing just as much during the transportation process from the farm to your grocery store? Frozen vegetables can be both cost-effective and make for a super-fast dinner, so feel free to keep your freezer stocked with some basics. And if you're buying fresh, farmers markets for the win—local, fresh, seasonal, *and* affordable.

As for cooked versus raw, this is really up to you, although some of you may find that raw vegetables are hard on your digestion, especially if you're not used to eating them. If you have a digestive condition like Irritable Bowel Syndrome (IBS) or find that too many salads make you feel gassy or bloated, try cooking most of your vegetables and see if that helps.

Some people are also sensitive to certain vegetables and fruits—those containing higher levels of FODMAPs (Fermentable Oligo-, Di-, Mono-saccharides, and Polyols). These short-chain carbohydrates and sugar alcohols are poorly absorbed in the small intestine, and pass along to the large intestine, where they are fermented by bacteria. This leads to gas, bloating, motility issues, and feeling like you might have an alien in your belly.

Not very pleasant, to say the least.

FODMAPs are common in grains and legumes, which are out for the program, but are also present in many vegetables and fruit. If you find that your Whole30 foods are still giving you digestive issues, try going low-FODMAP for a week and seeing if that helps. (You can download our low-FODMAP shopping list at whole30. com/pdf-downloads.) Refer to pages 129–130 for more digestive troubleshooting tips during your Whole30.

The vegetable and fruit side dishes we've given you here are delicious compliments to the meat, seafood, and egg recipes in previous sections. They also pair beautifully with simply prepared proteins, like our Perfect Steak (page 154) or Perfect Whole Roasted Chicken (page 157). Who says your greens can't be the star of the show?

We've also included dishes perfect for every season. While you can generally find most produce year-round these days, roasting butternut squash doesn't sound quite right in the July heat, and cold gazpacho may not be satisfying on a cold winter morning. We've given you substitutions for things like winter squashes if it's not

winter, and enough options (combined with our Perfect Vegetable tips starting on page 163) to see you through your Whole30 and then some.

Our mission? To help you discover a new vegetable or two, proclaim your love for a vegetable you used to dislike, and help you see that there is a whole world of delicious, nutritious veggie offerings besides mashed potatoes, peas, and corn.

Oh, but remember—technically, corn isn't a vegetable, it's a grain, so it's out for your Whole30. And peas are legumes, so they're out, too. (Same with lima beans, but no one ever complains about that.) However, potatoes of all varieties are *definitely* a part of our program, so really, our rules are a net win for you, because duck-fat roasted sweet potatoes > creamed peas.

That's not science, that's just common sense.

balsamic roasted sweet potatoes and brussels sprouts

SERVES 2

PREP TIME: 10 minutes
COOK TIME: 20 minutes
TOTAL TIME: 30 minutes

1 cup balsamic vinegar

1 sweet potato, peeled and cut into large dice

3 tablespoons melted ghee, clarified butter, coconut oil, or extra-virgin olive oil

½ pound Brussels sprouts, trimmed and cut in half

½ red onion, thinly sliced

3 cloves garlic, minced

½ teaspoon salt

¼ teaspoon black pepper

When it comes to sauces and dressings you might think more is better, but that's not the case with a balsamic glaze! The flavor is *so* strong, you really do only want a thin drizzle over your vegetables. Better to err on the side of caution and under-dress than to add too much and overwhelm the fresh flavors of this dish.

PREHEAT the oven to 400°F. Line a baking sheet with parchment paper.

BRING the vinegar to a boil in a small saucepan over medium-high heat. Turn the heat down to medium low and simmer until the balsamic is reduced by about half, 20 to 30 minutes. Remove from the heat, allow to cool, and reserve. (You can do this up to a week ahead of time; store in a covered container at room temperature.)

WHILE the glaze is reducing, combine the sweet potato and 1 tablespoon of the cooking fat in a medium bowl and stir or toss to coat evenly. Spread the coated sweet potatoes on the prepared baking sheet.

MEANWHILE, add the remaining 2 tablespoons of fat to a large skillet over medium-high heat and swirl to coat the bottom of the pan. When the fat is hot, add the Brussels sprouts and cook, shaking the pan occasionally as they start to brown, for 3 to 4 minutes. Add the onion and garlic and continue to cook, stirring, until the garlic is aromatic, an additional minute. Season with the salt and pepper.

ADD the Brussels sprout mixture to the sweet potatoes on the pan, spreading them evenly without crowding. Put the baking sheet in the oven and roast for 15 to 18 minutes, until the sweet potatoes are golden brown and soft and the sprouts are tender.

PLATE the Brussels sprouts and sweet potato mixture and drizzle with the balsamic sauce.

MAKE IT A MEAL: Make this a complete breakfast in no time! In the same skillet you used to cook the sprouts and onion, pan-fry some chicken sausage or eggs while the vegetables are roasting. This dish is also the perfect

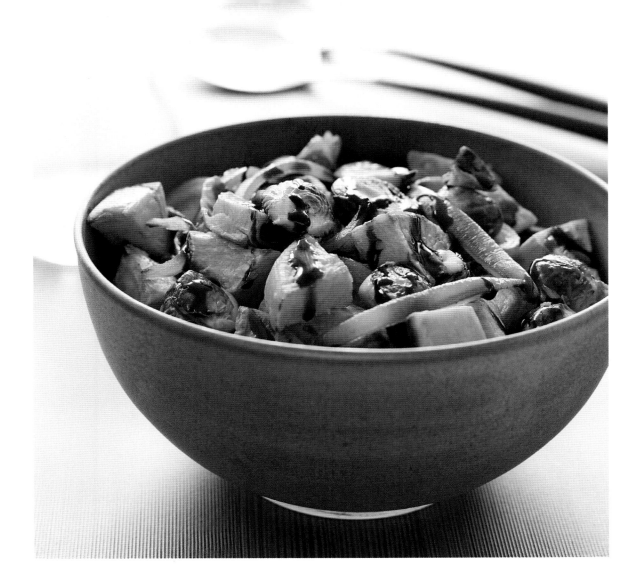

accompaniment to a whole roasted chicken (see page 157), Pork Chops with Spiced Applesauce (page 258), and Grilled Steak with Garlic-Shallot Puree and Avocado (page 216).

⭐ BRUSSELS SPROUT CHIPS *One of the best parts of roasted Brussels sprouts are the leaves that fall off the sprout and crisp up like a chip in the oven. You can "help" this process along by picking off a few outer leaves of each sprout after adding them to the baking sheet.*

broccoli, mushrooms, and yellow squash with red pepper sauce

SERVES 2

PREP TIME: 20 minutes
COOK TIME: 10 minutes
TOTAL TIME: 30 minutes

1 head broccoli, cut into florets

2 tablespoons coconut oil or extra-virgin olive oil

¼ small onion, finely chopped

½ pint button, cremini, or portabella mushrooms, quartered

1 medium yellow squash, cut into large dice

2 cloves garlic, minced

Salt and black pepper

½ cup Roasted Red Pepper Sauce (page 316)

Save prep time by making the Roasted Red Pepper Sauce up to 2 days ahead of time. You could also sprinkle 1 tablespoon red pepper flakes over the vegetables when you add the garlic, add your favorite Whole30-compliant salad dressing when serving, or top with the Ranch Dressing (page 316), Chimichurri (page 306), or Curry Sauce (page 307). Note, the squash and mushrooms will give off quite a bit of water while cooking, and will continue to "shed" even after you transfer them to a serving dish. To avoid a watery side dish, use a slotted spoon to remove the vegetables from the pan.

BRING 1 cup of water to a boil in a large pot. Place a colander or steamer inside the pot. Add the broccoli, cover, and steam until the broccoli is fork tender, 5 to 6 minutes. Remove the broccoli from the pot and set aside.

WHILE you wait for the water to boil, heat the oil in a large skillet over medium heat, swirling to coat the bottom of the pan. When the oil is hot, add the onion and mushrooms and cook, stirring occasionally, until the onion is translucent, 2 to 3 minutes. Add the yellow squash and garlic and continue to cook, stirring, until the squash is slightly softened, about 5 minutes. Remove the pan from the heat.

ADD the broccoli to the skillet and toss with the squash mixture. Lightly dust with salt and pepper, as the Roasted Red Pepper Sauce is also seasoned. Transfer the contents of the pan to a serving bowl or individual plates and top with the Roasted Red Pepper Sauce.

MAKE IT A MEAL: You could add just about any protein to this dish—it's the perfect "ingredient" meal, with a sauce that pulls it all together. It goes especially well with fried eggs (see page 149), burgers (see page 153), or Perfect Seared Chicken Breasts (page 157).

⭐ BROCCOLI *Don't waste those broccoli stems! You can use them to make a creamy, delicious soup. First, peel the stems and slice them into thin coins. Heat 1 tablespoon coconut oil, clarified butter, or ghee in a medium pot, then add half a chopped onion, 2 cloves minced garlic, 1 cup sliced mushrooms, and the broccoli stems. Cook for 10 minutes, stirring occasionally. Add 1 cup chicken broth and 1 cup full-fat coconut milk to the pot, stir, and pull the pot off the heat. Allow to cool for 5 minutes, then transfer the contents of the pot to a blender or food processor and blend until smooth, 20 to 30 seconds. Season with salt and pepper.*

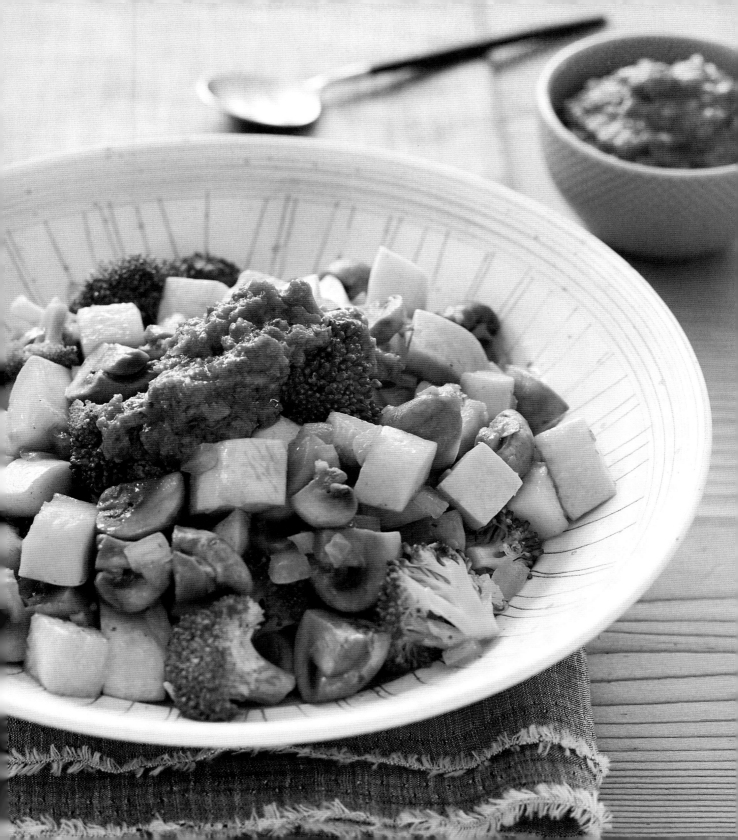

butternut squash soup

SERVES 2

PREP TIME: 15 minutes
COOK TIME: 30 minutes
TOTAL TIME: 45 minutes

---

3 tablespoons clarified butter, ghee, or coconut oil

½ cup diced onion

3 cups diced seeded peeled butternut squash

2 cloves garlic, minced

½ teaspoon ground ginger

4 cups chicken broth

1 teaspoon salt

½ teaspoon black pepper

Not sure how much squash to buy for this recipe? Generally, a 2-pound butternut squash yields 3 cups once the seeds are removed, but don't stress about having slightly more or less squash than the recipe calls for—this one is pretty forgiving. You can also buy pre-cut butternut squash and save yourself the guess work and 10 minutes of prep time, but that'll definitely add to your grocery bill.

IN a large pot, melt the cooking fat over medium heat, swirling to coat the bottom of the pot. When the fat is hot, add the onion and cook, stirring, until translucent, 2 to 3 minutes. Add the squash, garlic, and ginger and stir until the garlic becomes aromatic, about 1 minute.

ADD the chicken broth and bring to a boil over high heat. Boil until the butternut squash is soft, about 10 minutes. Remove the pot from the heat.

IN one or two batches, transfer the soup to a food processor or blender and blend on high speed until smooth in texture. Return the pureed soup to the pot.

HEAT the soup over medium-high heat until it thickens enough to coat the back of a wooden spoon, 7 to 10 minutes. Season with the salt and pepper.

MAKE IT A MEAL: To make this a complete meal, add cooked chicken, scallops, or hard-boiled eggs when returning the soup to the pot for the last 7 to 10 minutes of cooking. For extra greens, add two generous handfuls of spinach or kale in the last 3 minutes of cooking.

⭐ PREPPING SQUASH *Peeling and dicing squash isn't that tough if you have the right technique. First, cut a small amount off the bottom and top of the squash, to give it a flat surface. Next, use a vegetable peeler to peel the squash from top to bottom. Next, rest the squash on the flat bottom surface and cut in half from top to bottom, creating two long halves. Scoop the seeds from the middle of the squash with a large spoon. Finally, lay the two halves flat on the cutting board and cut strips lengthwise, then across, to create your dice. If some pieces are much thicker than others, cut in half again, so your cubes are all a relatively consistent size.*

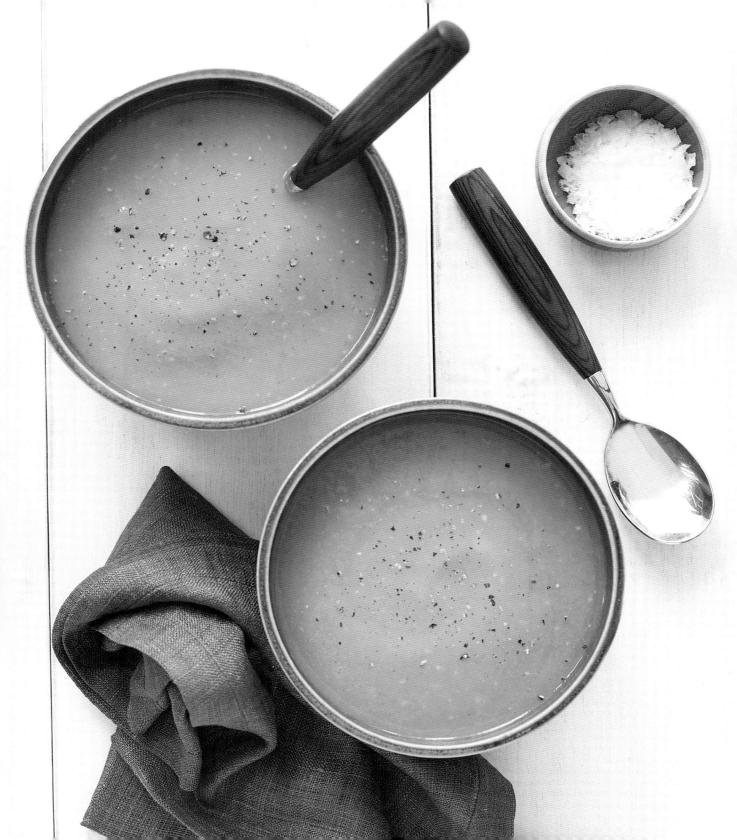

butternut squash with kale and swiss chard

SERVES 2

PREP TIME: 15 minutes

COOK TIME: 45 minutes

TOTAL TIME: 1 hour

---

2 cups large-diced seeded peeled butternut squash

1 tablespoon extra-virgin olive oil

1 bunch kale, stemmed, leaves cut into 1-inch ribbons

1 bunch Swiss chard, stemmed, leaves cut into 1-inch ribbons

3 tablespoons clarified butter, ghee, or coconut oil

1 clove garlic, minced

¼ cup raw sliced almonds

½ teaspoon chili powder

½ teaspoon salt

½ teaspoon black pepper

We've already said you can put a fried egg on anything, and this dish is no exception. If you have leftovers, this makes a quick, delicious breakfast. Just reheat your veggies in a pan or the microwave, slide a few fried eggs over the top, and serve.

PREHEAT the oven to 425°F. Line a baking sheet with parchment paper.

IN a large bowl, toss or mix the butternut squash with the olive oil until well coated. Place the squash on the prepared baking sheet and roast for 45 to 50 minutes, until fork-tender.

ABOUT 15 minutes before the squash is done, bring 2 cups of water to a boil in a large pot. Place a colander or steamer inside the pot. Add the kale and Swiss chard, cover, and steam until the kale is tender but not soft, 3 to 5 minutes. Remove the kale and chard from the pot and set aside. Drain the pot and wipe it out.

PLACE the same pot over medium heat, add the cooking fat, and swirl to coat the bottom. When the fat is hot, add the garlic and almonds and stir until the garlic is aromatic, about 1 minute. Raise the heat to high and add the steamed kale and Swiss chard. Toss for 20 to 30 seconds to combine, then remove from the heat and transfer everything from the pot to a serving dish.

COMBINE the roasted butternut squash with the kale and chard mixture. Add the chili powder, salt, and pepper, toss to combine, and serve immediately.

⭐ STEMMING GREENS *To remove the stems from kale and other hearty greens, hold the stem with one hand and place the pointer finger and thumb of your other hand around the stem just above the leaves. Pull your fingers along the stem, tearing the leaves off. (It's the same technique you use to remove rosemary or thyme leaves.) If you're having a hard time with this technique, or if your greens are too soft for this to work well, lay the leaf upside down on a cutting board and use a paring knife to cut the leaf free along both sides of the stem.*

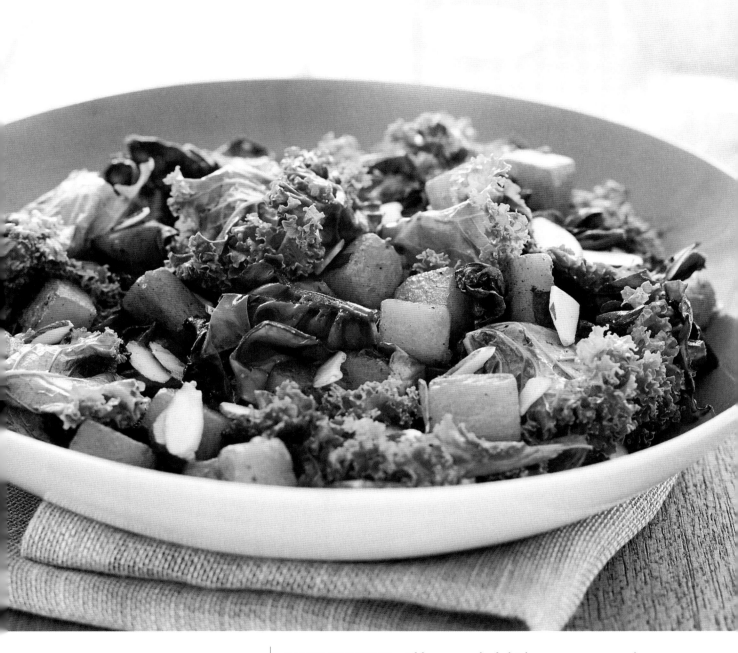

MAKE IT A MEAL: Add some cooked chicken sausage, ground beef, or roasted chicken just before serving to make a complete meal, or serve it alongside Perfect Oven-Baked Salmon (page 160) or Grilled Coconut-Curry Chicken (page 230).

cauliflower mash

SERVES 2

PREP TIME: 10 minutes
COOK TIME: 15 minutes
TOTAL TIME: 25 minutes

1 head cauliflower, cut into florets (about 4 cups)

2 cloves garlic, minced

½ cup coconut cream (see page 178)

2 tablespoons ghee or clarified butter

1 teaspoon salt

¼ teaspoon black pepper

½ cup chicken broth

1 tablespoon minced fresh parsley

This may be the most versatile recipe ever. It's a lighter substitute for mashed potatoes, and has dozens of variations to match nearly any style of cuisine. Add more chicken broth if you like it extra creamy, or keep the chicken broth to just a tablespoon or so if you prefer it really thick. Try topping with crumbled Whole30-compliant bacon or crispy prosciutto; add a blend of fresh herbs like rosemary, oregano, and thyme; kick it up a notch with 2 tablespoons of grated, peeled fresh horseradish root or 1 teaspoon chili powder; add a dollop of whole grain mustard (perfect alongside pork); or stir in shredded cabbage and kale sautéed in clarified butter or ghee.

BRING 2 cups of water to a boil in a large pot over medium-high heat. Add the cauliflower florets and garlic and simmer until the florets are fork-tender, about 15 minutes.

DRAIN the cauliflower and transfer to a food processor. Add the coconut cream, ghee, salt, and pepper and pulse until the cauliflower begins to turn smooth in consistency. Add the chicken broth one tablespoon at a time, pulsing to mix, until the desired consistency is achieved. Add the parsley and continue blending until completely smooth. Serve warm.

MAKE IT A MEAL: This dish goes well with anything. Seriously, anything. But if you made us pick a few favorites, we'd say Braised Beef Brisket (page 214), Chicken Meatballs (page 226), Halibut with Citrus-Ginger Glaze (page 240), and Walnut-Crusted Pork Tenderloin (page 252).

⭐ MASHING *You can use a variety of tools for this dish, depending on how you prefer the texture of your mash. If you prefer a silky smooth mash, the food processor is a must. If you like it really chunky, use a hand tool (like a potato masher or large kitchen fork) instead. If you like your mash somewhere in between, try using an immersion blender.*

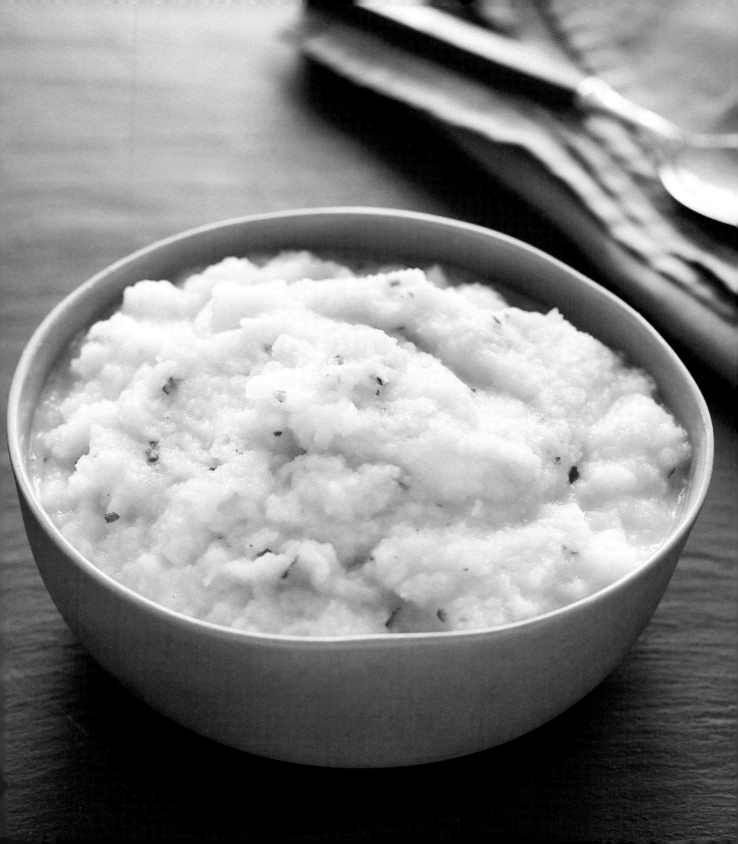

cauliflower rice

SERVES 2

PREP TIME: 15 minutes
COOK TIME: 15 minutes
TOTAL TIME: 30 minutes

---

1 large head cauliflower, cut into florets

3 tablespoons ghee or clarified butter

½ onion, finely chopped

1 carrot, peeled and finely chopped

2 cloves garlic, minced

½ cup chicken broth

1 tablespoon minced cilantro

½ teaspoon salt

½ teaspoon black pepper

This is another incredibly versatile recipe. Make a Moroccan-style rice by adding ¼ cup slivered almonds or pine nuts, ½ cup raisins, ½ teaspoon ground cumin, ¼ teaspoon ground turmeric, and ¼ teaspoon ground cinnamon. Make rice Asian-style by adding 2 tablespoons coconut aminos (a soy sauce substitute, see page 320 for details), 1 teaspoon sesame oil, and 2 minced green onions. Or make this a complete meal by adding a serving of your favorite chopped protein (like chicken, shrimp, flank steak, or pork) and any leftover sautéed vegetables you have in your fridge.

TO "rice" the cauliflower, place half of the florets in a food processor and pulse into a rice-like consistency, 15 to 20 pulses. (Don't over-crowd the cauliflower in the food processor, and don't over-pulse or the florets will get mushy.) Repeat to rice the remaining florets.

IN a large skillet, melt the ghee over medium heat and swirl to coat the bottom of the pan. When the ghee is hot, add the onion and carrot and cook, stirring, until the onion is translucent, 2 to 3 minutes. Stir in the garlic and cook until the garlic is aromatic, about 1 minute.

ADD the riced cauliflower to the skillet and mix thoroughly with the rest of the vegetables. Add the chicken broth, cover the pan with a lid, and steam until you've arrived at a rice-like consistency, 10 to 12 minutes. (The cauliflower should be tender, but not mushy or wet.)

REMOVE the pan from the heat and mix in the chopped cilantro. Adjust the seasoning with the salt and pepper.

MAKE IT A MEAL: Like its mashed counterpart, this cauliflower dish goes with anything. Try it with meals that include a sauce, like Grilled Coconut-Curry Chicken (page 230), Romesco Garlic Shrimp (page 244), and Pulled Pork Carnitas (page 254).

⭐ GRATING *If you don't have a food processor, you can use a box grater to shred the cauliflower into rice. Patience, however, as it will take quite a while! You can also make fried "rice" by omitting the chicken broth, adding more cooking fat to the pan, and pan-frying the rice until tender, about 5 minutes. For an even more authentic fried rice experience, stir two egg whites into the cauliflower while pan-frying.*

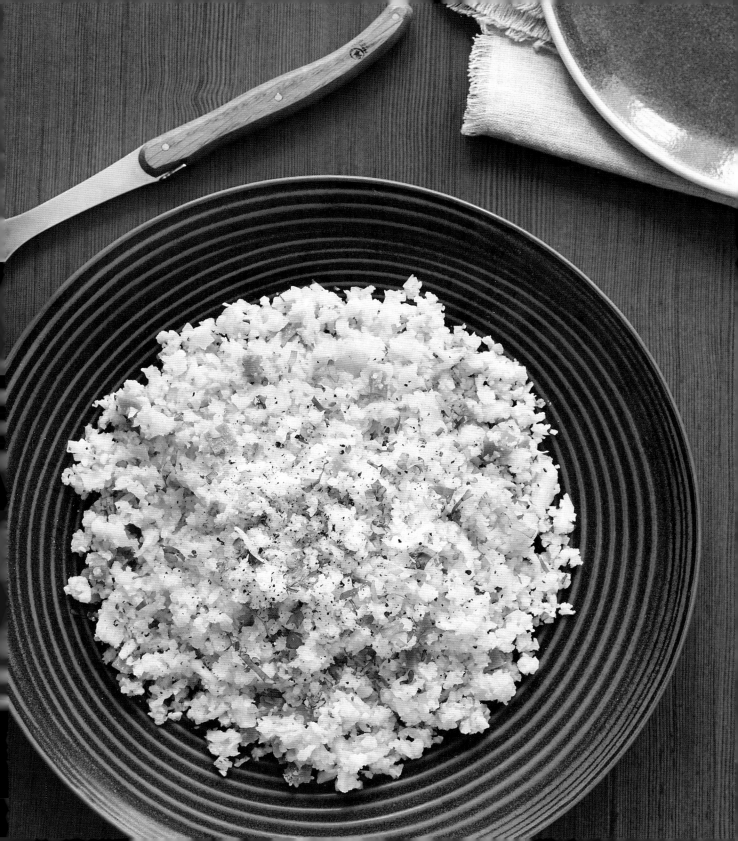

cold thai salad

SERVES 2

PREP TIME: 25 minutes
CHILL TIME: 30 minutes
TOTAL TIME: 55 minutes

---

2 small zucchini

1 small cucumber

2 carrots, peeled and shredded

½ cup mung bean sprouts (optional)

¼ cup chopped cashews

¼ cup chopped fresh cilantro

½ cup Sunshine Sauce (page 320)

Skip the 30 minutes of chill time by placing the zucchini, cucumber, carrots, and bean sprouts in the fridge the night before you prepare this dish—or just skip it altogether, if you don't mind your salad at room temperature. If you feel like a lighter dressing, try tossing the vegetables with our Asian Vinaigrette (page 330) or the creamy Cilantro-Lime Mayonnaise (page 310) instead of the Sunshine Sauce.

PEEL the zucchini with a regular peeler. Then, using a julienne peeler, make long slices along one side of one zucchini, until you get down to the seeded core. Rotate the zucchini and continue to peel until you've done all four sides. Repeat the process with the remaining zucchini and the cucumber. You should have about 2 cups of "noodles." (If you have a spiral slicer, you can use that instead of a julienne peeler.) Discard the cores.

PLACE the zucchini and cucumber noodles in a medium mixing bowl. Add the shredded carrots, bean sprouts if using, most of the chopped cashews, and most of the cilantro. Chill for 30 minutes.

ADD a tablespoon (or more) of water to the Sunshine Sauce to thin it out to the consistency of a creamy dressing and pour over the chilled salad, stirring well to combine. Garnish with the remaining cashews and cilantro and serve.

MAKE IT A MEAL: Add cooked shrimp, chicken, or hard-boiled eggs to the salad before chilling to make it a complete meal. Or serve alongside Halibut with Citrus-Ginger Glaze (page 240), Thai Cucumber Cups with Turkey (page 234), or Chimichurri Beef Kabobs (page 218).

⭐ THAI SOUP *You could easily turn this cold dish into a hot soup. Heat 4 cups of beef or chicken broth in a large pot. While that's warming, place a small skillet over medium heat and add the cashews. Toast them in the pan, shaking often, until golden brown, 3 to 4 minutes. Remove the cashews from the pan and set aside. Once the broth is warm, add the zucchini, carrots, and bean sprouts to the pot and allow to soften, 2 to 3 minutes. Transfer to individual serving bowls, add the toasted cashews, and top with the fresh cilantro. Serve alongside sliced cucumbers and Sunshine Sauce for dipping.*

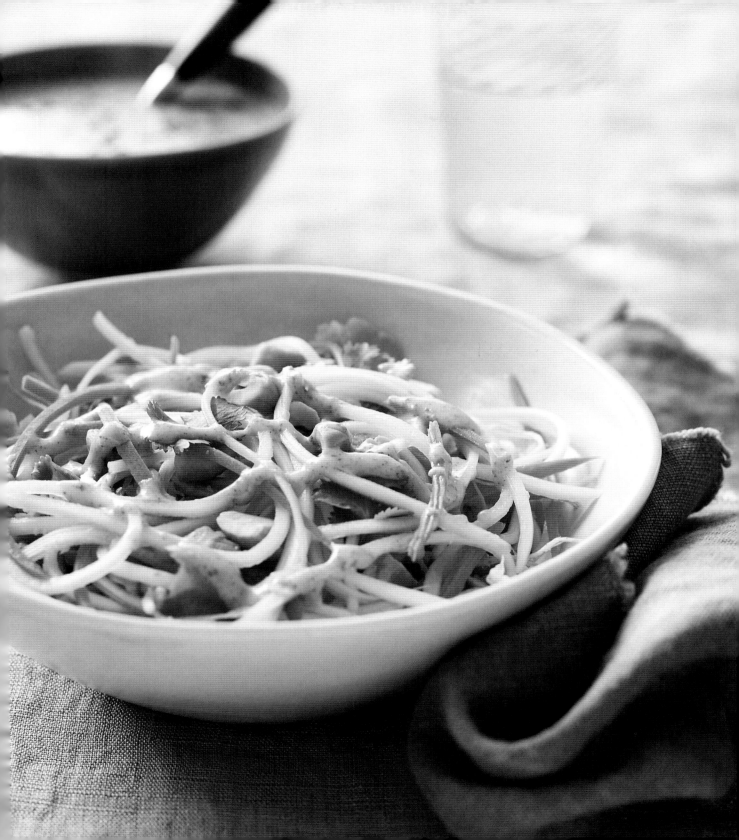

gazpacho

PREP TIME: 20 minutes
CHILL TIME: 30 minutes
TOTAL TIME: 50 minutes

---

1 medium cucumber, peeled and roughly chopped

2 medium tomatoes, peeled, seeded, and roughly chopped

1 red bell pepper, seeded, ribs removed, and roughly chopped

½ small onion, roughly chopped

2 cloves garlic, minced

1½ cups canned crushed tomatoes

1½ teaspoons red wine vinegar

1 tablespoon extra-virgin olive oil

½ teaspoon salt

½ teaspoon black pepper

If you don't have a food processor, you can chop each of these ingredients by hand, and then use a blender or immersion blender to mix the chopped ingredients with the tomatoes, vinegar, and olive oil. If you have some kind of vegetable chopper, that would make this job even quicker. (See page 140 for our recommendations.)

PULSE the cucumber in a food processor until finely chopped. Transfer to a bowl. Repeat this process with the chopped tomatoes, bell pepper, and onion, adding each item to the same bowl after chopping. (If you try to blend all the ingredients at once, they will mush instead of chop.) Stir in the garlic and return the contents of the bowl to the food processor.

ADD the crushed tomatoes, vinegar, olive oil, salt, and pepper to the food processor and blend until you achieve a smooth consistency.

REFRIGERATE the gazpacho for at least 30 minutes before serving—overnight is even better, as the flavors will continue to develop.

MAKE IT A MEAL: You can make this a complete meal by adding cooked shrimp and sliced avocado to the soup just before serving. Gazpacho also tastes great with a Kitchen Sink Scrambled Eggs (page 202), Mexican Tuna Boats (page 238), and Chicken Meatballs (page 226).

⭐ VARIATIONS *For even more flavor, add chopped fresh parsley, cilantro, or other leafy fresh herbs just before serving. To give the gazpacho a kick, add 2 tablespoons of your favorite hot sauce and ¼ teaspoon cayenne pepper. For a sweeter version, pulse the flesh from two mangoes in the food processor, then blend with the rest of the ingredients.*

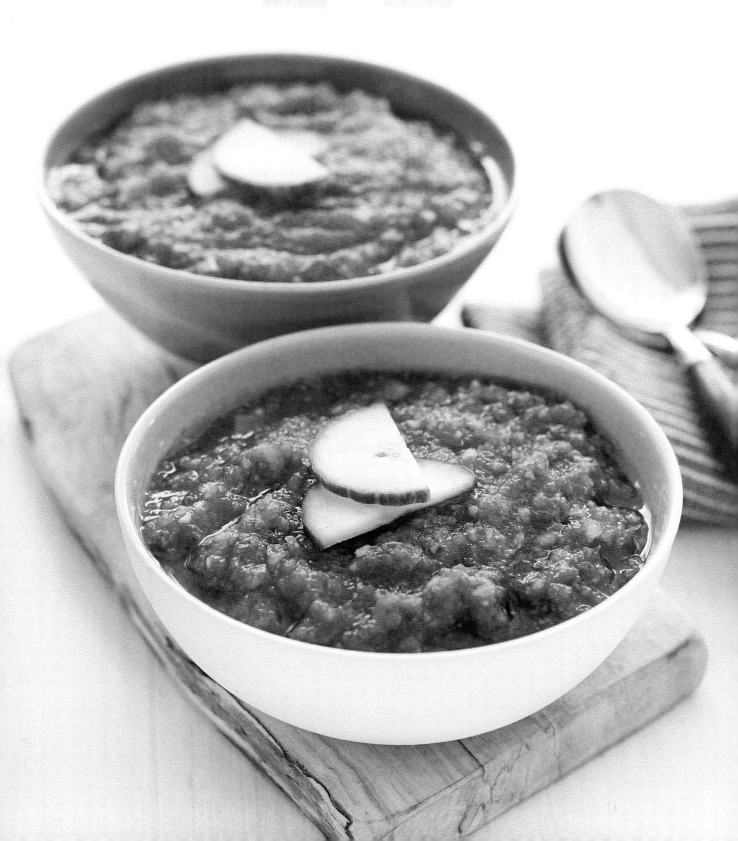

greek salad

SERVES 2

PREP TIME: 15 minutes

---

1 head romaine lettuce, chopped

4 tomatoes, seeded and cut into large dice

1 cucumber, peeled and cut into large dice

½ red onion, thinly sliced

30 pitted Kalamata olives, halved

¼ cup extra-virgin olive oil

2 tablespoons red wine vinegar

1 clove garlic, minced

¼ teaspoon salt

¼ teaspoon black pepper

Juice of ½ lemon

Give this hearty salad even more heft with canned artichoke hearts (quartered), sundried tomatoes, pepperoncini, or roasted red peppers, or top it with a creamy version of our Herb Citrus Vinaigrette (page 326).

COMBINE the lettuce, tomatoes, cucumber, onion, and olives in a large serving bowl.

COMBINE the olive oil, vinegar, garlic, salt, and pepper in a small bowl and whisk together.

POUR the dressing over the salad ingredients and top with the lemon juice.

MAKE IT A MEAL: Add canned tuna, hard-boiled eggs, cooked chicken or shrimp, or Whole30-compliant salami or prosciutto to make this a complete meal. Or serve with the Perfect Grilled Steak (page 154), Perfect Burger (page 153), or Perfect Grilled Shrimp (page 158).

⭐ PITTING OLIVES *You can buy pitted black olives (they don't have to be Kalamata), but pitting your own isn't that hard with the right technique. Lay the olive on a cutting board. Place the flat side of a large kitchen knife over the olive, and press down carefully on the knife until you feel the olive "give." Remove the knife—you should have a nice little seam in the olive, and the pit should be loose inside. Simply remove the pit with your fingers and discard. You can pit 2 to 3 olives at a time with this technique if your knife is big enough.*

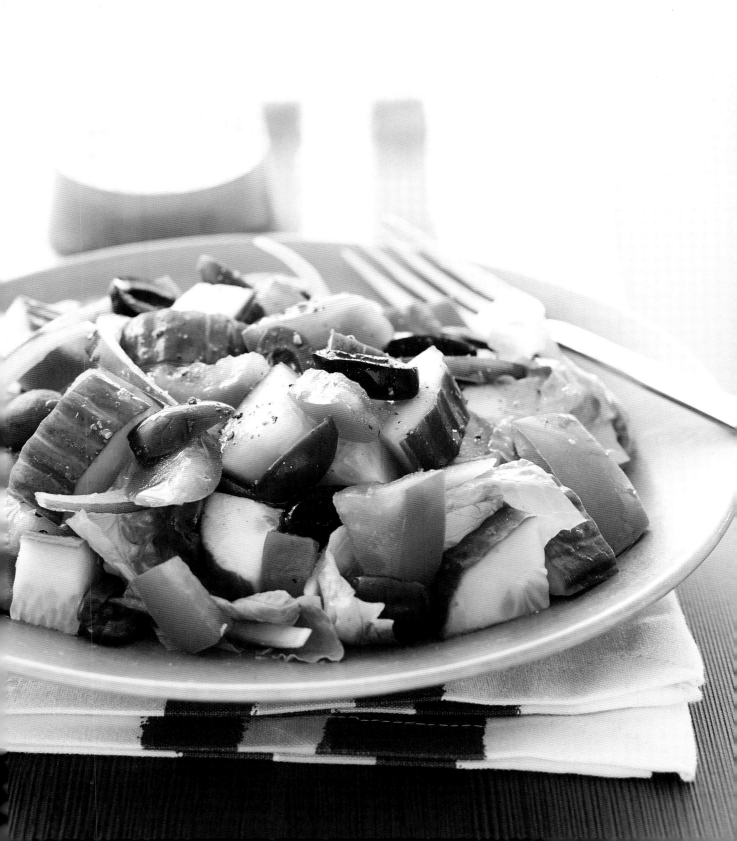

green beans with onions, mushrooms, and peppers

SERVES 2

PREP TIME: 15 minutes
COOK TIME: 15 minutes
TOTAL TIME: 30 minutes

---

2 cups ice

2 tablespoons plus ¼ teaspoon salt

1 pound green beans, ends trimmed

3 tablespoons clarified butter, ghee, or coconut oil

½ cup thinly sliced white onion

½ cup thinly sliced button, cremini, or portabella mushrooms

½ red bell pepper, seeded, ribs removed, and sliced into strips

¼ teaspoon black pepper

The quick cooking (blanching) ensures the green beans retain their crisp texture and vivid color when you cook them. Shocking them in cold water halts the cooking process (no more mushy green beans), and locks in the flavor, texture, and color. Properly shocked beans will be cold, bright green, and still have a firmness when snapped.

CREATE an ice bath for "shocking" the green beans by filling a large bowl halfway with cold water, then adding the ice.

BRING 3 cups of water and 2 tablespoons of the salt to a boil in a large saucepan over high heat Add the green beans and blanch for 20 seconds. Remove from the pot using kitchen tongs or a slotted spoon and shock them immediately in the ice bath. As soon as the green beans are chilled (about 1 minute), transfer to a colander and drain.

HEAT the cooking fat in a large skillet over medium-high heat, swirling to coat the bottom of the pan. When the fat is hot, add the onion and cook, stirring, until translucent, 2 to 3 minutes. Add the mushrooms and cook, stirring, for 2 minutes. Add the bell peppers and cook until the peppers and mushrooms have softened, about 2 minutes.

TURN the heat to high. Add the green beans to the skillet and toss with the other vegetables. Cook, shaking the pan often, until the beans are tender, about 2 minutes. (The easiest way to test is by tasting one!) Transfer the vegetables to a serving dish and season with the remaining ¼ teaspoon salt and the pepper.

MAKE IT A MEAL: Serve this colorful side dish with a Spinach Frittata (page 206), Stuffed Peppers (page 222), Halibut with Citrus-Ginger Glaze (page 240), or Chicken Meatballs (page 226).

⭐ HARICOTS VERTS *You might also see beans called haricots verts (French for "green beans") in the produce aisle. French green beans are longer and thinner than regular green beans, are more tender, and have a more complex flavor. They also tend to cook up faster, so if you're using haricots verts in this recipe, blanch for same amount of time, but cook, stirring, for just 1 minute in the last step.*

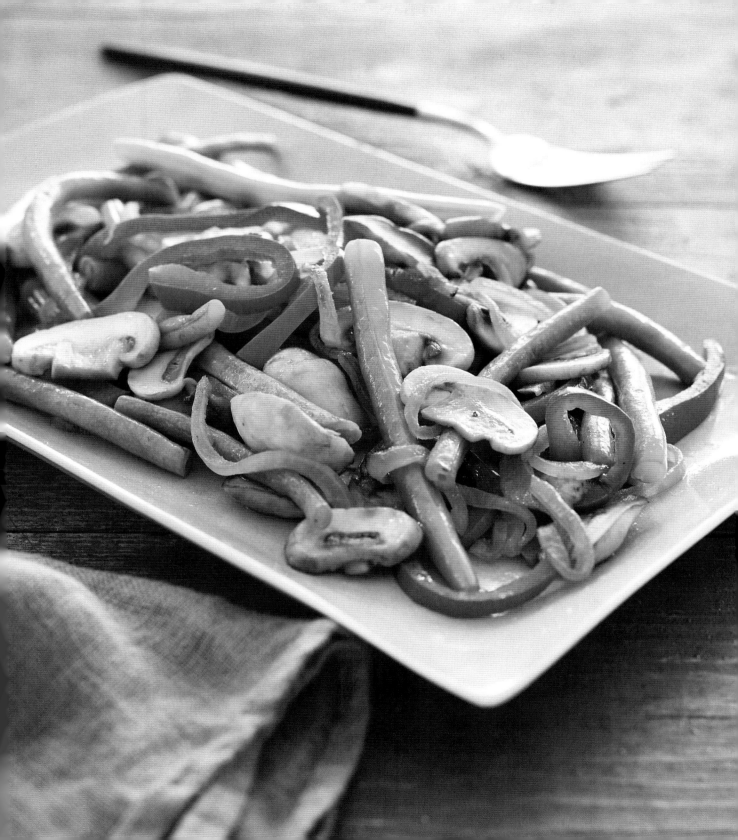

green cabbage slaw with lemon oil

SERVES 2

PREP TIME: 20 minutes

1 clove garlic, minced

Juice of 1 lemon

¼ cup extra-virgin olive oil

1 medium head green cabbage, finely shredded

1 cup shredded carrots

2 tablespoons chopped cashews

1 teaspoon sesame seeds

½ teaspoon salt

½ teaspoon black pepper

1 tablespoon ribbon-chopped fresh basil

Save time and use 4 cups of packaged shredded cabbage, or use 2 cups of packaged shredded cabbage mixed with 2 cups broccoli slaw. Adding a thinly sliced Granny Smith apple would also give the slaw a bite of tartness. A mayo-based dressing would contribute a bit more creaminess—just replace the olive oil with ¼ cup Basic Mayonnaise (page 179). Finally, for a fun variation, make a spicy slaw! Instead of lemon oil, mix the slaw with a dressing of ¼ cup apple cider vinegar, ¼ cup Whole30 Ketchup (page 323), and 1 teaspoon hot sauce (see page 403).

WHISK the garlic and lemon juice in a mixing bowl. While whisking, slowly add the olive oil in a steady stream until fully blended.

IN a large bowl, combine the cabbage, carrots, cashews, and sesame seeds. Mix with a wooden spoon to combine, then toss with the lemon oil. Adjust the seasoning with the salt and pepper and top with the basil.

MAKE IT A MEAL: This crisp, fresh dish goes well with just about anything. It's a great partner to the warmth of a Perfect Grilled Steak (page 154), is light enough to complement our Poached Salmon with Cucumber Dill Sauce (page 246), and is a cool companion for our Chimichurri Beef Kabobs (page 218). Or top it with cooked (cold) shrimp, salmon, chicken, or hard-boiled eggs to make it a complete meal.

⭐ SHREDDING CABBAGE *Shredding cabbage is really fast and easy if you have the right technique. First, cut the cabbage in half, then in half again. Take each quarter and remove the core of the cabbage (the thick white stem) by cutting it out with a sharp knife. Lay each quarter on a flat side and cut crosswise into thin slices, working from top to bottom. You'll end up with thin ribbons of cabbage, perfect for slaw. (Shredding carrots is easy too—just use the largest holes in your cheese grater until your carrot is down to a sliver!)*

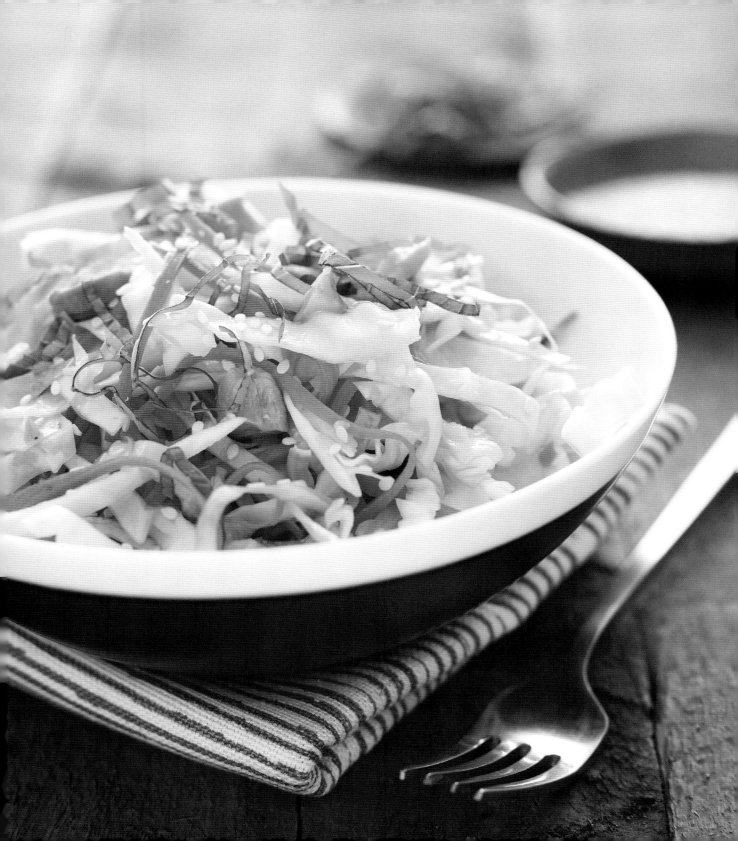

grilled asparagus with lemon zest

SERVES 2

PREP TIME: 3 minutes

COOK TIME: 5 minutes

TOTAL TIME: 8 minutes

---

1 pound asparagus, trimmed

1 tablespoon clarified butter, ghee, or coconut oil, melted

½ teaspoon salt

Grated zest and juice of 1 lemon

To make grilling the asparagus a bit easier, try threading four or five asparagus spears cross-wise on two wooden or metal skewers before seasoning them, or place them in a grill basket or in foil on the grill. This will keep the asparagus from accidentally falling through the grill grates. If you don't have a grill, cook the asparagus in a large skillet over medium-high heat in 1 tablespoon of cooking fat for 10 minutes, stirring occasionally to cook all sides evenly.

PREHEAT a grill to medium-high heat (400°F). Line a baking sheet with foil.

PLACE the asparagus on the baking sheet, drizzle with the melted cooking fat, and sprinkle with the salt. With tongs, transfer the asparagus to the grill, laying the spears horizontally across the grate, and grill until tender, 4 to 6 minutes.

TRANSFER the asparagus to a serving plate. Drizzle the lemon juice over the top and sprinkle with the lemon zest just before serving.

MAKE IT A MEAL: Since you're out there anyway, pair this with the Perfect Burger (page 153), Perfect Grilled Shrimp (page 158), or Grilled Coconut-Curry Chicken (page 230). It's also a hearty enough side to stand up to our Baby Back Ribs with Tangy BBQ Sauce (page 256), and goes great with Seared Salmon Benedict (page 210).

⭐ TRIMMING ASPARAGUS *The tougher parts of the asparagus stalk need to be removed before cooking. The easiest way to do this is to simply grasp the lighter colored root end and bend until it snaps. The asparagus will automatically break in just the right spot, so don't overthink it! You can even grab your asparagus in a small bundle and break the ends off all at once to save some time.*

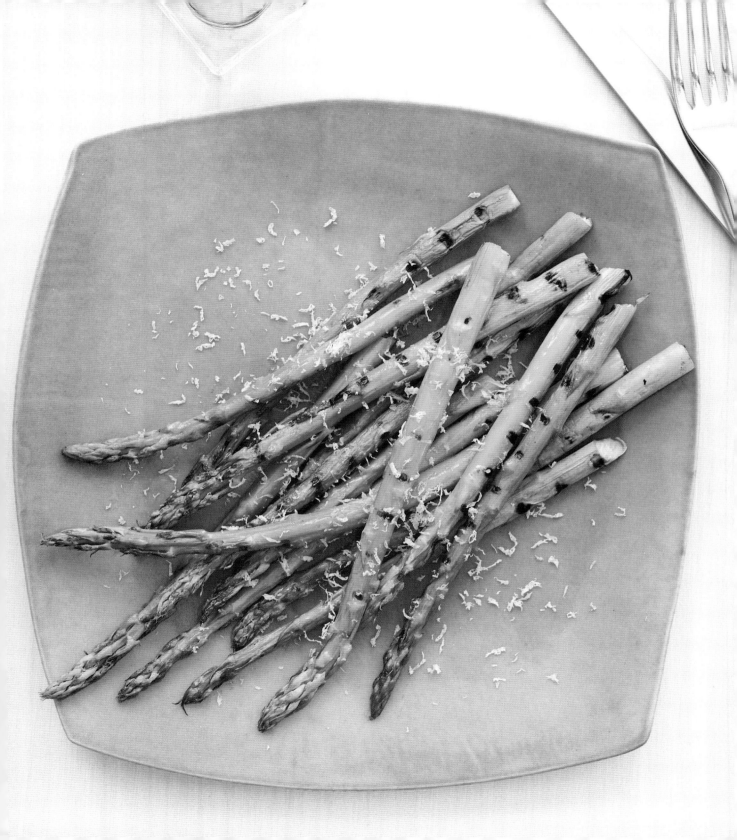

pan-roasted brussels sprouts and squash

SERVES 2

PREP TIME: 15 minutes
COOK TIME: 25 minutes
TOTAL TIME: 40 minutes

3 tablespoons extra-virgin olive oil

½ pound Brussels sprouts, trimmed and cut in half

½ red onion, cut into 1-inch pieces

1 teaspoon dried sage

½ teaspoon nutmeg

½ teaspoon black pepper

¼ teaspoon salt

3 cups diced peeled butternut squash

One large squash usually yields 2½ to 3 cups, so just buy a big one and call it good—no need to measure precisely for this recipe. You can also substitute any winter squash for butternut: this dish would be great with delicata, acorn, kabocha, or buttercup. Not winter squash season? Use 2 peeled, large-diced sweet potatoes or apples instead. Serving company? Add crumbled Whole30-compliant bacon or prosciutto and pomegranate seeds as a garnish.

HEAT the olive oil in a large skillet over medium heat and swirl to coat the bottom of the pan. When the oil is hot, add the Brussels sprouts and onion and season with the sage, nutmeg, pepper, and salt. Cover and cook, shaking the pan occasionally, until the sprouts begin to brown, 5 to 7 minutes. Turn the sprouts and add the squash and cook everything until the squash is fork-tender, an additional 7 to 10 minutes.

TRANSFER to a serving dish or plates and serve immediately.

MAKE IT A MEAL: When you add the squash to the pan, add cooked sausage, chicken sausage, or chicken to make it a complete meal. Or serve with Steak Salad (page 220), Grilled Coconut-Curry Chicken (page 230), or Walnut-Crusted Pork Tenderloin (page 252).

⭐ OVER-ROASTED SPROUTS AND SQUASH *You can also make this meal in the oven and free your stovetop for other dishes. First, skip cutting the Brussels sprouts in half—just trim the ends and leave them whole. Preheat the oven to 350°F. In a large mixing bowl, combine the Brussels sprouts, onion, and butternut squash. Add the olive oil and stir or toss until all the vegetables are well coated. Spread the vegetables on a parchment paper–lined baking tray and sprinkle with the sage, nutmeg, pepper, and salt. Roast in the oven for 30 to 40 minutes, until the Brussels sprouts and squash are fork-tender.*

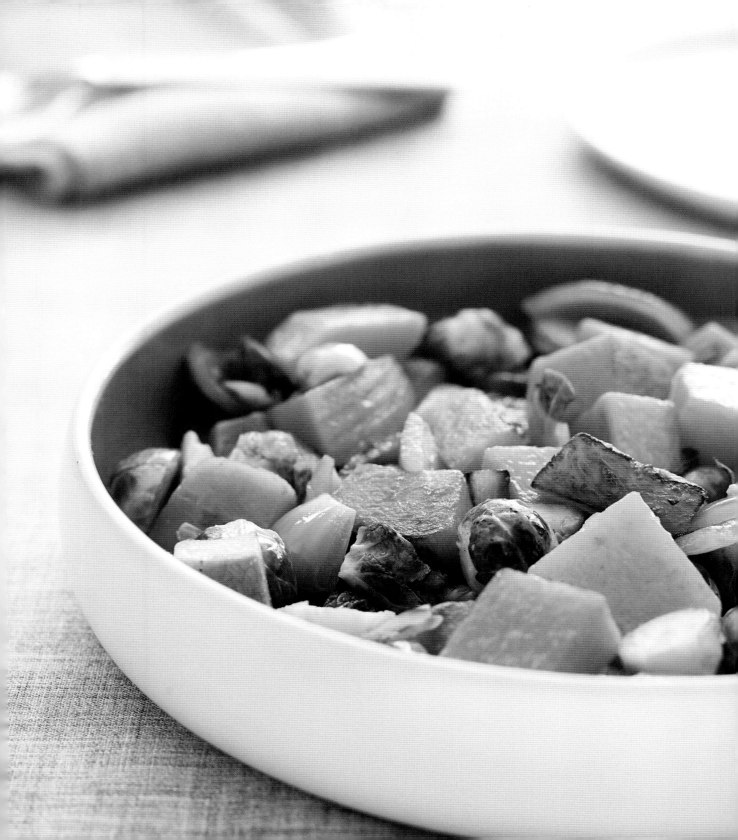

ratatouille

SERVES 2

PREP TIME: 20 minutes
COOK TIME: 35 minutes
TOTAL TIME: 55 minutes

¼ cup coconut oil or extra-virgin olive oil

¼ onion, finely chopped

1 cup diced zucchini

1 cup diced yellow squash

1 cup diced eggplant

½ teaspoon salt

½ teaspoon black pepper

½ cup finely diced green bell pepper

½ cup finely diced red bell pepper

2 cloves garlic, minced

1 cup Tomato Sauce (page 324)

1 teaspoon balsamic vinegar

3 fresh basil leaves, roughly chopped
(optional)

Got leftovers? You will if you double this recipe! Ratatouille is equally delicious cold. Serve with eggs the next morning for breakfast, or mix in some cooked chicken or shrimp for an easy lunch.

IN a medium pot, heat the oil over medium heat, swirling to coat the bottom of the pot. When the oil is hot, add the onion and cook, stirring, until translucent, 2 to 3 minutes. Add the zucchini, yellow squash, and eggplant and season with the salt and pepper. Cook for 2 minutes, stirring often. Add the green and red bell peppers and continue to cook for 2 to 3 minutes, stirring often. Add the garlic and cook until aromatic, about 1 minute. Add the tomato sauce and ½ cup water. Mix completely and bring to a simmer over low heat. Cook, stirring occasionally, until all the vegetables are tender, about 25 minutes.

TRANSFER to a serving dish, casserole dish, or individual plates, sprinkle with the vinegar, and garnish with the basil, if desired.

MAKE IT A MEAL: Make this a complete meal by adding homemade sausage (see page 162) or pre-cooked diced chicken during the last 10 minutes of cooking. Or serve with Perfect Poached Eggs (page 150), Chicken Meatballs (page 226), or Stuffed Peppers (page 222).

⭐ GRILLED RATATOUILLE *You can make ratatouille right on the grill. Preheat a grill to medium high (400°F) and prep all the vegetables, cutting the onion, green pepper, and red pepper into quarters and slicing the zucchini, squash, and eggplant into long, thin strips. In a large bowl, coat the vegetables with the oil and season with salt and pepper. Place the eggplant on the grill first, cooking for 3 minutes. Then add the peppers and onion and cook for another 2 minutes. Finally, add the zucchini and squash and cook until everything is slightly charred and tender, about 5 more minutes. (Flip each vegetable once during cooking.) Place on a serving dish, top with warmed tomato sauce and basil, and serve.*

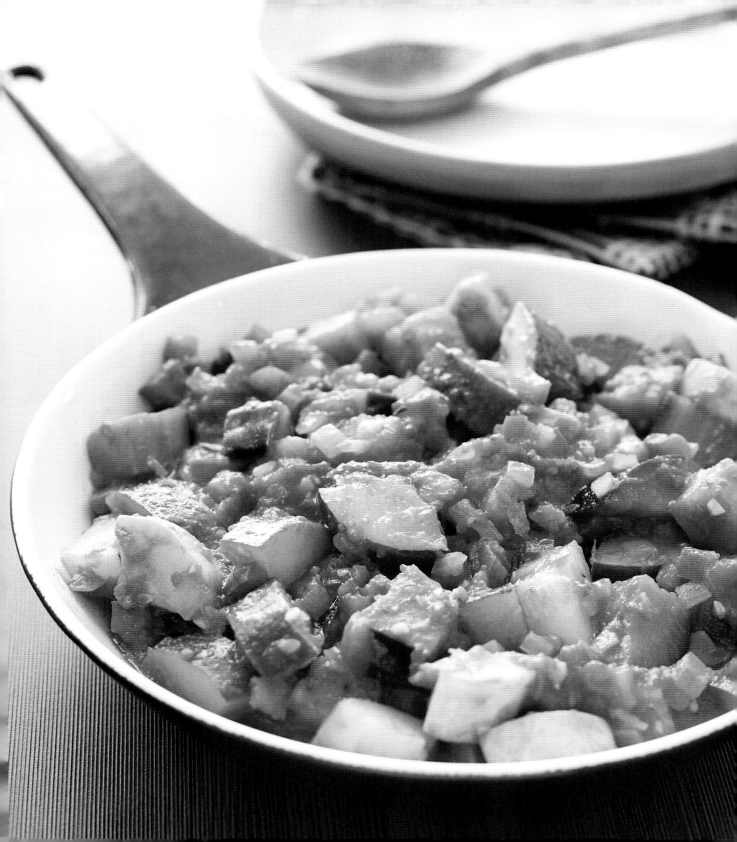

roasted beet, orange, and avocado salad

SERVES 2

PREP TIME: 10 minutes

COOK TIME: 35 to 60 minutes

TOTAL TIME: 45 minutes to 1 hour 10 minutes

---

2 medium beets

2 tablespoons extra-virgin olive oil

1 tablespoon balsamic vinegar

1 orange, halved, one half zested and juiced, one half peeled and cut into segments

½ teaspoon salt

¼ teaspoon black pepper

1 avocado, split lengthwise, pitted, peeled, and diced

If you're planning to double this recipe for leftovers, double everything *but* the avocado. The dressed beets and orange slices will hold up well in the fridge for a day or two, but avocado tends to turn brown and mushy. Your best bet is to add a fresh avocado to your leftovers right before serving. We also love adding delicate greens such as pea shoots or frisée to give the salad a little added texture.

PREHEAT the oven to 425°F.

RINSE the beets thoroughly and carefully stab all sides with a fork. Place in a medium bowl and add 1 tablespoon of the olive oil, tossing or mixing to thoroughly coat. Wrap the oiled beets in aluminum foil, pinching the top closed to create a seal. Place the beets in the center of a baking sheet and roast for 35 minutes. Check them by carefully opening the foil and sticking a thin knife into the center of a beet: If it goes in easily, the beets are done. If there's resistance, close them back up and put back into the oven for 10 minutes. Repeat until the knife slides into the center of the beet easily. Let rest until cool enough to handle.

REMOVE the skin from the beets—you may want to wear gloves and an apron, as beet juice will stain your skin and clothes. Dice the beets into 1-inch pieces and place in a serving bowl.

IN a small bowl, combine the remaining 1 tablespoon olive oil with the vinegar, orange juice, salt, and pepper and whisk until combined.

ADD the orange segments and avocado to the beets. Drizzle with the dressing, sprinkle on the orange zest, toss to coat, and serve.

MAKE IT A MEAL: This fresh salad tastes great in all seasons. Serve with Perfect Whole Roasted Chicken (page 157), Beef Brisket (page 214), or Halibut with Citrus-Ginger Glaze (page 240).

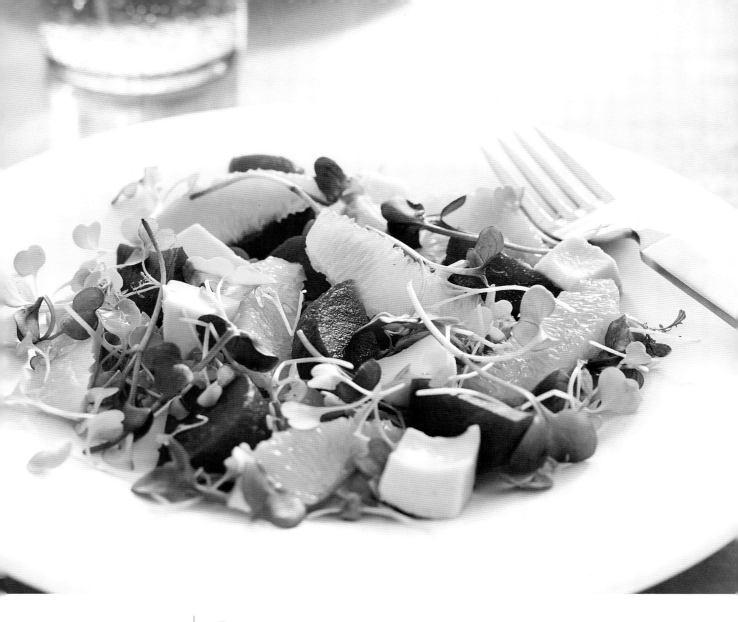

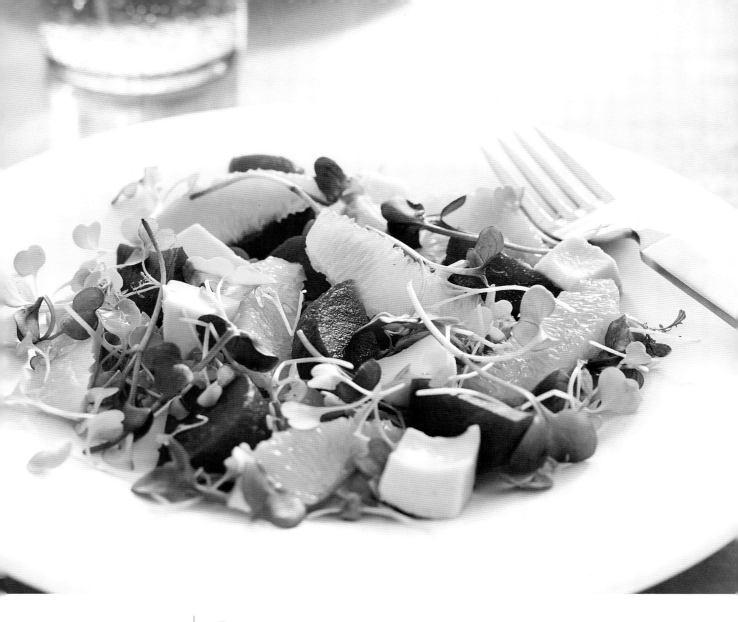 BEETS *If you get whole beets with the stems still on, remove them before roasting. Cut them about an inch above the root, not any closer. You don't want to risk cutting into the beet itself, as that will allow juice and flavor to leak out while roasting. Beets can vary in their cooking times, so don't be surprised if yours require a full hour to fully roast. Plan ahead, or roast them on your meal prep day—they'll keep in the fridge for 3 to 4 days. Make sure you peel them before storing, though—they're easier to peel when they're still warm.*

roasted root vegetables in curry sauce

SERVES 2

PREP TIME: 15 minutes

COOK TIME: 35 minutes

TOTAL TIME: 50 minutes

---

1 cup peeled diced potato (any variety)

1 cup peeled diced rutabaga

1 cup peeled diced turnips

1 cup peeled diced parsnips

1 cup peeled diced carrots

¼ cup cooking fat

½ cup Curry Sauce (page 307)

Mix and match some of the heartier vegetables based on what's in season, available at your local grocery store, or what you feel like eating. They don't have to be roots, either! Beets, celery root, kohlrabi, eggplant, Brussels sprouts, broccoli, cauliflower, salsify, or cassava (yuca) would all work well with the curry sauce.

PREHEAT the oven to 400°F. Line 2 baking sheets with parchment paper.

MELT the cooking fat (if necessary), combine with all the vegetables in a large mixing bowl, and toss or mix to thoroughly coat. Spread the vegetables in one layer on the 2 baking sheets. Do not crowd the vegetables or they'll steam instead of roast.

ROAST for 30 to 40 minutes, until the vegetables are lightly browned on the outside and fork-tender. Transfer to a serving bowl or individual plates and top with the Curry Sauce.

MAKE IT A MEAL: You could add cooked sausage, chicken sausage, chicken, or sliced beef to the vegetable mixture just before serving to make this a meal—just heat your protein in a pan or microwave before mixing with the hot vegetables. You can also pair this dish with Perfect Fried Eggs (page 149), Perfect Seared Chicken Breast (page 157), or Chicken Meatballs (page 226).

⭐ PEELING RUTABAGA *Rutabaga is a direct cross between a cabbage and a turnip, and when cooked, tastes both sweet and savory. It can be tough to peel, though—your standard kitchen peeler (especially if it's dull) may not work. If your standard peeler isn't getting the job done, use a paring knife. First, cut the rutabaga in half. Place each half flat-side down on a cutting board and, using a sharp paring knife, carefully slice the skin off in 2-inch increments. (You may need a few passes to get to the lighter colored flesh underneath.) Repeat on the other half.*

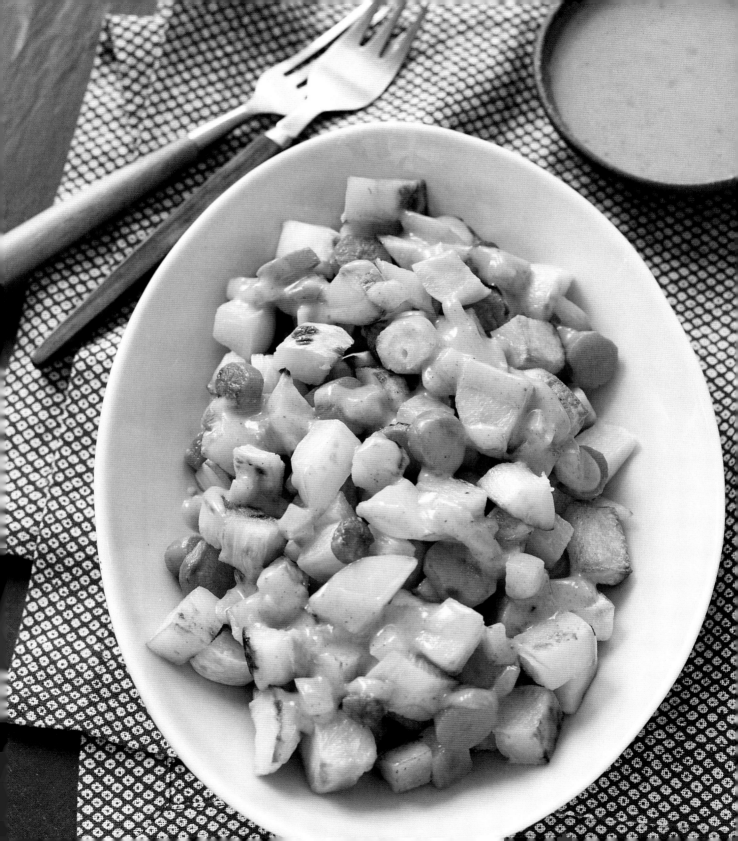

roasted spaghetti squash

SERVES 2

PREP TIME: 10 minutes
COOK TIME: 1 hour
TOTAL TIME: 1 hour 10 minutes

---

1 whole spaghetti squash

2 tablespoons extra-virgin olive oil

2 teaspoons fresh thyme leaves
(or ¼ teaspoon dried)

½ teaspoon salt

¼ teaspoon black pepper

You can roast the spaghetti squash whole if you puncture the sides with a fork first, but your noodles turn out softer and wetter, as they steam more inside the full squash. We recommend cutting it in half and undercooking it slightly so it has that al-dente pasta texture. You can check for doneness by poking a sharp knife through the skin of the upside-down squash—if it slides through easily, it's probably done. You can also use an oven mitt to flip one half of the squash over and run a fork down the side of the squash. If it comes away from the side in a nice spaghetti texture easily, you're good. If your "noodles" are too firm or don't easily scrape, flip it back over, put it back in the oven for 5 to 10 minutes, and check again. (The ultimate doneness check? Taste it! Your "spaghetti" should be tender: not too firm, but not mushy.)

PREHEAT the oven to 425°F. Line a baking sheet with foil or parchment paper.

CUT the squash in half lengthwise and remove the seeds with a large spoon. Drizzle the insides evenly with the olive oil. Place the squash flesh-side down on the baking sheet.

ROAST the squash for 1 hour, until fork-tender. Carefully turn the squash flesh-side up and let cool until cool enough to handle.

USE a fork to gently scrape out the flesh; the squash will come out in noodle-like strands. Season evenly with the thyme, salt, and pepper, and serve immediately.

MAKE IT A MEAL: It's supremely easy to turn this vegetable side into a complete meal. Top with a meaty Tomato Sauce (page 324); add cooked sausage, roasted tomatoes, sautéed onions, and our Pesto (page 315); or mix leftovers with steamed spinach and top with a few fried eggs for a quick and easy breakfast.

⭐ CUTTING SQUASH *Cutting a spaghetti squash in half might be the most difficult part of this recipe. Melissa Joulwan, author of the* Well Fed *cookbook series, suggests using a paring knife to "score" a groove in the skin first, then following that groove with a large kitchen knife. You can see a video of her entire technique at www.w30.co/cutsquash.*

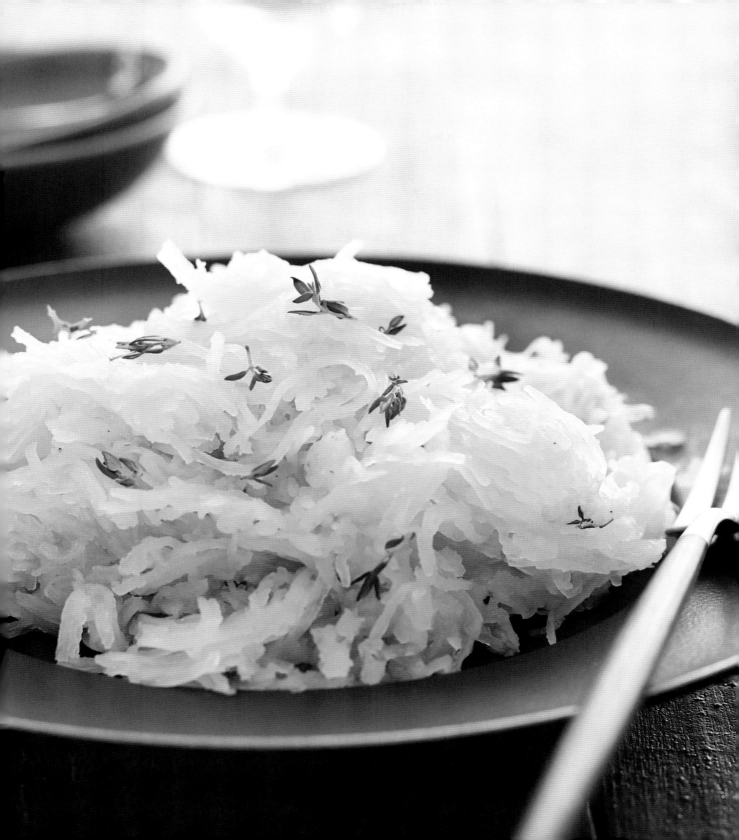

roasted sweet potatoes

SERVES 2

PREP TIME: 10 minutes

COOK TIME: 30 to 60 minutes

TOTAL TIME: 40 minutes to 1 hour 10 minutes

---

2 medium sweet potatoes

2 tablespoons extra-virgin olive oil

2 tablespoons clarified butter, ghee, or coconut butter

Salt and black pepper

You can also slice your sweet potatoes into long "spears" before roasting—these are perfect for dipping! Add the spears to a bowl with the olive oil and mix to coat. Place the spears in one layer on a parchment paper–lined baking sheet and roast as directed, about 40 minutes, until the edges are brown but not burned. These pair well with Ranch Dressing (page 316), Garlic Aioli (page 309), or Sunshine Sauce (page 320).

PREHEAT the oven to 375°F.

WASH the sweet potatoes thoroughly and pat dry. With a fork or paring knife, carefully puncture all sides of each potato. Rub the olive oil evenly over the skin.

WRAP each sweet potato securely in foil, sealing the foil on top. Place on a baking sheet and roast for 30 minutes. Starting at the 30 minute mark, insert a fork or knife into the center of the potato every 5 minutes; they are done when they are very soft and tender. (Depending on the size of the potatoes, this may take up to 1 hour.)

REMOVE the foil and cut the sweet potatoes open lengthwise. Keeping the skin on, add 1 tablespoon of butter to each sweet potato, scraping the flesh gently with a fork so the butter melts into the flesh. Season to taste with salt and pepper.

MAKE IT A MEAL: This simple but delicious side goes well with just about anything. We think it complements Braised Beef Brisket (page 214), Grilled Coconut-Curry Chicken (page 230), Cod with Mushroom and Red Pepper Relish (page 242), or Pork Chops With Spiced Applesauce (page 258). Or, stuff a roasted sweet potato with Pulled Pork Carnitas (page 254) and top with our Avocado Mayonnaise (page 310).

⭐ COMPOUND BUTTER *A compound butter (see page 181) would be a delicious addition to this simple side dish. Some combinations to consider: 2 teaspoons chopped rosemary leaves and ¼ cup chopped, toasted pecans; ½ teaspoon each cinnamon and nutmeg, ¼ cup chopped toasted walnuts, and ¼ cup chopped raisins; or 2 cloves minced garlic with 2 teaspoons each chopped rosemary, thyme, and sage.*

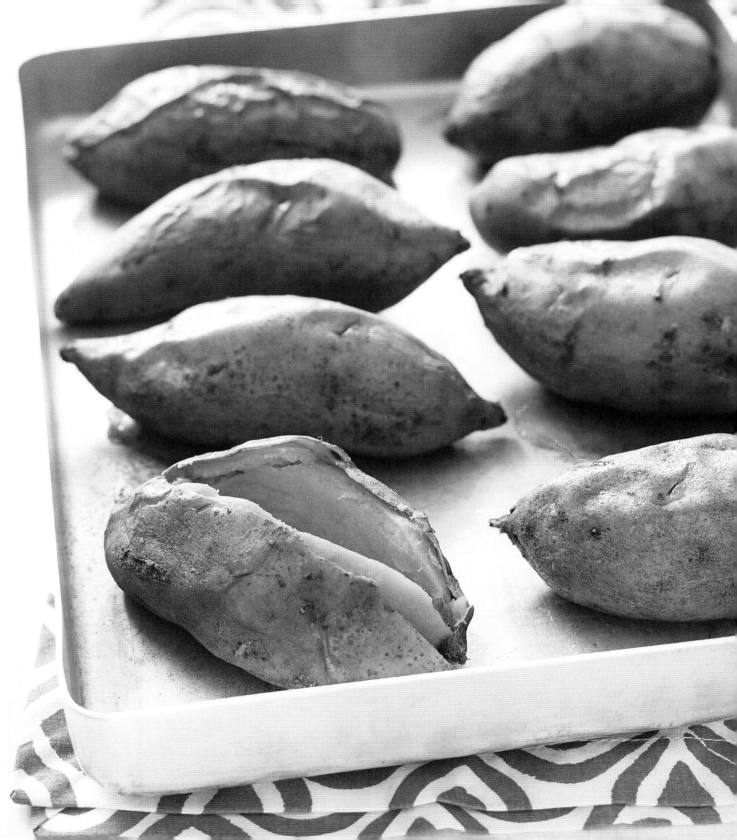

sautéed kale with almonds

SERVES 2

PREP TIME: 10 minutes

COOK TIME: 5 minutes

TOTAL TIME: 15 minutes

---

1 head kale, stemmed, leaves cut into 1-inch ribbons

3 tablespoons cooking fat

1 clove garlic, minced

¼ cup raw sliced almonds

½ teaspoon salt

½ teaspoon black pepper

Grated zest and juice of ½ lemon

Kale is one vegetable that *really* needs to be washed before cooking, as it can taste pretty gritty au naturel. Your best bet is to wash it and then spin in a salad spinner until the leaves are really dry. This is especially important for baked kale chips (see the tip). Alternatively, you can wash and pat the leaves with a dish towel or paper towels until they're totally dry.

BRING 1 cup of water to a boil in a large pot. Place a colander or steamer inside the pot. Add the kale, cover, and steam until the kale is tender but not soft, 3 to 5 minutes. Remove the colander or steamer from the pot and transfer to a dish towel to catch any dripping water.

HEAT the cooking fat in a large skillet over medium-high heat, swirling to coat the bottom of the pan. When the fat is hot, add the garlic and almonds and cook until the garlic is aromatic, about 1 minute. Increase the heat to high, add the kale, and cook for 1 minute, tossing to combine the kale with the garlic and almonds. Transfer to a serving dish and season with the salt, pepper, and lemon juice. Top with the lemon zest and serve.

MAKE IT A MEAL: This hearty green is the perfect match for our Spinach Frittata (page 206), Stuffed Peppers (page 222), or Baby Back Ribs (page 256).

⭐ KALE CHIPS *Want to double your kale consumption today? Make kale chips in the oven while this dish is cooking on the stovetop. Preheat the oven to 300°F. Line a large baking sheet with parchment paper. Stem a head of kale and tear the leaves into large pieces. Add the pieces to a large mixing bowl along with ½ tablespoon extra-virgin olive oil and massage well to thoroughly coat the leaves. Lay them out in one layer on the baking sheet and sprinkle with salt. (If you have too much kale for one baking sheet, use two. Don't crowd the kale, or the leaves will steam instead of crisp.) Bake for 20 to 25 minutes, until the edges are brown but not burned. Allow to cool on the baking sheet for 5 minutes, and enjoy!*

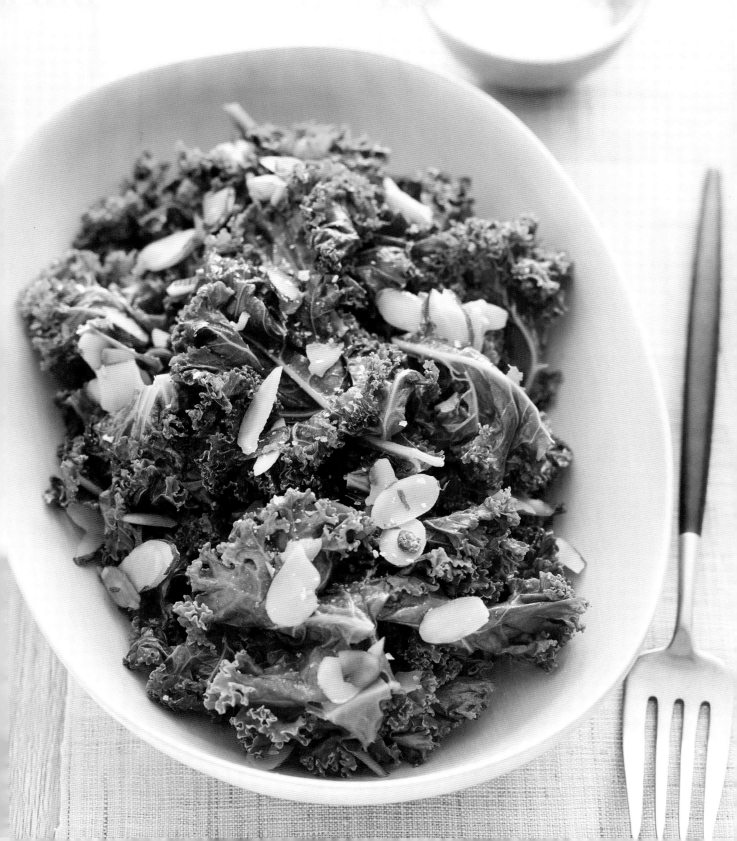

sweet potato soup

SERVES 2

PREP TIME: 10 minutes
COOK TIME: 25 minutes
TOTAL TIME: 35 minutes

---

2 tablespoons cooking fat

2 large-diced peeled sweet potatoes

½ teaspoon ground ginger (or
2 tablespoons minced fresh ginger)

1 pinch ground cinnamon, plus extra
for garnish

1 cup full-fat coconut milk

½ teaspoon salt

¼ teaspoon black pepper

For a more savory soup, use ½ teaspoon garlic powder, ½ teaspoon onion powder, and 1 tablespoon fresh thyme leaves in place of the cinnamon, and add some fresh sliced mushrooms when you return the soup to the pot for the final stage of cooking. For more of a traditional fall flavor, use a sugar-free apple pie spice mixture in place of the cinnamon, add some finely diced sweet onion and apple in the final stage of cooking, and top with chopped pecans. For a thinner soup, simmer for just 1 to 2 minutes, then add compliant chicken broth one tablespoon at a time until you reach the desired consistency.

IN a Dutch oven or large pot, heat the cooking fat over medium heat, swirling to coat the bottom of the pot. When the fat is hot, add the sweet potatoes, stirring to coat them with the fat. Add the ginger and cinnamon and stir for 15 seconds. Add 3 cups of water and the coconut milk and bring to a boil. Simmer until the sweet potatoes become soft, about 15 minutes. Remove the pot from the heat.

IN one or two batches, puree the sweet potato mixture in a food processor or blender to a smooth consistency, or use an immersion blender to mix it right in the pot. Return the soup to the pot. Cook the soup to your desired thickness over medium-low heat—the longer it simmers, the thicker the soup will become. Season to taste with the salt and pepper, garnish with extra cinnamon, and serve.

MAKE IT A MEAL: You could add any pre-cooked meat to this soup and make it a complete meal—try grilled chicken, sausage, ground beef, or scallops. Or, serve alongside our Stuffed Peppers (page 222), Thai Cucumber Cups (page 234), or Mexican Tuna Boats (page 238).

⭐ FRESH GINGER *Peeling and mincing fresh ginger can be a difficult task—watch your fingertips! First, peel the ginger root by scraping the skin off with the edge of a spoon or a vegetable peeler. (Don't worry if you miss a few spots in the corners.) From there, you can mince the ginger by hand by cutting the root into coins, then cutting the coins into matchsticks, then dicing the matchsticks a few times until you have a very fine mince. Or, use a Microplane (like a mini-cheese grater) to grate the ginger. Do this over a bowl or plate to catch the juices as you grate.*

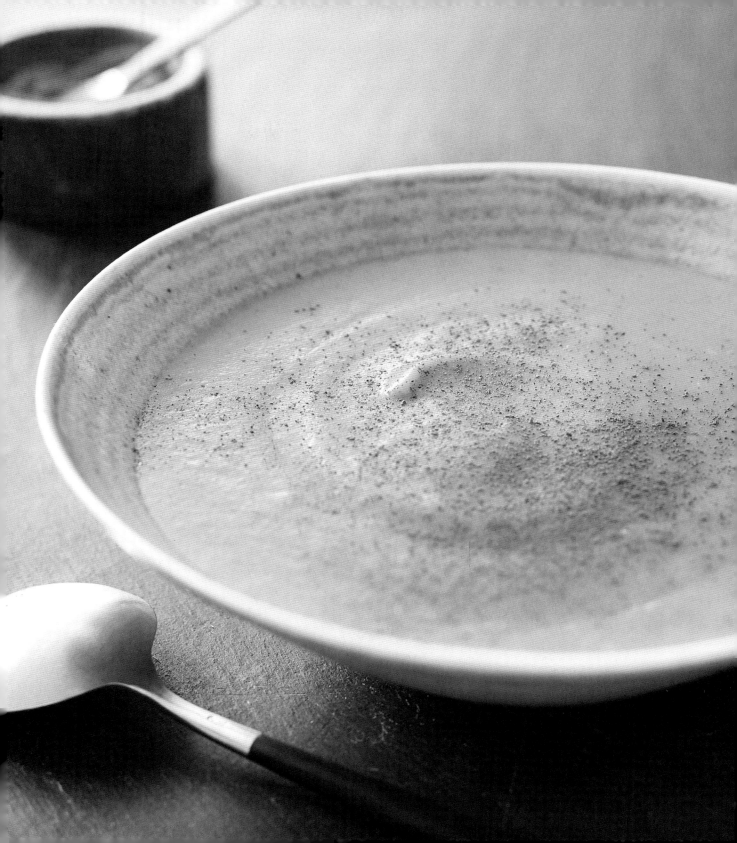

DRESSINGS, DIPS, AND SAUCES

IF THERE'S ONE SECTION OF THIS BOOK that you want to become intimately familiar with, it's this one. In fact, you could cook *just* using our Kitchen Fundamentals tips and these dressings, dips, and sauces for the entirety of your Whole30 and never get bored with your food.

Dressings, dips, and sauces are literally the spice of your Whole30 life. They transform plain old meat and veggies into cohesive, flavorful meals; change Mexican-themed dinners into Asian-inspired lunches; and give you an easy way to turn one roasted chicken into three days of totally different meals. Take our Broccoli, Mushroom, and Summer Squash recipe on page 264. Without the red pepper sauce, this dish is pretty ho-hum . . . cooked veggies with garlic, salt, and pepper. Keep making sides like this and you'll be bored out of your Whole30 mind in no time. But *with* the pesto, presto! You've got a delicious dish exploding with flavor and texture—so much so that it could easily be the star of your dinner show, served alongside any basic protein.

The more you play around with these recipes, the more you'll see that the variations are limitless! Just look at our Basic Mayonnaise* variations on page 309. One five-minute recipe can be transformed any number of ways, adding depth, dimension, and creamy, dreamy goodness to your dishes.

Wait, you don't like mayo? Oh, but you haven't tried *our* mayo.

Let's be honest—the store-bought stuff tends to be gloopy, slimy, and tastes, well, kind of funny. But our mayo, made from scratch with just five ingredients, is light and fluffy. It tastes clean and neutral, with no aftertaste. And once you mix it up with hot sauce, avocado, fresh herbs, or wasabi, you may just find yourself scraping the bowl and licking the spoon after you make yet another batch.

We're convinced mayo is the new cake batter.

Including dressings or sauces in your regular meal planning also makes your meal prep easier, as most of these can be made in advance, prepared in extra-big batches, or frozen for later use. So for those of you new to cooking, let's lay out a game plan for three nights of Whole30 dinners based around dressings and sauces.

Find some recipes in this section that look delicious, and prepare three or four in advance. For example, let's prepare a batch of Basic Mayonnaise (page 179), our Chimichurri (page 306),

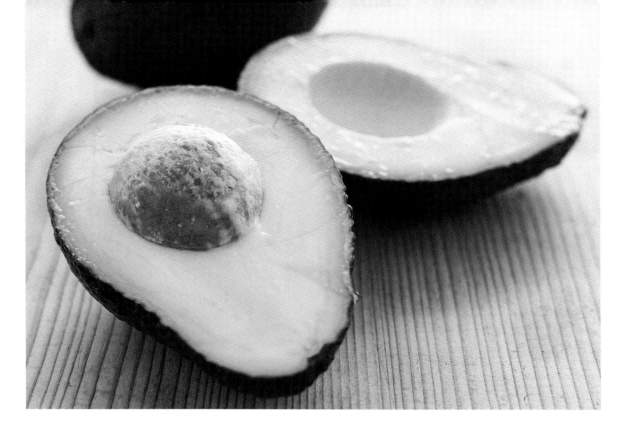

Sunshine Sauce (page 320), and Curry Sauce (page 307). Next, plan your dinners for the week, shopping for simple ingredients specifically designed to go with the sauces you've already prepared.

At dinnertime, use our Whole30 Cooking Fundamentals (starting on page 146) to prepare your basic protein and vegetables. Let's say you've planned on a grilled steak with mashed sweet potato and steamed spinach; a seared chicken breast with roasted carrots and fresh garden salad; and oven-baked salmon with sautéed broccoli, pepper, onions, and mushrooms.

Now, the magic . . . top your meat and veggies with one of your sauces or dressings—the steak would be delicious with Chimichurri, the chicken tastes great drizzled with Sunshine Sauce, your garden salad can be dressed in a

mayo-based Balsamic (page 328), and our Curry Sauce is perfect over salmon and veggies.

See what just happened there? You've got dinner in 20 minutes or less, and a family who thinks you're some kind of culinary genius. Plus you made enough leftover sauce from each meal to make your next few meals exciting, too—eggs topped with Chimichurri for breakfast, raw celery dipped in Sunshine Sauce with lunch, ground beef mixed with Curry Sauce for dinner, and enough mayo left over to make a big batch of Protein Salad (page 161) for on-the-go days. Whoa. We practically came to your house and cooked this all for you. Aren't you lucky! For more meal planning ideas, turn to page 194.

*If you can't eat eggs, don't worry—we've given you an egg-free version of our Basic Mayonnaise on page 180, so you won't miss out on all of the dressing and sauce variations in this section.

buffalo sauce

MAKES 2 CUPS

PREP TIME: 5 minutes
COOK TIME: 2 minutes
TOTAL TIME: 7 minutes

½ cup coconut oil

½ cup ghee or clarified butter

1 cup hot sauce

2 tablespoons apple cider vinegar

1 clove garlic, minced

Want to kick your heat up a notch?
Add ¼ teaspoon cayenne to the mix—
more if you're feeling feisty. You can
also mix the buffalo sauce into ground
beef for a spicy twist on a burger. Top
with a fried egg, some avocado, and
a little more of the sauce mixture.

IN a small saucepan, gently melt the coconut oil and ghee over medium-low heat until completely liquefied.

COMBINE the hot sauce, vinegar, and garlic in a medium mixing bowl and whisk until thoroughly blended. While whisking, drizzle in the melted coconut oil and ghee. The sauce should have a smooth, consistent texture.

STORE this sauce in an airtight container in the fridge for up to 7 days. (Note, the coconut oil and ghee will solidify in the cold, so pull it out of the fridge, let it come back to room temperature before serving, and gently stir to reblend.)

⭐ BUFFALO WINGS *For the perfect buffalo wings, fire up the grill! Preheat the grill to medium-high heat (400°F). Add a pound of wings to the grill and close the lid. Turning the wings every few minutes, cook until lightly charred and the skin starts to bubble, 15 to 20 minutes. Toss the wings with the buffalo sauce in a large bowl immediately after removing them from the grill—then let them sit in the sauce for a few minutes before serving with a side of celery and carrots and our Ranch Dressing (page 316). (You can also preheat the oven to 375°F and, following the same technique, have golden, crispy wings in about an hour.)*

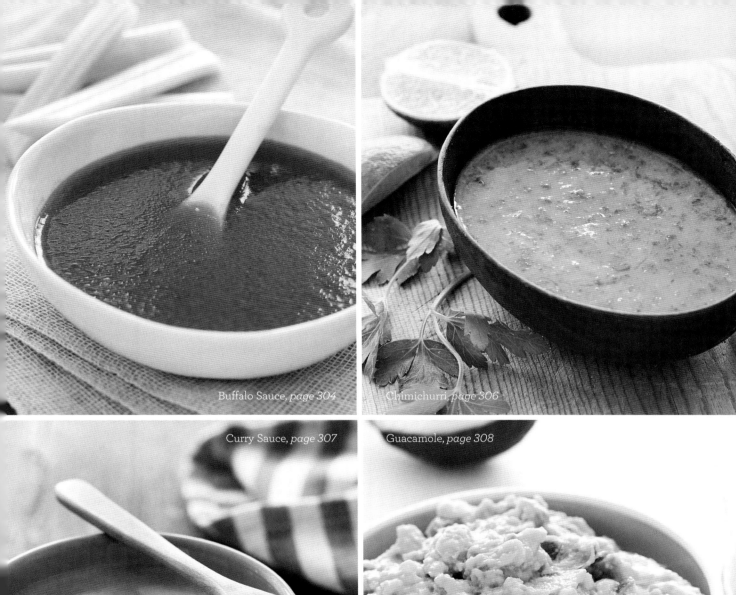

Buffalo Sauce, *page 304*

Chimichurri, *page 306*

Curry Sauce, *page 307*

Guacamole, *page 308*

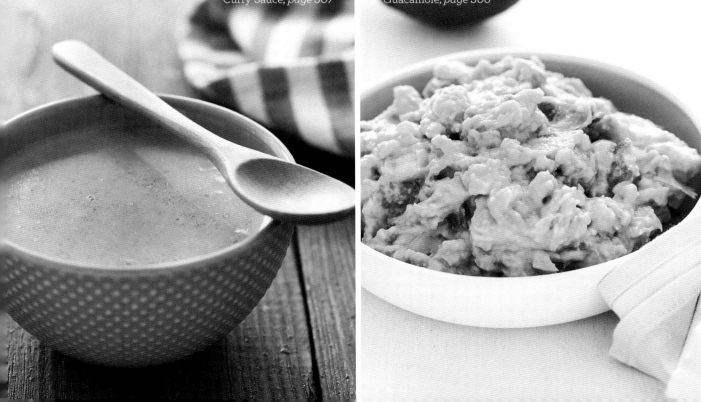

chimichurri

MAKES 2½ CUPS

PREP TIME: 10 minutes

¼ cup red wine vinegar

¼ cup lime juice

2 cloves garlic, minced

½ shallot, minced

1 ½ cups extra-virgin olive oil

¼ cup fresh cilantro

¼ cup fresh parsley leaves

½ teaspoon salt

½ teaspoon black pepper

Versatile chimichurri is a great topping for steak, lamb chops, chicken, and eggs, and is fantastic drizzled over grilled vegetables. You can also use it to marinate meat (like a flat-iron or skirt steak) before grilling.

COMBINE the vinegar, lime juice, garlic, and shallot in a food processor and mix on low speed. Drizzle in the olive oil while mixing; the dressing will begin to emulsify. Add the cilantro, parsley, salt, and pepper and continue to mix on low until the dressing is uniform in texture and the herb pieces are chopped quite small.

CHIMICHURRI will last 2 to 3 days in the refrigerator. If making ahead, bring it to room temperature before serving. If the dressing has separated, gently whisk to reblend.

⭐ STORING CHIMICHURRI *If you make a big batch of chimichurri, you can freeze portions in ice cube trays. That makes it easy to pop out just what you need for your next meal or recipe. Spoon the chimichurri into the trays (don't over-fill), then cover the top tightly with plastic wrap. When the sauce is frozen, remove the plastic wrap, pop out the cubes, and transfer them to a resealable plastic bag. These will keep for up to 6 months in the freezer, and each cube is about 1 ounce.*

curry sauce

MAKES 2 CUPS

PREP TIME: 15 minutes

COOKING TIME: 15 minutes

TOTAL TIME: 30 minutes

1 tablespoon cooking fat

½ onion, diced

1½ teaspoons minced fresh ginger

1 clove garlic, minced

1½ teaspoons yellow curry powder

½ teaspoon red curry powder

2 cups full-fat coconut milk

Grated zest and juice of ½ lime

½ teaspoon salt

¼ teaspoon black pepper

Like your curry on the hotter side? Substitute ½ teaspoon cayenne pepper for the red curry powder, or simply add the same amount of cayenne along with the curry powder. This sauce is delicious on salmon, white fish, chicken, and roasted vegetables.

HEAT the cooking fat in a medium skillet over medium heat. When the fat is hot, add the onion and cook until translucent, 2 to 3 minutes. Add the ginger and cook for 1 minute, stirring quickly. Add the garlic and cook for another minute while continuing to stir.

ADD both curry powders and stir quickly for 30 seconds to open up the flavor of the spices. Once fragrant, add the coconut milk. Turn the heat down to low and allow the mixture to simmer (not boil) until the mixture thickens a bit, 8 to 10 minutes. (It will continue to thicken as it cools.) Season with the lime zest and juice, salt, and pepper.

KEEP warm and serve right away, or let the flavors develop even further in the refrigerator; it'll keep for about 5 days. (Note, the coconut milk will solidify in the cold, so pull it out of the fridge and let it come back to room temperature before serving.)

⭐ CITRUS ZEST *You'll notice that many recipes in this book use citrus zest. Don't skip this step! Zest (the colored part of the peel) from lemon, lime, grapefruit, or orange adds an abundance of flavor to your dish, makes for an attractive garnish, and contains even more micronutrients than the juice. You won't regret investing in a good zester—they're inexpensive, and will save you precious time in the kitchen. However, you can get the same effect by rubbing your citrus over the small holes of a grater or Microplane; or using a vegetable peeler, then chopping your zest finely with a knife. When zesting, make sure you only remove the brightly colored skin, and don't peel all the way down into the bitter white pith.*

guacamole

MAKES 3 CUPS

PREP TIME: 15 minutes

3 ripe avocados, split lengthwise, pitted, and peeled

Juice of 1 lime

1 teaspoon salt

½ onion, finely diced

1 tomato, finely diced

½ jalapeño, seeded and finely diced

3 tablespoons chopped fresh cilantro

1 clove garlic, minced

Guacamole is one of the most versatile condiments. Use it as a dip with carrots, celery, peppers, and jicama; drop a healthy dollop on your burger, chicken breast, or eggs; use it in place of mayo in tuna or chicken salad; or mix it with salsa for an easy Mexican-inspired salad dressing. Feel free to customize your guacamole too—add more lime juice and a dash of zest, make it spicy with ¼ teaspoon cumin and ¼ teaspoon cayenne pepper, or take a nontraditional approach and add chopped pineapple and mango, strawberries, pomegranate seeds, or kale to the mixture.

IN a medium bowl, mix together the avocados, lime juice, and salt. Mash with a fork or potato masher if you like it chunky; use an immersion blender or food processor if you prefer a creamy texture. Mix in the onion, tomato, jalapeño, cilantro, and garlic.

SERVE immediately, or store in an airtight container and refrigerate before serving. Your guacamole will keep in the fridge for up to 3 days.

⭐ STORING GUACAMOLE *Even if you store your guacamole in an airtight container, you're likely to notice it turning brown on the top after a day in the fridge. This isn't mold and won't affect the taste, but it is kind of unsightly. You have two options here—either scrape off the top layer before serving, or mix it all up with a spoon until the brown color disappears. You can also try this tip from thekitchn.com for preventing the brown in the first place: pack your guacamole down tight into the container with the back of a spoon, pressing out any air bubbles. Then, pour a thin layer of lukewarm water over the top, making sure the entire surface area is covered. The water won't let any air come into contact with the guacamole—no air contact, no browning.*

mayonnaise variations

These mayo-based dipping sauces, dressings, and marinades all use our Basic Mayonnaise (page 179) or Egg-free Mayonnaise (page 180) as a base. By mixing and matching additional ingredients, you can totally change the flavor and feel of just about any dish. All variations take about 5 minutes to prepare, and make about 1 cup.

Your mayonnaise is good until about 7 days after your egg expiration date, so note the date on the carton, add a week, and write that date on your mayo storage container.

garlic aioli

1 cup Basic Mayonnaise (page 179)

2 cloves garlic, minced

Juice of ½ lemon

To make the aioli even more flavorful, roast the garlic before adding it to the mayo (see the tip on page 322). This is the perfect dipping sauce for raw or roasted vegetables. You can also mix it into a Protein Salad (page 161) or Cauliflower Mash (page 270), or thin it a bit to make a creamy dressing for our Greek Salad (page 278).

MIX all the ingredients in a small bowl until fully incorporated.

wasabi mayonnaise

1½ tablespoons wasabi powder

1 cup Basic Mayonnaise (page 179)

Wasabi mayo is a great topping for salmon, tuna, and other fish, a nice binder for tuna or potato salad, a tasty dipping sauce for baked "fries," and a nice drizzle for our Grilled Asparagus with Lemon Zest (page 284).

MIX the wasabi powder and 1½ tablespoons of water together in a small bowl until it forms a firm paste. (If it's too dry, add a little more water.) Mix the wasabi paste and the mayo in a small bowl until fully blended. Add more of the wasabi mixture if you like it spicier, but note that wasabi takes 5 to 10 minutes to "activate"— so wait and taste-test before adding more.

cilantro-lime mayonnaise

¾ cup Basic Mayonnaise (page 179, replacing the lemon juice with lime juice)

¼ cup minced fresh cilantro

1 clove garlic, minced

This variation is used in our Steak Salad (page 220), and also works well with shrimp and scallops, as a dipping sauce for raw or roasted vegetables, and atop the Perfect Burger (page 153). You can also use it as a creamy dressing for our Cold Thai Salad (page 274).

COMBINE all ingredients in a bowl and mix well.

avocado mayonnaise

1 avocado, split lengthwise, pitted, and peeled

½ cup Basic Mayonnaise (page 179)

Juice of ½ lime

If you want a smooth, creamy texture, use a food processor or immersion blender. If you want it chunky, use a fork to mash and mix. This makes a great binder for tuna, salmon, chicken, or egg salad, a delicious dipping sauce for raw and roasted vegetables, and a creamy topping for a Mexican-inspired Perfect Ground Meat (page 152).

IN a small bowl or food processor, mash the avocado with a fork, potato masher, or immersion blender; or mix in the food processor on low. Add the mayo and lime juice and mix or blend until fully incorporated.

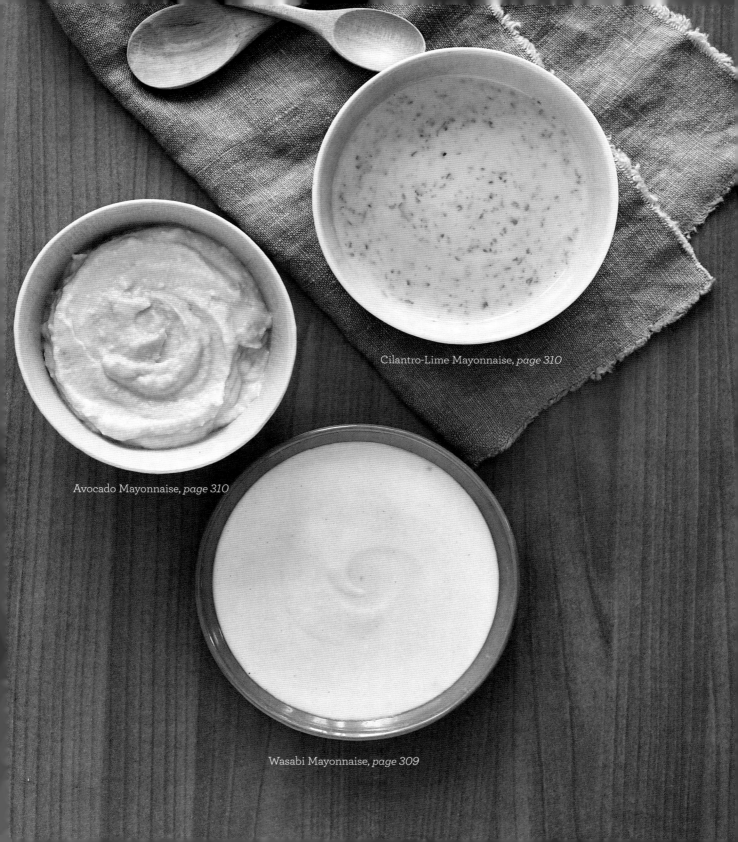

Cilantro-Lime Mayonnaise, *page 310*

Avocado Mayonnaise, *page 310*

Wasabi Mayonnaise, *page 309*

herb mayonnaise

1 cup Basic Mayonnaise (page 179)

2 tablespoons minced mixed herbs

1 clove garlic, minced

Juice of ½ lemon

⅛ teaspoon cayenne pepper

Try a mix of fresh herbs (we like rosemary, basil, thyme, parsley, and chives) and use the mayo to top a Perfect Chicken Breast (page 157) or to mix into tuna, salmon, or egg salad. It'd also be a great topping for our Roasted Sweet Potatoes (page 296). Or, add a little water and shake it up to create a creamy salad dressing.

COMBINE all the ingredients in a bowl and mix well.

roasted red pepper mayonnaise

¾ cup Basic Mayonnaise (page 179)

¼ cup Roasted Red Pepper Sauce (page 316)

This is a great way to change up a leftover dressing or sauce. This variation would be delicious on a Perfect Burger (page 153), Perfect Grilled Steak (page 154), over Perfect Scrambled Eggs (page 150), and as a dipping sauce for raw or roasted vegetables.

MIX the mayo and sauce together in a small bowl until fully incorporated.

tartar sauce

1 cup Basic Mayonnaise (page 179)

2 tablespoons minced fresh dill leaves

1 tablespoon minced dill pickles

2 teaspoons minced chives

Juice of ½ lemon

¼ teaspoon black pepper

Tartar sauce is traditionally served with fish (like our Perfect Oven-Baked Salmon on page 160), but it's also delicious mixed into a Protein Salad (page 161) or served as a dip for roasted sweet potato spears (see page 296).

COMBINE all ingredients in a small bowl and mix until blended.

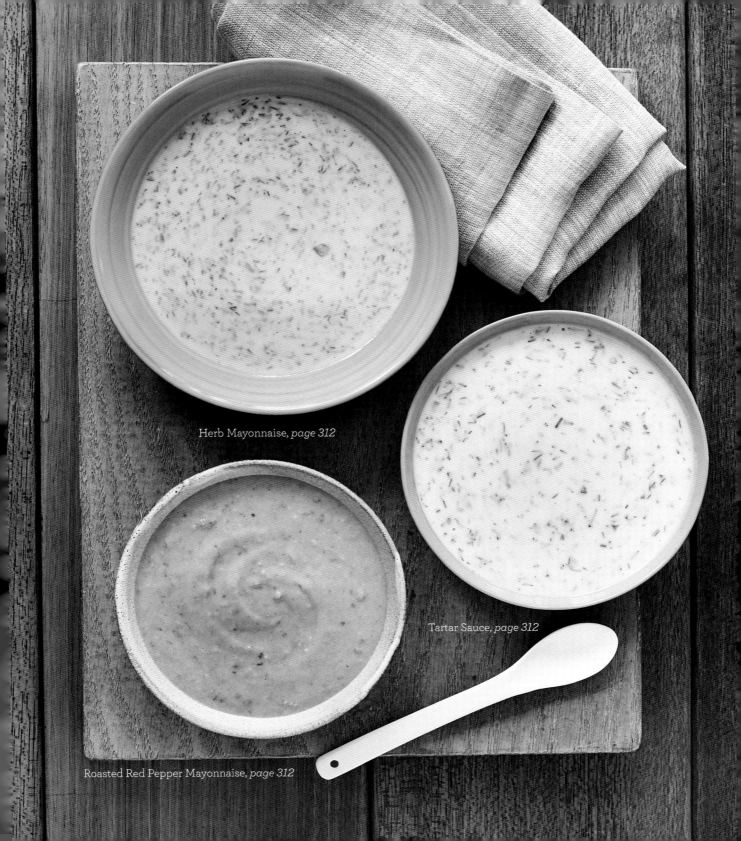

Herb Mayonnaise, *page 312*

Tartar Sauce, *page 312*

Roasted Red Pepper Mayonnaise, *page 312*

hollandaise

MAKES 2 CUPS

PREP TIME: 15 minutes

---

1 ½ cups clarified unsalted butter or ghee

4 large egg yolks

2 tablespoons lemon juice

1 teaspoon salt

⅛ teaspoon cayenne pepper (optional)

Most people think of hollandaise as a topping for poached eggs (see page 150), but it's also great over grilled fish, smoked salmon, and vegetables like asparagus, green beans, Brussels sprouts, and potatoes.

IN a medium saucepan over low heat, melt the butter or ghee until warm but not bubbling.

COMBINE the egg yolks, lemon juice, salt, and cayenne pepper (if you like) in a food processor or blender and pulse 10 to 15 times to combine. Slowly drizzle in the warm butter or ghee while mixing on low speed, until the sauce emulsifies and thickens. If the sauce becomes too thick, blend in a tablespoon of warm water.

SERVE the sauce immediately, or hold covered in a small saucepan on the lowest heat setting for up to an hour. Make your hollandaise fresh every time you serve it, as it doesn't store well in the refrigerator.

⭐ IT'S IMPORTANT *that your butter or ghee is warm but not hot—if it's too hot, the sauce could curdle. If you made clarified butter with salted butter, skip the salt in this recipe. You can always add a dash after tasting if it needs more.*

pesto

MAKES 2 CUPS

PREP TIME: 10 minutes

½ cup walnuts

3 cloves garlic, minced

3 cups packed fresh basil leaves

1 cup spinach leaves

Juice of ½ lemon

1 ½ cups extra-virgin olive oil

½ teaspoon salt

½ teaspoon black pepper

Use this pesto in place of tomato sauce; try it mixed in with our Italian-inspired Perfect Ground Meat (page 152), or drizzled over Stuffed Peppers (page 222). Another one of our favorite "ingredient" meals is to make Roasted Spaghetti Squash (page 294), add sun-dried tomatoes and Whole30-compliant sausage or chicken sausage, and top with pesto and a sprinkle of pine nuts. It's also delicious on eggs, or mixed into your favorite Protein Salad (page 161).

HEAT a dry skillet over medium-high heat. When the pan is hot (sprinkle some water on the dry pan—if it sizzles, it's hot), add the walnuts in a single layer and stir or shake frequently until lightly browned, about 2 minutes.

COMBINE the walnuts and garlic in a food processor and pulse a few times to combine. Add the basil and spinach and pulse until coarsely chopped. Add the lemon juice. While mixing on low speed, add the olive oil in a slow stream until all the ingredients are fully blended. Add the salt and pepper and pulse a few more times to combine.

STORE in the refrigerator for up to 2 to 3 days, or freeze in ice cube trays (see technique on page 306).

⭐ PESTO NUTS *Traditional pesto uses pine nuts, but these can be expensive. We've used walnuts instead, but free to substitute whatever nuts you have on hand—pecans or almonds would work just as well.*

ranch dressing

MAKES 1½ CUPS

PREP TIME: 15 minutes

1 cup Basic Mayonnaise (page 179)

¼ cup coconut cream (see page 178)

2 tablespoons red wine vinegar

1 tablespoon minced fresh parsley

½ teaspoon garlic powder

½ teaspoon onion powder

½ teaspoon black pepper

¼ teaspoon paprika

This thick and creamy, kid-approved ranch is great for basting chicken, fish, or pork; makes a great dipping sauce for raw vegetables; and is perfect on a fresh green salad.

WHISK together the mayo, coconut cream, and vinegar in a small bowl. Add the parsley, garlic powder, onion powder, pepper, and paprika and stir until thoroughly combined.

THIS dressing will keep in the refrigerator for 2 to 3 days.

⭐ SUPER SNACK *Prep our Buffalo Sauce (page 304), whip up our hot wings, cut up some carrot sticks and celery, and serve with the Ranch Dressing, and you've got yourself the perfect sports-watching, New Year–celebrating, or housewarming appetizer.*

roasted red pepper sauce

MAKES 2 CUPS

PREP TIME: 10 minutes

1 jar (16 ounces) roasted red peppers, drained

¼ cup extra-virgin olive oil

¼ onion, roughly chopped

2 cloves garlic, minced

2 tablespoons chopped fresh parsley

1 tablespoon capers, drained

Juice of ½ lemon

½ teaspoon salt

½ teaspoon black pepper

We tell you to pair this sauce with the Broccoli, Mushrooms, and Yellow Squash on page 264, but when we "road tested" the recipe, we ended up putting the sauce on *everything*—fried eggs in the morning, our burger at lunch, and roasted cauliflower at dinner. Double this recipe—you'll thank us.

COMBINE all ingredients in a food processor and pulse 5 to 10 times to combine, then blend on high speed until smooth.

STORE in the refrigerator for up to 5 days.

⭐ YOU COULD *easily change the flavor of this sauce by substituting the same amount of sundried tomatoes or roasted eggplant for the roasted red peppers, or try black olives to make a tapenade-like spread for vegetables or meat.*

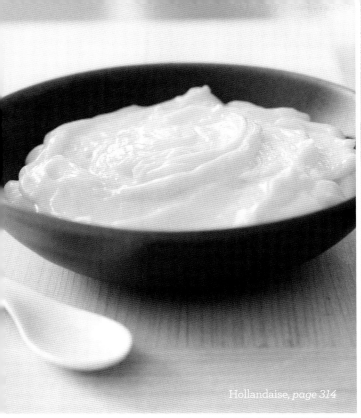
Hollandaise, *page 314*

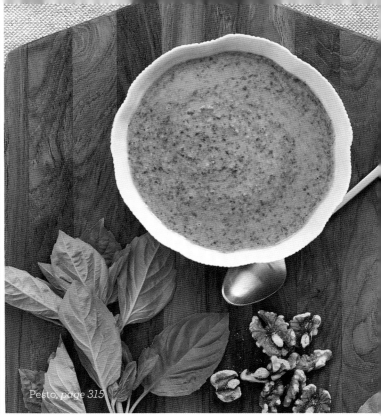
Pesto, *page 315*

Ranch Dressing, *page316*
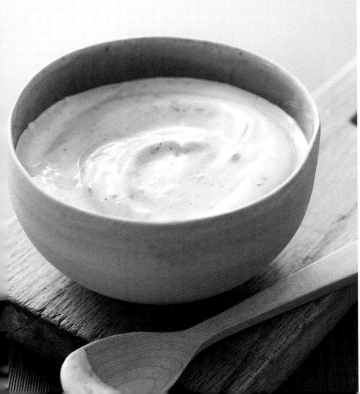

Roasted Red Pepper Sauce, *page 316*
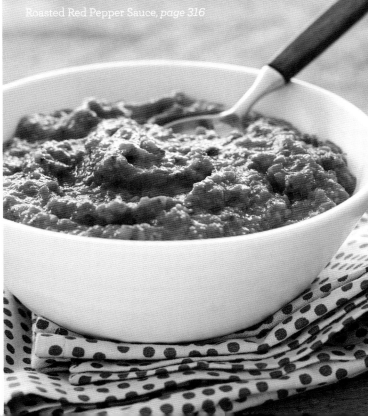

romesco sauce

MAKES 2 CUPS

PREP TIME: 15 minutes
COOK TIME: 10 minutes
TOTAL TIME: 25 minutes

---

2 tablespoons cooking fat

½ cup almonds, chopped

1 small onion, diced

3 cloves garlic, minced

1 teaspoon chili powder

1 teaspoon paprika

2 tomatoes, seeded and chopped

2 tablespoons extra-virgin olive oil

1½ teaspoons red wine vinegar

1 teaspoon salt

½ teaspoon black pepper

Romesco is a traditional garlicky nut- and red pepper–based sauce that originated in Spain, but we're giving it a twist by using tomatoes instead of peppers. This sauce pairs perfectly with our Garlic Shrimp and Zucchini Noodles (page 244), or serve with grilled meat or fish; over roasted cauliflower, broccoli, or Brussels sprouts; or as a burger spread.

MELT the cooking fat in a large skillet over medium-high heat. When the fat is hot, add the almonds and toast for 3 minutes, stirring often. Add the onion and cook, stirring, for 2 minutes. Add the garlic and cook until aromatic, about 1 minute. Add the chili powder and paprika and cook until the flavors open up, about 30 seconds. Finally, add the tomatoes, mix into the ingredients, and cook, stirring to bring up the tasty bits from the bottom of the pan, until the tomatoes are warmed through, about 2 minutes.

TRANSFER the sauce mixture to a food processor. Add the rest of the ingredients and blend on low speed until the sauce is smooth, then pour into a serving dish or glass storage container.

ALLOW to cool before refrigerating; the sauce will keep for up to 5 days.

⭐ SEEDING TOMATOES *Seeding a tomato can be messy if you try to dice it before removing the seeds. Try this method: place the tomato on a cutting board, stem facing up. Slice left-to-right across the middle of the tomato, creating two equal halves. Then, scrape out the seeds and white core with a small spoon. You'll be left with nothing but firm tomato flesh, far easier to slice and dice.*

salsa

MAKES 3 CUPS

PREP TIME: 15 minutes

6 tomatoes, cored, seeded, and diced

½ cup chopped fresh cilantro

½ onion, finely diced

3 cloves garlic, minced

1 jalapeño, finely diced

½ teaspoon salt

¼ teaspoon black pepper

Grated zest and juice of ½ lime

Salsa is a great replacement for ketchup, and livens up just about any ingredient. It's great on Perfect Scrambled Eggs (page 150), as a topping for a Perfect Seared Chicken Breast (page 157) or a Perfect Burger (page 153), or as a dip for raw celery, carrots, and jicama sticks. It's also a natural match for our Guacamole (page 308).

MIX all the ingredients together in a small bowl and stir gently to combine. Serve immediately, or allow the flavors to come together in the refrigerator for 1 to 3 hours.

STORE your salsa in the refrigerator for up to 1 week.

QUICK PREP *A vegetable chopper would cut your prep time in half, and ensure all of your dice were the same size. You can find them at any kitchen store, or on Amazon—they're generally between $12 and $30. You could use a food processor to carefully pulse each ingredient one at a time, but don't combine them all at once, or you'll end up with a bowl of mushy salsa.*

sunshine sauce

adapted from *Well Fed*, by Melissa Joulwan

MAKES 1 CUP

PREP TIME: 10 minutes

½ cup unsweetened sunflower seed butter

½ cup coconut milk

Juice of 1 lime

1 tablespoon coconut aminos (optional)

1 clove garlic, minced

½ teaspoon crushed red pepper flakes

½ teaspoon rice vinegar or apple cider vinegar

This dip (a universal favorite of Whole30ers everywhere) is fantastic with fresh, raw vegetables (carrots, bell peppers, celery, or broccoli), drizzled over roasted vegetables (carrots, parsnips, sweet potatoes), as a sauce for our Perfect Seared Chicken Breast (page157), and as a dressing for our Cold Thai Salad (page 274) and Green Cabbage Slaw (page 282). If you can't find compliant sunflower seed butter, you can use almond butter instead.

MIX all the ingredients together in a small bowl and stir to combine. Store in an air-tight container in the refrigerator for up to 3 days.

⭐ COCONUT AMINOS *Coconut aminos are a soy sauce substitute made from the fermented sap of the coconut tree. It tastes remarkably like soy sauce, and can open up a whole new world of Asian-inspired cooking. Many smaller health food stores carry coconut aminos, but you can also buy them online through Amazon or other retailers. They're not necessary for the Sunshine Sauce, but we think they're so versatile they're worth the $8 investment. (We even bring a bottle with us to our favorite sushi restaurant!)*

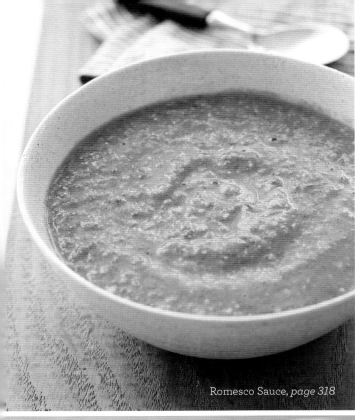
Romesco Sauce, *page 318*

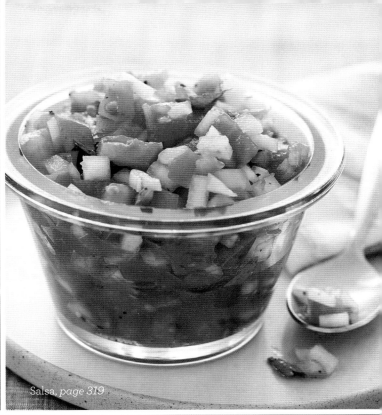
Salsa, *page 319*

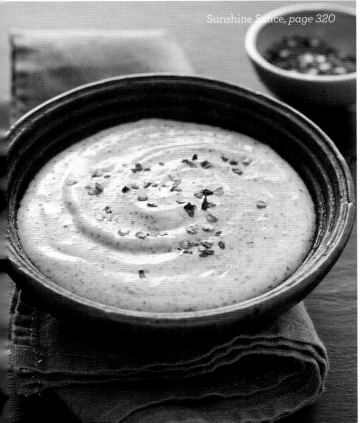
Sunshine Sauce, *page 320*

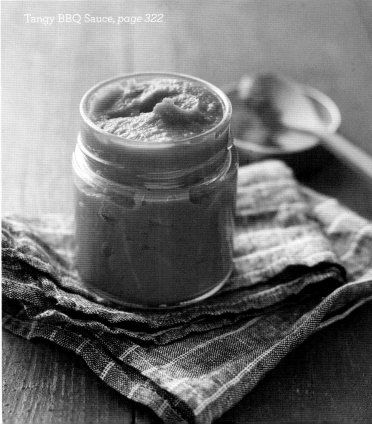
Tangy BBQ Sauce, *page 322*

tangy bbq sauce

MAKES 2 CUPS

PREP TIME: 15 minutes
COOK TIME: 1 hour 10 minutes
TOTAL TIME: 1 hour 25 minutes

2 tablespoons ghee or clarified butter

1 small onion, diced

3 cloves roasted garlic (see tip)

1 large sweet potato, peeled and cut into 1-inch dice

½ cup apple cider

1 can (3 ounces) tomato paste

1 tablespoon apple cider vinegar

1 teaspoon paprika

1 teaspoon salt

½ teaspoon chipotle powder

If you roast an entire head of garlic at once, you'll have leftovers to use in other recipes. Remove the skin from the leftover roasted cloves and place the garlic in an airtight container. Pour in enough extra-virgin olive oil to cover the cloves completely, and store in the refrigerator for up to 1 week. No need to reheat the cloves before adding them to a recipe—just toss them into the pot or pan cold and let them reheat with your dish.

HEAT the ghee in a medium skillet over medium heat. When the ghee is hot, add the onion and cook, stirring occasionally, until they start to brown and caramelize, 15 to 20 minutes.

MEANWHILE, combine the roasted garlic, sweet potato, and apple cider in a medium saucepan. Add enough water to just barely cover the sweet potatoes—do not over-cover. Bring to a boil, then reduce the heat to a simmer and cook until the sweet potato is fork-tender, about 15 minutes. Strain and reserve the liquid from the pan.

COMBINE the sautéed onion and sweet potato mixture in a food processor or blender. Add the tomato paste, vinegar, paprika, salt, and chipotle powder. Add ¼ cup of the reserved cooking liquid and blend on low to medium speed. If the mixture is still too thick, add more liquid, ¼ cup at a time, while blending until you arrive at the desired consistency. (The sauce should pour like ketchup.)

STORE in the refrigerator for up to 2 to 3 days.

⭐ ROASTED GARLIC *You could use raw garlic here, but you'll miss out on the sweeter, more mellow flavor of garlic when it's roasted. To roast garlic in the oven, preheat the oven to 400°F. Peel the loose outer skin from a large head of garlic and wrap in foil, closing off the top. Place on a baking sheet and roast for 45 minutes, until the bulb is lightly browned at the top and feels soft when you squeeze it. Remove the garlic bulb from the foil carefully, and set aside until it's cool to the touch. Peel each clove of garlic carefully, using the sharp tip of a paring knife to break open each individual clove—it may be easier to squeeze the garlic out.*

whole30 ketchup

MAKES 1 CUP

PREP TIME: 5 minutes

COOK TIME: 10 minutes

TOTAL TIME: 15 minutes

1 cup tomato paste

½ cup apple cider

½ cup apple cider vinegar

1 teaspoon garlic powder

½ teaspoon salt

⅛ teaspoon ground cloves (optional)

Don't expect the familiar "Heinz 57" from this recipe—grocery store ketchup is thick and sweet thanks to sugar—nearly 4 grams per tablespoon. In fact, Heinz 57 uses both high-fructose corn syrup *and* corn syrup to sweeten their paste. We could use date paste to make our ketchup sugary, but that's not really in line with the spirit of the Whole30. This ketchup will have more of a lighter vinegar flavor, different but still delicious on eggs, burgers, and baked potato "fries."

HEAT a medium saucepan over medium heat. Add the tomato paste, apple cider, and vinegar. Stir completely and let it come to a simmer, but do not allow to boil.

ADD the garlic powder, salt, and cloves and cook, stirring frequently to prevent scorching—you may need to turn the heat down to low or simmer here. Simmer until the ketchup has thickened enough to evenly coat the back of a spoon, 5 to 8 minutes. Remove from the heat and allow to cool. Serve when cool, or store refrigerated in an air-tight container; it'll keep for up to 2 weeks.

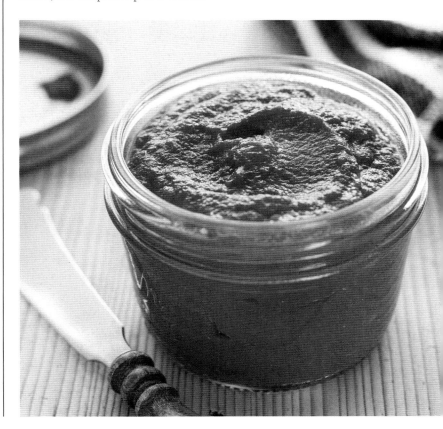

tomato sauce

MAKES 3 CUPS

PREP TIME: 15 minutes
COOK TIME: 1 hour
TOTAL TIME: 1 hour 15 minutes

1 tablespoon cooking fat

1 onion, finely chopped

2 celery stalks, finely chopped

1 carrot, peeled and finely chopped

2 cloves garlic, minced

1 can (28 ounces) crushed tomatoes

1 teaspoon fresh thyme

1 teaspoon fresh oregano

1 bay leaf

1 teaspoon salt

1 teaspoon black pepper

If you're serving this sauce fresh, you can substitute about 6 fresh tomatoes for the canned. You can also quickly turn this into a meat sauce: Just add 1 pound of leftover Perfect Ground Meat (page 152) and 1 cup of beef broth in the last ten minutes of simmering. Serve over Roasted Spaghetti Squash (page 294), steamed zucchini noodles (see page 244), or a pile of wilted spinach for a quick, easy, complete meal.

HEAT the cooking fat in a large pot over medium heat. When the fat is hot, add the onion, celery, and carrot and cook, stirring, until the onion becomes translucent, 2 to 3 minutes. Add the garlic and stir until aromatic, about 1 minute. Add the tomatoes, thyme, oregano, bay leaf, salt, and pepper.

REDUCE the heat to a simmer, cover, and cook over low heat, stirring every 20 minutes, until the sauce is thick and smooth, about 1 hour. Discard the bay leaf.

STORE in the refrigerator for up to 5 to 7 days.

⭐ SAUCE STORAGE *If you plan to freeze the sauce, canned tomatoes will actually taste better. The sauce will keep in the freezer for 3 to 4 months, but because ice crystals will get inside the sauce, just a word of warning—it may come out runnier than it went in. You can always thicken it up again by adding another can of tomatoes while it's reheating.*

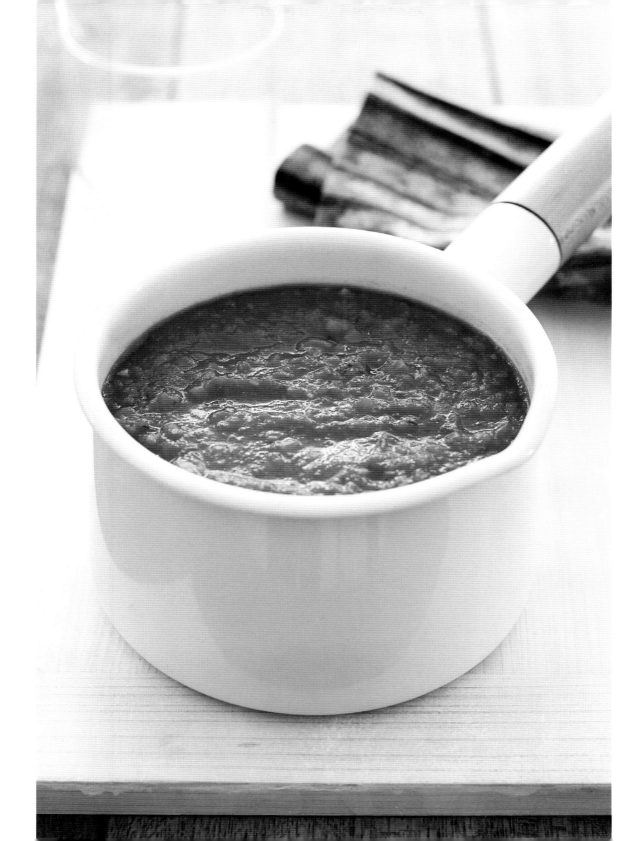

vinaigrette variations

These variations are all loosely based on our Basic Vinaigrette recipe (page 184). By mixing and matching additional ingredients, you can create unique flavors for your dressings or marinades. To make creamy vinaigrette, use Basic Mayonnaise (page 179) instead of the olive oil in any of the recipes. All variations take 5 to 10 minutes to prepare, and make 1 cup.

As all of these variations include fresh ingredients, store them in the fridge for no more than 3 to 4 days. You'll need to take your bottle out of the fridge about a half-hour before serving, as the olive oil will get hard and cloudy when cold. Just give it a shake before pouring.

herb citrus vinaigrette

1½ tablespoons orange juice

1½ tablespoons lemon juice

1½ tablespoons lime juice

2 cloves garlic, minced

2 teaspoons mustard powder

¾ cup extra-virgin olive oil

1 teaspoon fresh thyme leaves

1 teaspoon minced fresh cilantro

1 teaspoon minced fresh parsley

½ teaspoon salt

½ teaspoon black pepper

This dressing is great on our Stir-Fry Chicken (page 340), and also makes the perfect marinade or topping for fish, shrimp, or scallops, or a fresh green salad.

WHISK together the orange juice, lemon juice, lime juice, garlic, and mustard powder in a small mixing bowl. Drizzle in the olive oil while whisking steadily to emulsify. Add the thyme, cilantro, parsley, salt, and pepper and whisk until blended.

italian vinaigrette

¼ cup red wine vinegar

2 tablespoons minced fresh oregano (or 2 teaspoons dried)

1 clove garlic, minced

1 teaspoon mustard powder

¾ cup extra-virgin olive oil

½ teaspoon salt

¼ teaspoon black pepper

This is a great marinade for chicken or shrimp, or it can be used instead of the lemon oil in our Green Cabbage Slaw (page 282).

MIX together the vinegar, oregano, garlic, and mustard powder in a small bowl. Add the olive oil in a steady stream while whisking to emulsify. Adjust the seasoning with salt and pepper and whisk until fully incorporated.

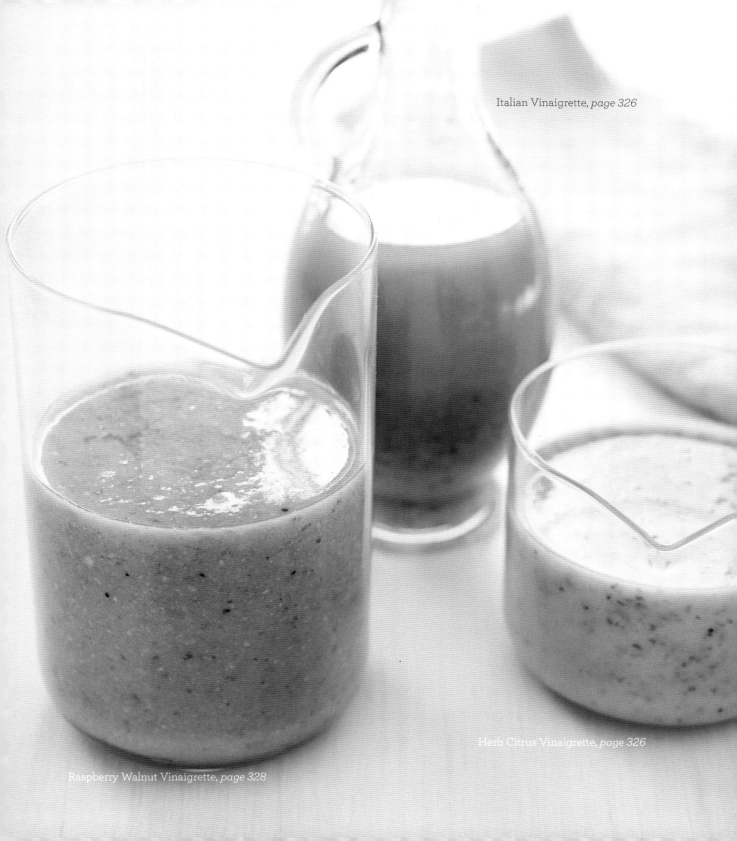

Italian Vinaigrette, *page 326*

Herb Citrus Vinaigrette, *page 326*

Raspberry Walnut Vinaigrette, *page 328*

raspberry walnut vinaigrette

½ cup fresh raspberries, finely chopped or smashed

¼ cup apple cider vinegar

2 tablespoons finely chopped walnuts

1 teaspoon minced fresh cilantro (or ¼ teaspoon dried)

¾ cup extra-virgin olive oil

Salt and black pepper

This dressing is used in our Harvest Grilled Chicken Salad (page 232), but it's also delicious on a summer salad of baby spinach, chopped berries (blueberries, blackberries, strawberries, and raspberries), and diced cucumbers, or mix it into any variation of a Protein Salad (page 161). You can also swap out the raspberries for a different berry in this recipe, or use crushed pomegranate seeds in the winter.

MIX together the raspberries, vinegar, walnuts, and cilantro in a small bowl. Drizzle in the olive oil while whisking steadily to emulsify. Adjust to taste with salt and pepper and whisk until fully blended.

balsamic vinaigrette

¼ cup balsamic vinegar

2 cloves garlic, minced

2 teaspoons mustard powder

¾ cup extra-virgin olive oil

1 teaspoon minced fresh cilantro (or ¼ teaspoon dried)

Salt and black pepper

This dressing is used in our Walnut-Crusted Pork Tenderloin (page 252), and also makes a great topping for grilled vegetables (see page 164), white fish, and salads. We also like to make a creamy variation (sub in Basic Mayonnaise, page 179, for the olive oil) and use it as a dip for a raw vegetable tray, drizzle it over Oven-Roasted Brussels Sprouts and Squash (page 286), or mix it into a Protein Salad (page 161).

MIX together the vinegar, garlic, and mustard powder in a small bowl. Add the olive oil in a steady stream while whisking to emulsify. Add the cilantro, adjust to taste with salt and pepper, and whisk until fully incorporated.

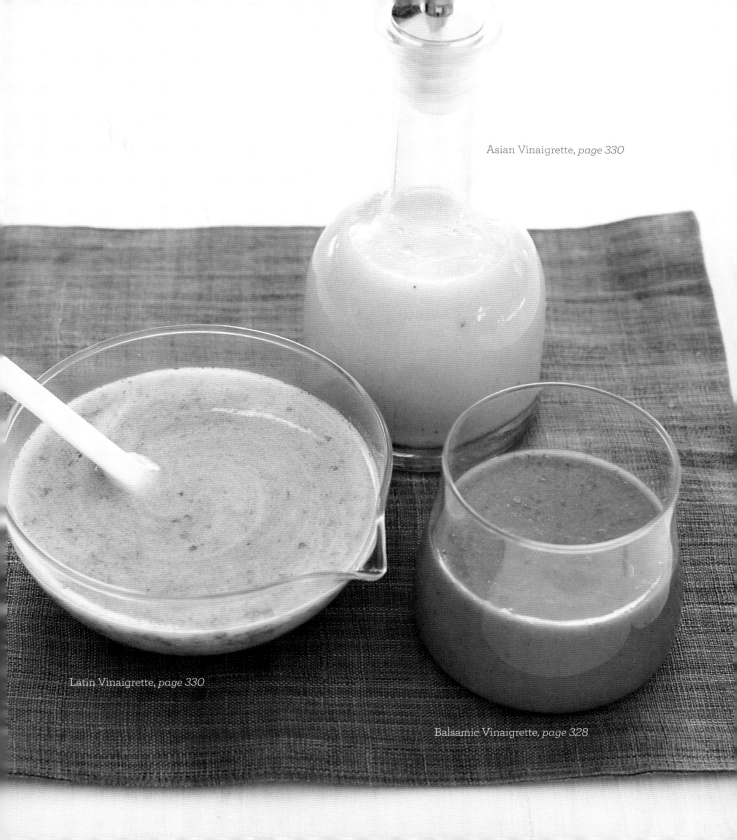

Asian Vinaigrette, *page 330*

Latin Vinaigrette, *page 330*

Balsamic Vinaigrette, *page 328*

asian vinaigrette

¼ cup rice vinegar

1 tablespoon sesame oil

1 clove garlic, minced

½ teaspoon minced fresh ginger

¾ cup extra-virgin olive oil

Red pepper flakes

Salt and black pepper

This makes a great alternative dressing for our Cold Thai Salad (page 274). A creamy variation (use Basic Mayonnaise, page 179, instead of olive oil) can be mixed into Cauliflower Rice (page 272) or spooned over Perfect Oven-Baked Salmon (page 160).

MIX together the rice vinegar, sesame oil, garlic, and ginger in a small bowl. Add the olive oil in a steady stream while whisking to emulsify. Adjust the seasoning with a pinch of red pepper flakes, salt, and pepper and whisk until fully incorporated.

latin vinaigrette

2 cloves garlic, minced

1 jalapeño, seeded and minced

Juice of 5 limes

¾ cups extra-virgin olive oil

2 tablespoons minced fresh cilantro

2 tablespoons minced fresh parsley

½ teaspoon salt

¼ teaspoon black pepper

WHISK together the garlic, jalapeño, and lime juice in a small mixing bowl. Drizzle in the olive oil while whisking steadily to emulsify. Add the cilantro, parsley, salt, and pepper and whisk until blended.

This is a delicious marinade for a Perfect Grilled Steak (page 154), Perfect Seared Chicken Breast (page 157), or Perfect Grilled Shrimp (page 158).

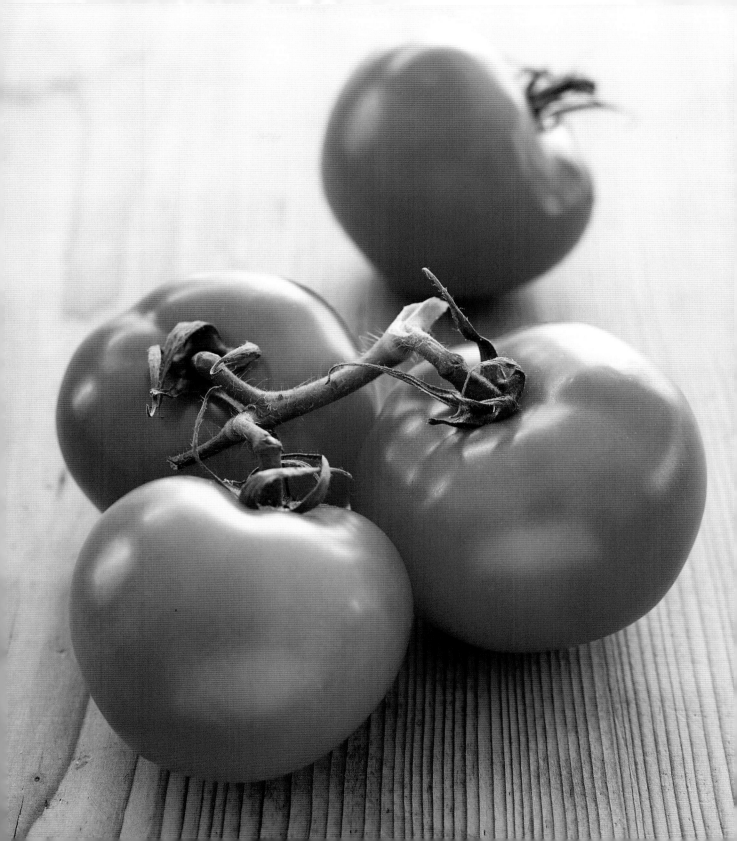

ONE POT MEALS

BEFORE YOU GET TOO EXCITED at the title of this section, we need to tell you something. You will be using more than one pot to prepare some of these dishes.

Okay, most of these dishes.

We know you were envisioning a two-minute clean-up after cooking from this section—just you, a sponge, and one pot (unlike the usual kitchen carnage that shows up after you prep, cook, and serve dinner). But the title of this section isn't really meant to represent your cooking vessels; rather, the fact that you'll be cooking a complete meal (protein, vegetables, and natural fats) all in one dish, with no need to find a side dish or dressing pairing.

So we are making it easier on you here. Just maybe not easier on your dishwasher.

If you feel like you're in "Good Food jail" (chained to your cutting board, stove, and sink) during this Whole30, let's talk about a few ways you can streamline the preparation, cooking, and clean-up process.

The first tip is to batch-prep your food. Set aside a few hours on a Sunday or thirty minutes on a weeknight after work and make some things ahead of time. Prepare a marinade or spice mixture you know you'll be using soon, make three or four dressings and sauces, and pre-chop your vegetables (they're fine stored in a covered container in the fridge for a few days). The less you have to do when you're rushing around to get dinner on the table, the cleaner your kitchen will be.

Place a "garbage bowl" on the counter for remnants like onion tops, apple cores, or herb stems. Limiting trips to and from the garbage can saves time and spills onto your kitchen floor.

Reuse kitchen tools as often as you can. If you're just chopping vegetables, there is no need to use more than one cutting board—just wipe the remnants of the vegetables off, then move to your next ingredient. Same with knives and measuring cups—you may need a quick rinse in between, but you certainly don't need a fresh tool for every ingredient. (Careful with raw meat, though—that should have its own cutting board, and any tools that come into contact with the meat should be washed thoroughly before using them again.)

Combine ingredients whenever you can. If you add the onions, the peppers, and the mushrooms to the pan all at the same time, leave them all on the same cutting board or hold them all in the same mixing bowl—no need to dirty extras. Same for spice mixtures; if you're combining all the spices in the pan anyway, just use one small dish to hold them all during your prep.

If you need to coat vegetables in oil before roasting them, you can put them in a bowl, add the oil, and mix . . . or you can do what we do, which is lay the vegetables out on your lined baking sheet, drizzle the oil evenly over the veggies, and toss with your hands until they are well coated. One less greasy bowl to wash = winning.

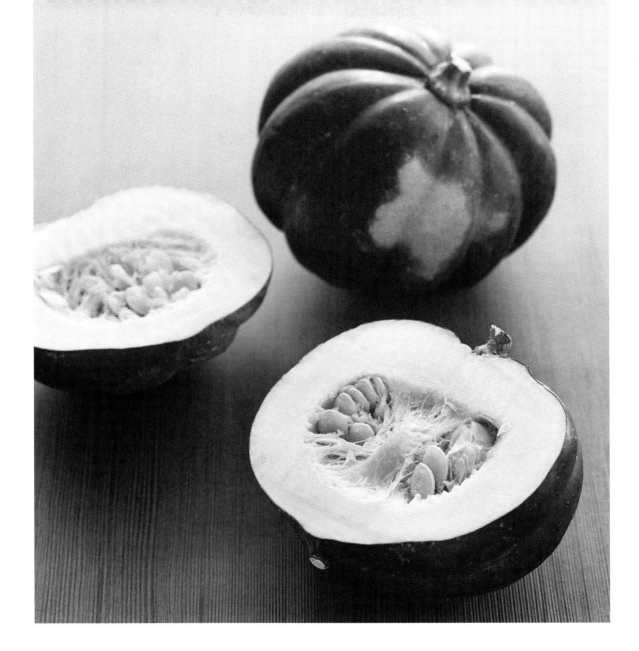

Finally, we know every cookbook will tell you to clean as you go, but you really should clean as you go. (Or at the very least, rinse.) If something is simmering for a few minutes, wash a bowl or two, wipe your counter down, or return your spices to the cabinet. If you can finish cooking your meal with a relatively clean kitchen, the clean-up post-dinner is a snap.

Especially if you make your spouse, partner, or roommate do it.

chicken cacciatore

ONE POT MEALS

SERVES 2

PREP TIME: 15 minutes
COOK TIME: 40 minutes
TOTAL TIME: 55 minutes

4 tablespoons cooking fat

1 pound chicken legs (bone-in, skin-on)

½ pound chicken thighs (boneless)

½ teaspoon salt

½ teaspoon black pepper

½ onion, minced

½ red bell pepper, finely diced

1 cup mushrooms, sliced

2 cloves garlic, minced

1 tablespoon capers, drained

1 14.5-ounce can diced tomatoes

1 cup chicken broth or water

1 tablespoon fresh basil leaves, rough chopped

While you could make this dish with boneless, skinless everything, you'd be missing out. The chicken skin holds the fat, and fat equals flavor. Plus, skin-on chicken retains the sauce better, and gives a warm, rustic look to the dish. While it's not an official rule, we'd recommend purchasing pastured and/or organic chicken, especially when you are making dishes that include the chicken skin.

IN a large skillet with high edges, heat 2 tablespoons of the cooking fat over medium-high heat, swirling to coat the bottom of the pan. Season the chicken with the salt and pepper and place in the pan. Sear the chicken until golden brown, about 3 minutes on each side. Remove the chicken from the pan and set aside.

WITH the same pan still on medium-high heat, add the remaining 2 tablespoons of cooking fat, onions, and peppers and sauté for 2 to 3 minutes, until the onion becomes translucent. Add the mushrooms and continue to cook, stirring for 2 minutes. Add the garlic and stir until aromatic, about 1 minute. Add the capers and diced tomatoes.

RETURN the chicken to the pan and cover everything with the chicken broth or water. Reduce the heat to medium and bring everything to a simmer. Turn the heat down to low and continue to simmer (not boil) until the chicken reaches an internal temperature of 160°F, about 30 minutes.

GARNISH with the chopped basil and serve.

⭐ **WITH A LITTLE PLANNING,** *you could buy a 2½ to 3 pound whole chicken and use it to make this entire dish. First, roast the chicken using the technique on page 157. Strip the meat from the legs and thighs (keep the skin!) and refrigerate for later. Then, take the chicken carcass and make broth using the technique on page 177. When you're ready to make this meal, start at the cacciatore instructions above, adding the roasted meat to the sauce and simmering for just 10 minutes to heat it all the way through. This reduces the cooking time to just 15 minutes, and makes the most of the whole chicken.*

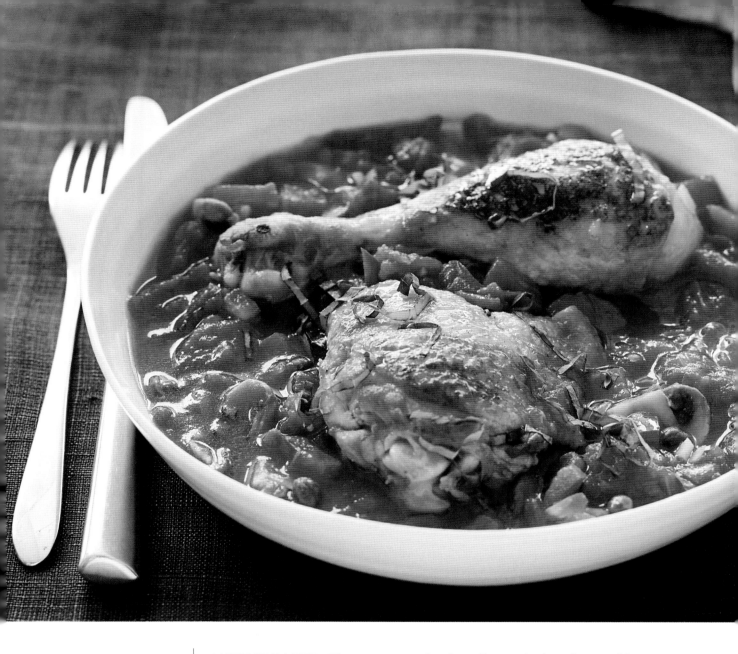

MAKE IT A MEAL: This one-pot meal technically stands alone, but to add even more nutritional power, serve over Cauliflower Rice (page 272), a plate of fresh baby spinach leaves, or a thin layer of mashed potatoes. For more of an Italian feel, serve over zucchini noodles (see technique on page 272) or Roasted Spaghetti Squash (page 294).

chicken chowder

SERVES 2 (WITH LEFTOVERS)

PREP TIME: 20 minutes

COOK TIME: 25 minutes

TOTAL TIME: 45 minutes

½ teaspoon salt

½ teaspoon cumin

¼ teaspoon paprika

⅛ teaspoon cayenne

1 pound chicken thighs (boneless)

1 quart chicken or vegetable broth

2 medium sweet potatoes, 1-inch cubed

1 head broccoli cut into 1-inch pieces (save stems)

2 cloves garlic, minced

1 jalapeño, finely diced (optional)

1 14.5-ounce can coconut milk

1 tablespoon fresh cilantro, minced

1 lime, juiced

½ small red onion, finely chopped

Want to add a different flavor to this meal? Try grilling your chicken instead of roasting it, substitute chicken for shrimp or hard-boiled eggs, or use cauliflower instead of broccoli. You can also turn this into a chicken "noodle" or "rice" chowder by adding pre-cooked Cauliflower Rice (page 272), Roasted Spaghetti Squash (page 294), or zoodles (page 244) just before the final reheat.

PREHEAT the oven to 350°F.

MIX the salt, cumin, paprika, and cayenne in a small bowl. Season the chicken thighs evenly with the spice mixture. Place the chicken in a baking pan and roast for 20 minutes. Remove the chicken from the oven and let it rest for 5 minutes on a cutting board. Cut the chicken into 1-inch cubes.

WHILE the chicken is roasting, add the broth to a medium-sized pot. Bring to a boil, then add the sweet potatoes. Cook over high heat until the sweet potatoes are fork-tender, about 10 minutes. Remove the sweet potatoes from the broth with a slotted spoon and set them aside.

ADD the broccoli stems, garlic, and jalapeño (if you want the extra kick) to the broth. Reduce the heat to medium high and boil for 15 minutes. Add the broccoli florets and coconut milk, and continue to boil until the broccoli is very tender, about 5 minutes. Remove the pot from the heat.

TRANSFER the broth and vegetables from the pot to a food processor or blender and blend until smooth. Place the blended mixture back into the pot and add the cooked chicken, sweet potatoes, and cilantro. Return the pot to medium heat, stir well, and cook for 2 to 3 minutes to reheat the chicken and sweet potatoes. Serve immediately.

GARNISH the chowder with the fresh lime juice and finely chopped red onion.

⭐ YOU CAN *bring this dish to work for a hot lunch even if you don't have a microwave. Before you leave for the day, heat the soup on medium-low heat until it's hot but not boiling, then place in a double-walled thermos. The thermos will keep it hot until lunchtime.*

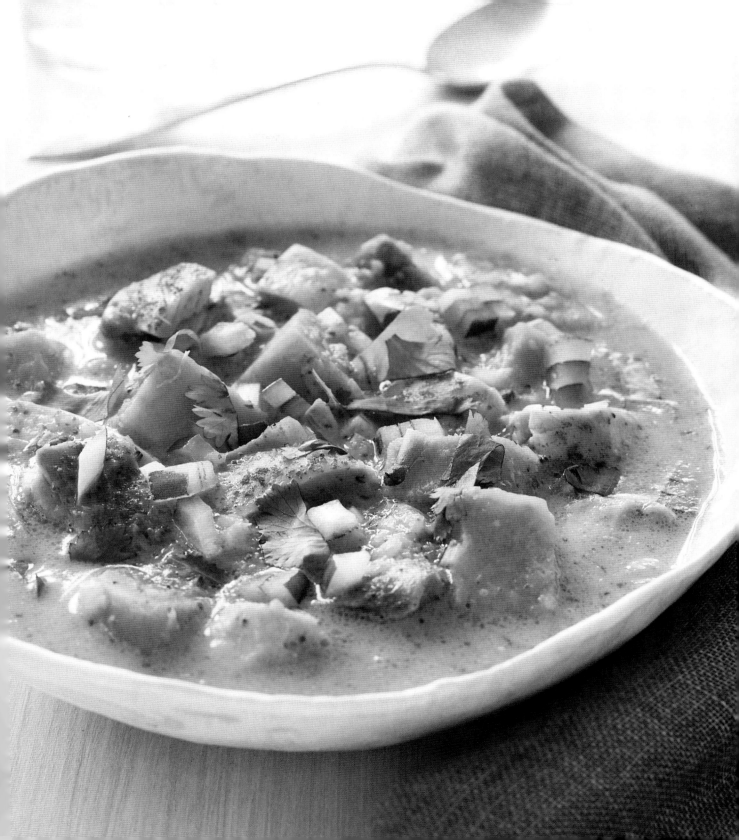

chicken primavera

SERVES 2 (WITH LEFTOVERS)

PREP TIME: 15 min
COOK TIME: 27 min
TOTAL TIME: 42 min

---

2 tablespoons cooking fat

½ cup diced onions

2 cloves garlic, minced

1 teaspoon minced fresh oregano

1 teaspoon fresh thyme

3 cups diced seeded tomatoes (about 3 large tomatoes)

1 pound boneless, skinless chicken thighs, 1-inch diced

2 cups green beans, cut into 1-inch pieces

1½ cups medium-diced zucchini

1½ cup medium-diced yellow squash

¼ teaspoon red pepper flakes

1 teaspoons salt

½ teaspoon black pepper

1 to 2 tablespoons minced fresh basil leaves

This meal is just begging to be spooned over vegetable noodles. Serve over Roasted Spaghetti Squash (page 294), zucchini noodles (page 244), or use your spiral slicer and steam some sweet potato or carrot noodles.

IN a large pot or Dutch oven, heat the cooking fat on medium-high heat and swirl to coat the bottom of the pan. Add the onions, garlic, oregano, and thyme and cook until the onions are translucent and the garlic is fragrant, 2 to 3 minutes.

ADD the tomatoes and chicken to the pot and cook, stirring occasionally, until the tomatoes have softened, 3 to 4 minutes. Add the green beans, zucchini, and squash and cook, stirring occasionally, until the vegetables are crisp-tender and the chicken is cooked through (with no pink remaining in the center), 5 to 6 minutes. Add the red pepper flakes, salt, and pepper, sprinkle on the basil, stir for 30 seconds to incorporate, and serve immediately.

⭐ TAKE SOME SHORTCUTS *Take 5 minutes off your prep time by using a 28-ounce can of diced tomatoes instead of fresh. (Don't drain them—just toss the whole can in the pot in step 2.) And while fresh herbs really make a flavor difference here, if you're short on time, substitute ½ teaspoon each of dried oregano and thyme, and 1 to 2 teaspoons of dried basil.*

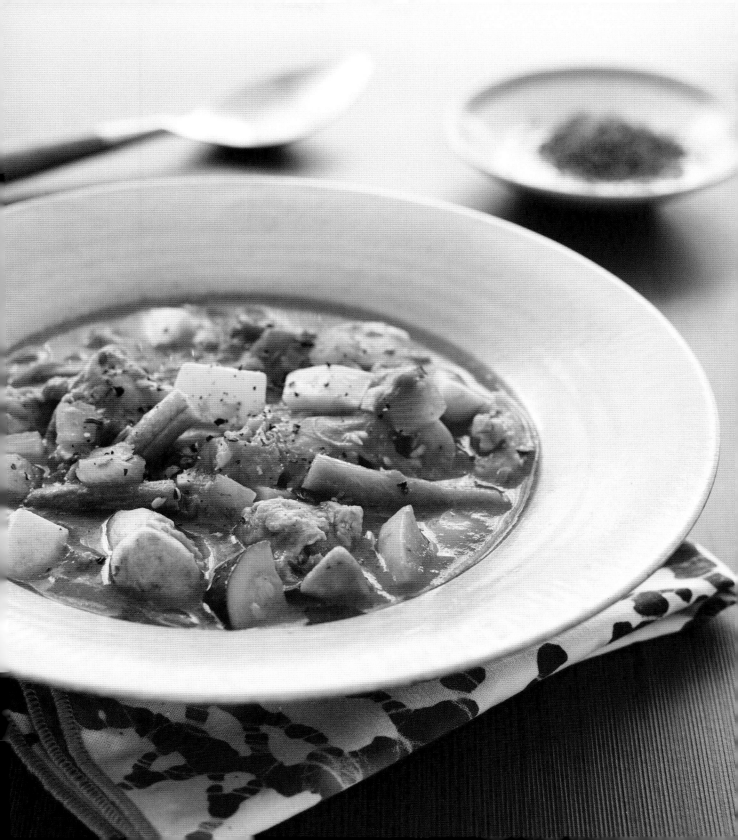

stir-fry chicken

SERVES 2

PREP TIME: 10 minutes

COOK TIME: 10 minutes

TOTAL TIME: 20 minutes

---

3 tablespoons cooking fat

1 pound chicken breast or thighs (boneless, skinless)

1 clove garlic, minced

1 tablespoon ginger, grated

1 head broccoli florets

2 cups mushrooms, sliced

2 carrots, julienned

½ pound green beans, cut into 1-inch pieces

2 green onions, minced

½ lime, juiced

1 tablespoon minced fresh cilantro

This simple dish is the perfect base for your favorite dressing or sauce (page 302). Double the recipe, select two different dressings, and you've got dinner and tomorrow's lunch covered. Hot stir-fry also goes well over a crisp, cold salad. Use your favorite sturdy salad greens (try Boston, Bibb, butter, or romaine), thinly sliced cabbage, or a pre-cut cole slaw mix and top with our Herb Citrus Vinaigrette (page 326) or Latin Marinade (page 330). Want something other than chicken? Try using thinly sliced flank steak or shrimp instead.

HEAT 2 tablespoons of the cooking fat in a large skillet over medium heat, swirling to coat the bottom of the pan. Place the chicken in the pan and sear until the outside is browned and it lifts easily from the bottom of the skillet, about 3 minutes on each side. Add the garlic and ginger. Cook and stir until aromatic, about 1 minute. Remove the chicken from the pan and slice into thin strips. Set the sliced chicken aside.

WIPE the pan clean and dry.

HEAT the remaining 1 tablespoon of cooking fat in the skillet over medium-high heat. Add the broccoli, mushrooms, carrots, and green beans and quickly stir-fry until the vegetables begin to soften, 2 to 3 minutes. Add the chicken strips to the pan; mix, and continue to cook for 2 to 3 minutes until everything is heated through.

TOP with the green onions, lime juice, and cilantro. Serve immediately.

⭐ CUT YOUR PREP AND COOK TIME *in half by using pre-cooked chicken or shrimp and replacing the fresh vegetables with a frozen vegetable mix. Let the vegetables thaw in the fridge while you're at work—when it's time to cook, follow the instructions above, stir-frying until everything is heated through.*

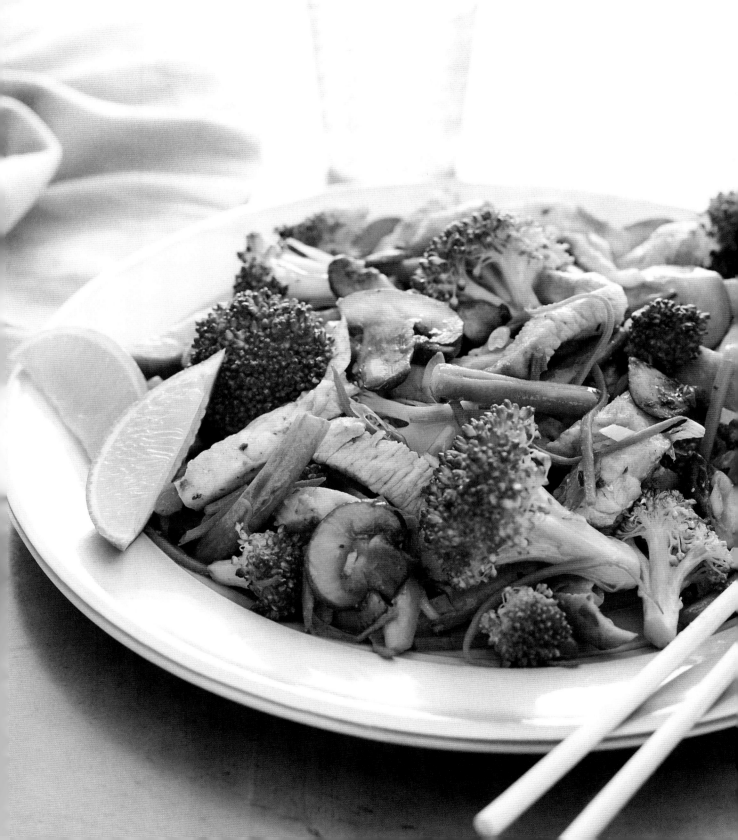

classic chili

PREP TIME: 20 minutes

COOK TIME: 1 hour 15 minutes

TOTAL TIME: 1 hour 35 minutes

---

1 pound ground meat (beef, lamb, bison)

1 onion, finely chopped

3 cloves garlic, minced

1 teaspoon cumin

1 teaspoon chili powder

½ teaspoon paprika

½ teaspoon mustard powder

½ teaspoon salt

1 red bell pepper, finely chopped

1 green bell pepper, finely chopped

1 can (14.5 ounces) diced tomatoes

2 cups beef broth

Different garnish options can really change the flavor of this dish. Try topping with fresh cilantro, jalapeños, crushed red pepper, or a drizzle of Ranch Dressing (page 316). If you're active and need to eat more carbohydrates, cut some potatoes or butternut squash into small cubes and add them to the pot just before simmering, or serve your chili in a "bowl" of roasted acorn squash halves.

HEAT a large pot or high-walled skillet over medium-high heat (without cooking fat). Add the ground meat and cook until the meat is fully browned, 7 to 10 minutes. Remove the meat from the pot with a slotted spoon and transfer it to a side dish, keeping the leftover fat in the pot.

ADD the onions, garlic, cumin, chili powder, paprika, mustard powder, and salt to the pot. Reduce the heat to medium low and cook until the onions are translucent, 4 to 5 minutes.

ADD the bell peppers, tomatoes, and broth and return the meat to the pot. Turn the heat up to high. When the chili reaches a boil, reduce the heat to low and simmer uncovered for 1 hour.

⭐ THIS RECIPE *can easily be made in a slow cooker. Follow all of the directions exactly as above, up to the point when your onions are translucent. At that point, transfer the contents from the pot to your slow cooker. Add the bell peppers, tomatoes, and broth and set to low heat, cooking for 6 to 8 hours.*

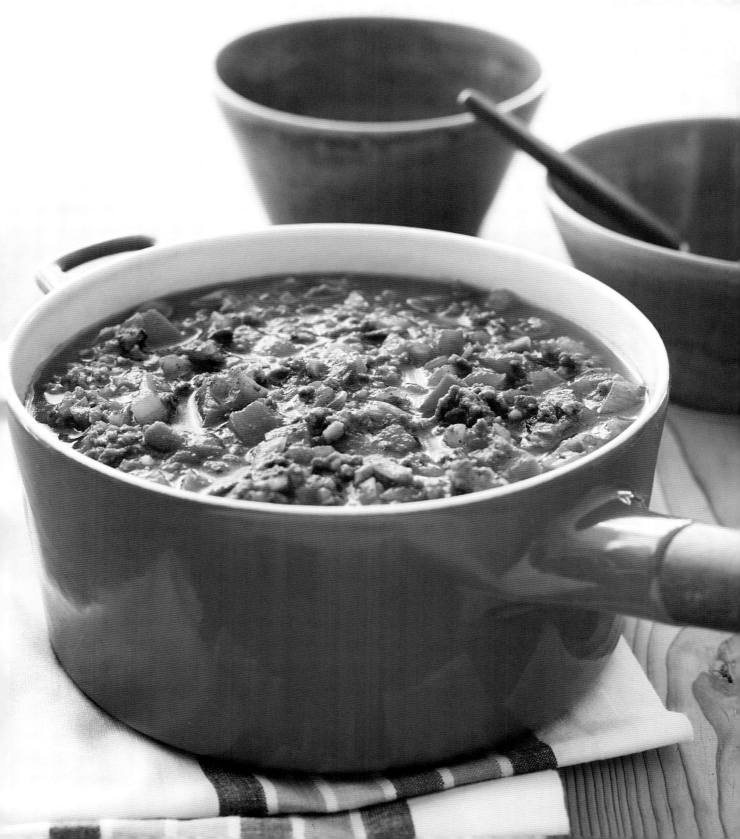

roasted pork shoulder with butternut squash, kale, and tomatoes

SERVES 2 (WITH LEFTOVERS)

PREP TIME: 10 minutes
COOK TIME: 3 hours
TOTAL TIME: 3 hours 10 minutes

---

2 teaspoons paprika

1 teaspoon chili powder

1 teaspoon garlic powder

1 teaspoon onion powder

1 teaspoon salt

½ teaspoon black pepper

½ lime, juiced

1½ pounds pork shoulder (boneless)

1 butternut squash, 1-inch diced

1 bunch kale, stems removed, leaves chopped

1 cup diced tomatoes

If you have leftover pork or if you make a double batch, freeze the pork in 1-cup servings so you can easily thaw it for future meals. You can serve the leftover pork with our Tangy BBQ sauce (page 322) in lettuce cups, over a salad with our Latin Vinaigrette (page 330), topped with fried eggs and Chimichurri (page 306), or added to a Vegetable Frittata (page 206). If butternut squash isn't in season, substitute two diced sweet potatoes.

PREHEAT the oven to 300°F.

MIX the paprika, chili powder, garlic powder, onion powder, salt, and pepper in a small bowl. Add the lime juice and stir. Place the pork in a Dutch oven or deep roasting pan and coat all sides of the pork with the spice mixture. Add 1 cup of water and cover tightly with a lid or aluminum foil. Cook in the oven, turning the pork shoulder in the pan every 45 minutes.

AFTER 2 hours and 15 minutes, add the butternut squash and ½ cup of water to the Dutch oven or pan. Cook for 30 more minutes, then add the kale and tomatoes. Place back in the oven for 15 minutes more.

REMOVE the pan from the oven and leave covered until you are ready to serve. With tongs or a slotted spoon, arrange the vegetables on plates, then break the pork apart into generous chunks and place over the vegetables. Spoon the braising liquid from the pan over the pork.

⭐ PORK SHOULDER *cuts also include Pork Butt, Boston Butt, and Picnic Shoulder Roast. These cuts all come from the same area, but include different sizes and portions of the shoulder muscles. If you can't find a cut labeled specifically "pork shoulder," any of these cuts would work.*

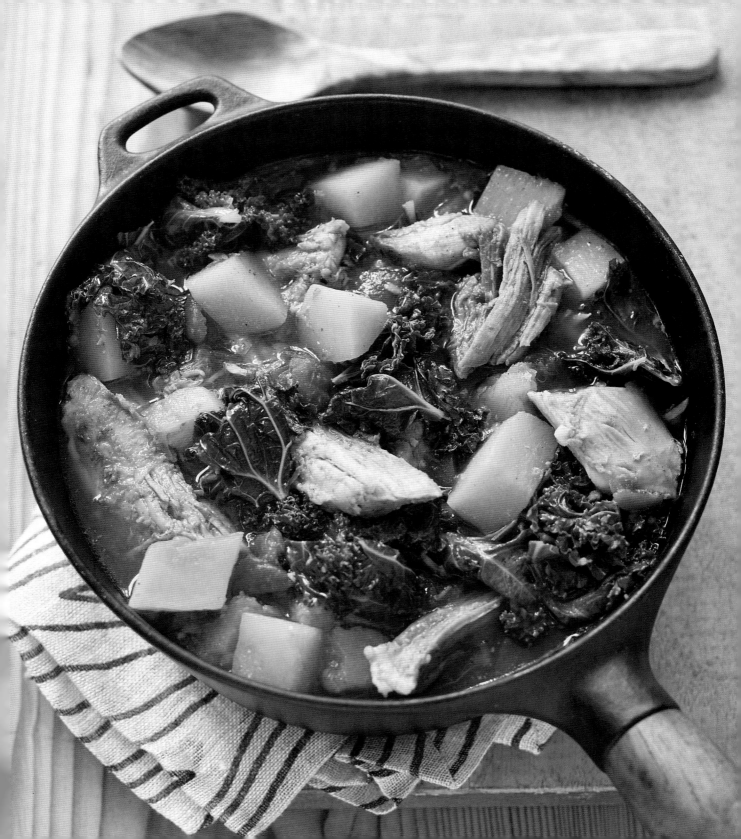

no-fuss salmon cakes

created by Melissa Joulwan for *It Starts With Food*

SERVES 2

PREP TIME: 15 minutes
COOK TIME: 30 minutes
TOTAL TIME: 45 minutes

---

3 6-ounce cans wild-caught salmon (boneless, or bones removed)

1 cup canned sweet potatoes

1 egg

½ cup almond flour

2 scallions, thinly sliced, plus extra for garnish

2 tablespoons fresh parsley, minced (or 2 teaspoons dried)

2 tablespoons fresh minced dill (or 2 teaspoons dried)

1 teaspoon salt

½ teaspoon paprika

¼ teaspoon ground black pepper

2 tablespoons clarified butter, ghee, or coconut oil, melted

Lemon wedges for serving (optional)

While these salmon cakes are a complete meal on their own (especially topped with the Tartar Sauce on page 312), they pair well with sautéed green beans and a fresh garden salad, our Grilled Asparagus with Lemon Zest (page 284), or Roasted Sweet Potatoes (page 296). They also reheat beautifully, so make a double-batch and enjoy these for breakfast the next day—top two cakes with some wilted spinach and a fried egg.

PREHEAT the oven to 425°F and cover a large baking sheet with parchment paper.

DRAIN the liquid from the salmon and crumble the fish into a large mixing bowl, removing the bones and flaking the fish with a fork. Add the sweet potato, egg, almond flour, scallions, parsley, dill, salt, paprika, and pepper and mix well with a wooden spoon.

BRUSH the parchment paper with the melted fat, then use a ⅓-cup measuring cup to scoop the cakes and drop them onto the parchment. Flatten the patties with your hand until they are uniform in thickness.

BAKE for 20 minutes, then flip each patty with a spatula and return to the oven. Bake until golden brown, about 10 more minutes.

SERVE with sliced scallions and lemon wedges for squeezing over the top, if desired.

⭐ YOU CAN FIND *de-boned canned salmon at your local health food store—that will save you about 10 minutes of prep time. Look for wild-caught to ensure you're getting the highest level of nutrition, especially anti-inflammatory omega-3 fatty acids like EPA and DHA. These fatty acids come from the food wild salmon eat, like algae and krill. Farmed salmon don't eat these foods, so they don't contain the same healthy fats.*

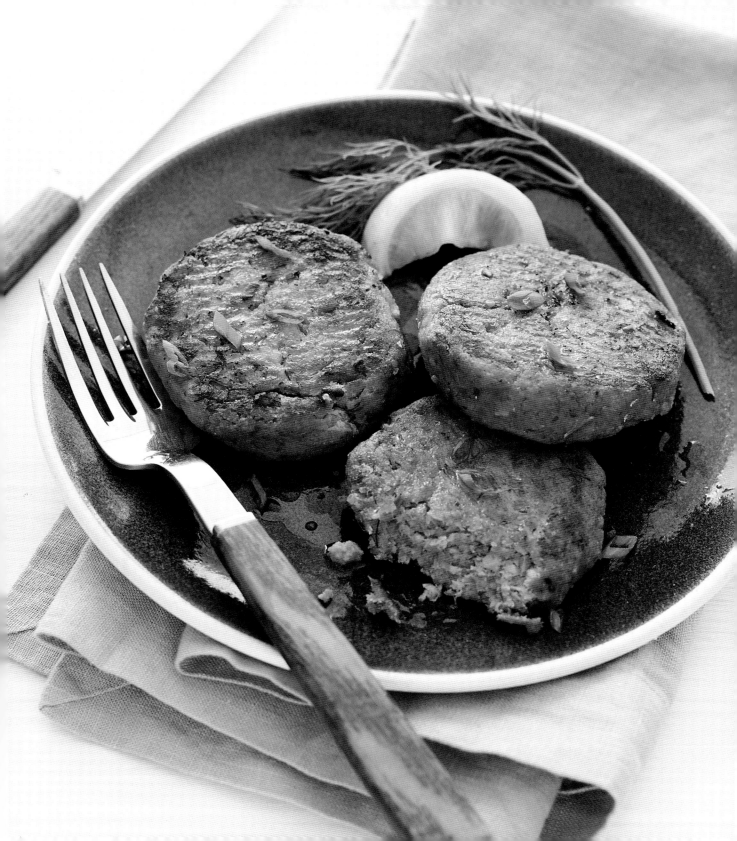

pot roast

SERVES 2 (WITH LEFTOVERS)

PREP TIME: 15 minutes
COOK TIME: 6 to 8 hours
TOTAL TIME: 6 to 8 hours

1½ pounds beef roast (chuck, boneless short ribs, brisket, top round, rump)

1 teaspoon salt

½ teaspoon black pepper

1 onion, sliced

3 carrots, unpeeled and cut into 2-inch pieces

3 stalks celery, cut into 1-inch pieces

1 small butternut squash, peeled and large-diced

2 cloves garlic

2 sprigs thyme

2 cups beef broth or water

If you have the time, you can add even more flavor to your roast by browning the meat, onions, and carrots before adding to the slow cooker. Set the slow cooker to low heat, and season your roast with salt and pepper. Melt 2 to 3 tablespoons of clarified butter or coconut oil in a large pot (or Dutch oven) over medium-high heat. Add the onions and (without stirring), sear them for 1 minute on one side, then flip using a wide spatula and sear the other side for 1 minute. (Onions should be slightly browned.) Remove from the pan, add the carrots, repeating the process, until carrots are also browned. Add 1 tablespoon of cooking fat, and add the roast to the pan. Sear it for 1 minute on all sides, until browned. Follow the rest of the above instructions.

SET your slow cooker to low heat, and season your roast with the salt and pepper.

ADD the beef roast, onions, carrots, celery, butternut squash, garlic, and thyme sprigs to the slow cooker. Top with the broth or water (or enough to cover the roast halfway) and leave the roast to cook for 6 to 8 hours. The roast should be fork-tender when done.

REMOVE the roast, transfer to a large plate or serving dish, and cover with foil. Allow the meat to rest for 15 minutes before serving.

REMOVE the thyme springs from the broth and discard. Slice the roast against the grain. Divide the meat and vegetables on individual plates, and ladle broth over the top.

⭐ JUST LIKE WOOD, *meat also has grain—muscle fiber bundles that are thicker and more prominent in harder-working muscle meat like the cuts that go into a beef roast. Cutting parallel to the grain (along the same lines as the grain) can make your meat much tougher. Instead, cut against the grain (perpendicular to those lines), to naturally soften up the meat and retain a much more tender texture.*

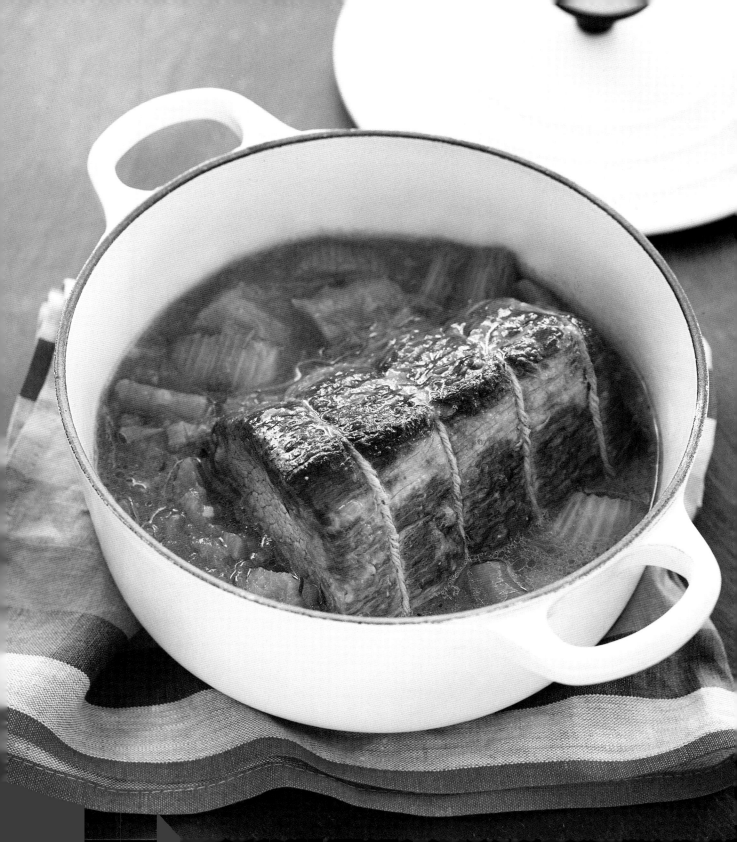

shepherd's pie

SERVES 2 (WITH LEFTOVERS)

PREP TIME: 10 minutes
COOK TIME: 50 minutes
TOTAL TIME: 1 hour

---

2 medium sweet potatoes, peeled and large-diced

4 cups cold water

4 tablespoons clarified butter or ghee

½ cup coconut milk

1 onion, finely chopped

2 stalks celery, finely chopped

1 carrot, peeled and finely chopped

1 pound ground meat (beef, lamb, bison)

2 cloves garlic, minced

1 teaspoon salt

½ teaspoon black pepper

1 sprig fresh thyme leaves (or ¼ teaspoon dried thyme)

2 teaspoons fresh oregano leaves (or ½ teaspoon dried)

For a lighter dish, use Mashed Cauliflower (page 270) instead of sweet potato for the top layer. You can also use mashed white potatoes for a more traditional feel. Crumble some crispy prosciutto or Whole30-compliant bacon (see page 404) over the top, or serve with our Whole30 Ketchup (page 323) for a kid-friendly meal. This dish freezes and reheats beautifully, so consider doubling the recipe, making one to eat and one to freeze.

PREHEAT the oven to 375°F.

IN a large pot, place the sweet potatoes in the cold water and bring to a boil. Boil until the potatoes are fork-tender, about 10 minutes. Drain the water from the pot, add 2 tablespoons of the butter and the coconut milk (away from the heat). Mash the potatoes with a potato masher, large kitchen fork, or immersion blender, or blend them in a food processor for a creamier texture. Transfer the potatoes to a bowl and set aside.

RETURN the same pot to the stove on medium heat, and melt the remaining 2 tablespoons of butter. Add the onions, celery, and carrots and cook, stirring, for 5 minutes. Add the ground meat and garlic. Cook, stirring often, until the meat is browned, 7 to 10 minutes. Season with the salt, pepper, thyme leaves, and oregano. Remove from the heat and let the meat and veggies cool in the pot for 5 minutes.

SPOON the meat and vegetable mixture evenly over the bottom of a casserole dish or 9x12-inch glass baking dish. Carefully spread the mashed sweet potatoes over the top of the meat and vegetable mixture. Roast in the oven for 30 minutes, letting the top brown slightly. Cut into slices and serve.

⭐ MOVE YOUR OVEN RACK *up one slot from the middle position to create more of a golden-brown crust on the mashed potatoes. Want to really fancy it up? Use the tines of a fork to press a design into your sweet potato before cooking.*

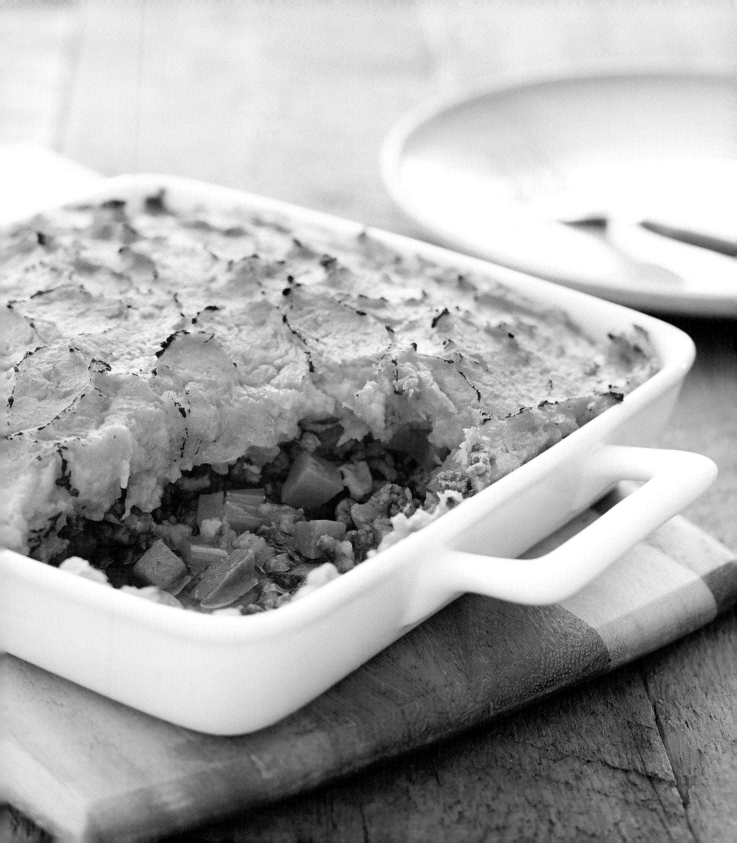

thai coconut soup

SERVES 2

PREP TIME: 20 minutes

COOK TIME: 40 minutes

TOTAL TIME: 1 hour

---

2 quarts chicken or vegetable broth (see page 177)

1 stalk lemongrass, cut into 2-inch pieces

1 small ginger root, peeled and cut into 1-inch pieces

1 shallot or 1 small red onion, diced

1 jalapeño, seeded and halved

3 limes, halved + 1 lime, zested, halved, and juiced

1 pound chicken thighs (boneless), cut into 1-inch cubes

1 14.5-ounce can coconut milk

3 cups mushrooms, quartered

1 red bell pepper, diced

1 parsnip, cut into ¼-inch coins

1 carrot, cut into ¼-inch coins

1 teaspoon salt

1 green onion, finely chopped

1 tablespoon finely chopped fresh cilantro

Want more spice? De-seed and finely dice another jalapeño and toss it in when you add the chicken. Craving some seafood? Use shrimp, scallops, or a firm white fish instead. Need more greens? Add a bag of baby spinach or a few handfuls of zucchini noodles just as you're pulling it off the stove, letting them wilt in the hot broth before garnishing and serving.

IN a large pot, bring the broth, lemongrass, ginger, shallot, jalapeño, and 6 of the lime halves to a boil. Reduce the heat to medium and let simmer uncovered for 15 minutes.

STRAIN the lemongrass, ginger, shallot, jalapeño, and limes from the broth. Add the chicken, coconut milk, mushrooms, bell pepper, parsnip, carrot, and salt to the broth. Cook over medium-high heat until the chicken is cooked through and the carrots and parsnips are tender, about 25 minutes.

SPOON into bowls and garnish with the green onion, cilantro, and zest and juice from the remaining lime.

⭐ DON'T BE INTIMIDATED *by lemongrass. This woody plant with a lemony scent is a common addition to Thai recipes. To use it, cut off the lower bulb and remove the tough outer leaves, leaving just the yellow center. Find this (and lots of other interesting herbs and spices) at your local health food store or Asian market—but if you can't find it, just add more ginger root and half of the lime zest to the broth instead.*

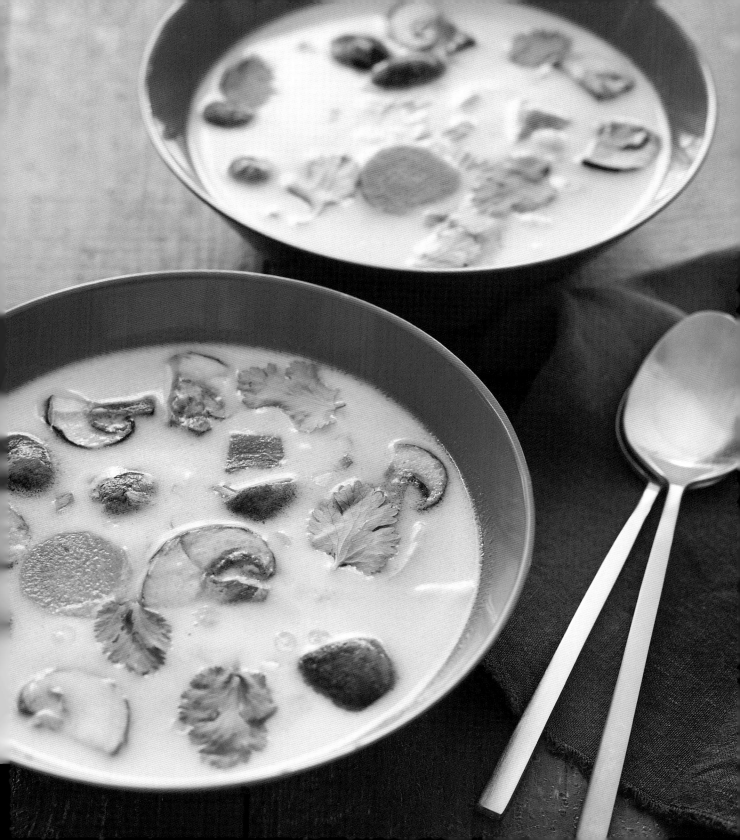

FANCYPANTS MEALS

AT SOME POINT during your Whole30, you're probably going to want to entertain. Maybe it's your turn to cook a family dinner, or there's a birthday smack in the middle of your Whole30, or maybe you just want to silence family and friends who keep saying, "You can't eat anything! You must feel so deprived. I could never eat like that."

Whatever the reason, we've got you covered.

Each of these fancypants meals are complete, start to finish—your main course, plus side dishes. (Some even have appetizers.) We'll give you a game plan for each one, helping you figure out prepping and planning so you're not ignoring your guests, distracted by a smoking frying pan.

Unless you're an experienced cook, we recommend saving these meals until you're a week or two into your Whole30, and have some experience planning, prepping, and cooking several dishes at once. However, don't wait too long! Pulling off a meal like this will boost your kitchen confidence, and assure your loved ones that no, you're not starving, deprived, or miserable while on the Whole30.

In fact, if you didn't tell your guests you just served them a Whole30 meal, we doubt anyone would even notice—which might open the door to conversations like, "Did you like it? Oh, it was delicious, was it? Well guess what? That entire meal was Whole30. So now that you know the food is amazing and understand that you're not deprived in any way. What's stopping you from trying it, Mom?"

Sharing the Good Food word via sneak attack is a totally valid strategy in our book.

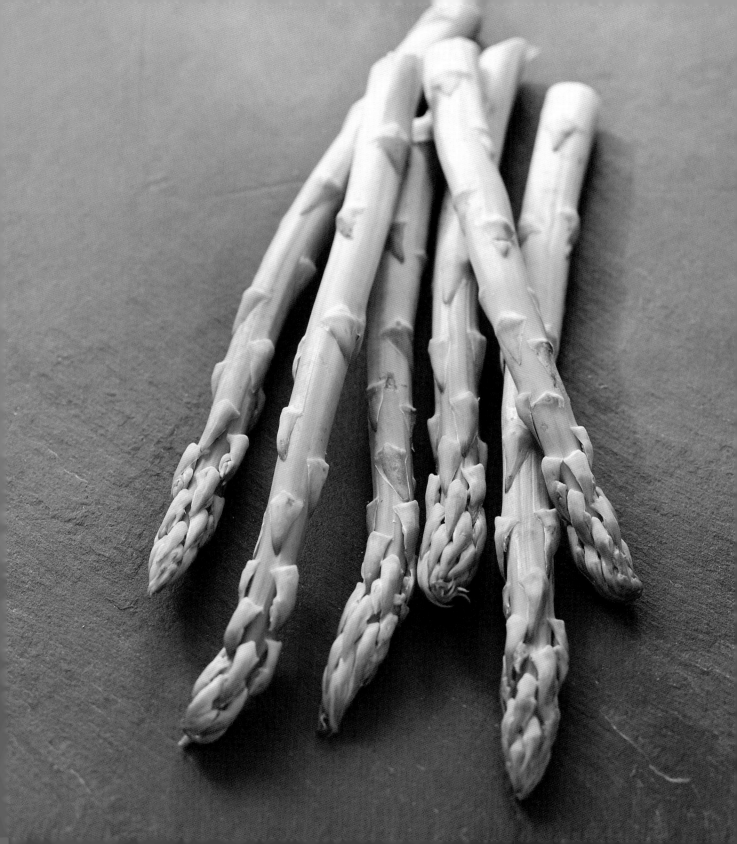

backyard barbecue

NOTHING SAYS SUMMERTIME like a backyard barbeque, but your food game has stepped up significantly since the days of burned hot dogs, soggy potato chips, and cans of soda. Have the family or friends over for our cookout and they'll be impressed with your creative menu without even realizing they've eaten their first Whole30 meal.

MENU

Dallas's Watermelon Salad

Pesto Shrimp with Cherry Tomatoes

Dry-Rubbed Grilled Steak

Grilled Vegetables with Balsamic Glaze

Sneaky, right?

This meal demands some prep ahead of time, though. First, unless you've got major grill experience, you may want to cook a few practice steaks before the big event. It's likely that your guests will all want their steaks cooked to different temperatures, and every grill is different, and our recommended cooking times may be slightly off for your particular set up—so get in there a week or two before the event and make some test steaks. (It's not so bad—you get to eat your practice runs.)

You'll also want to invest in some good grill tools, including a wire brush, a set of long tongs, and that grill basket we mentioned on page 145. Yes, you could cook veggies right on the grate of the grill using the technique we outlined on page 164, but we guarantee you'll have casualties, and a grill basket is so much easier.

Finally, make sure your grill is clean before the big day. A dirty grill makes your food stick, preventing that nice sear you're trying to achieve, and can put off a lot of smoke—or fire! A few days before the event, heat your grill to high and, once it's hot, clean the grates with a wire brush. (You can also do this the next time you actually cook something out there.) Then, apply a very light coating of extra-virgin olive oil to protect the grates until the next use.

- Prepare the pesto

- Prepare the balsamic glaze

- Make the watermelon salad

- Mix the spices for the dry rub

- Chop all the veggies for the grill basket

- OPTIONAL: Mix up a pitcher of mocktails (see pages 391–392)

- OPTIONAL: Make your favorite dipping sauce (starting on page 309) and cut some raw veggies

STORE everything in covered containers in the fridge, except the balsamic glaze and the spice mixture—those you can leave on the counter.

AS FOR TIMING, these dishes are pretty easy to manage. First, pull the pesto out of the fridge and start marinating the steaks in the dry rub about an hour before guests arrive. Begin cooking the shrimp 15 to 20 minutes before your party's starting time, so you can lay out your appetizer as people are walking in the door.

WHEN YOU'RE ABOUT 30 MINUTES FROM MEAL-TIME, preheat the grill and oven, then sear the steaks on the grill. Hand the steaks off to someone to stick in the oven while you transfer the grill basket full of vegetables to the grill. The veggies may take longer than the steaks to cook (especially if you like your steaks rare), but allowing them to rest a few more minutes won't hurt.

DON'T FORGET ABOUT THE WATERMELON SALAD! It may just be the best part of the whole meal. (Dallas created it after tasting a similar dish at a Mexican restaurant in Seattle.) Leave it in the fridge until just before serving, as it's tastiest when it's cold.

SERVE EVERYTHING FAMILY STYLE, inviting your guests to bring their plates to the food. (This is a barbeque! No need to be formal.) You can simply point out which steaks are done to which temperature, and let guests help themselves to the side dishes.

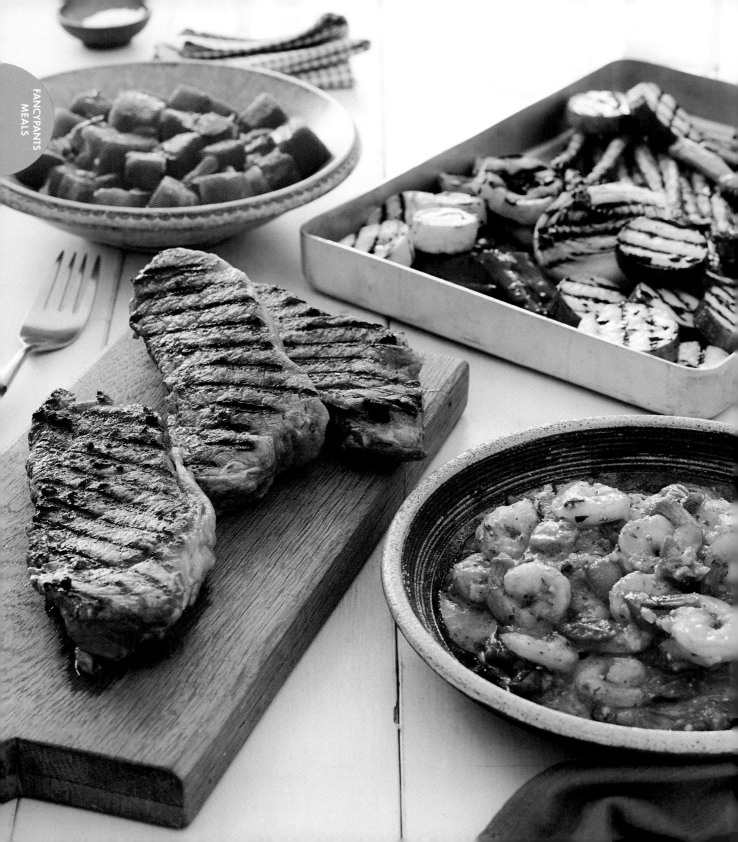

dallas's watermelon salad

SERVES 4

PREP TIME: 10 minutes

CHILL TIME: 20 minutes

TOTAL TIME: 30 minutes

---

2 pounds watermelon, cut into large dice

2 tablespoons extra-virgin olive oil

Juice of 2 limes

Leaves from 4 sprigs fresh mint, finely chopped

½ serrano chile pepper, seeded, finely sliced (optional)

PLACE all of the ingredients in a large non-reactive bowl and use a wooden spoon to combine. Cover and chill in the refrigerator for at least 20 minutes before serving. The salad can also be made up to one day ahead of time.

pesto shrimp with cherry tomatoes

SERVES 4

PREP TIME: 25 minutes

COOK TIME: 10 minutes

TOTAL TIME: 35 minutes

---

2 tablespoons cooking fat

¼ onion, finely chopped

1 clove garlic, minced

¾ pound (21 to 25) raw shrimp, peeled and deveined

2 cups cherry or grape tomatoes, cut in half

1 cup Pesto (page 315)

HEAT the cooking fat in a large skillet over medium heat. When the fat is hot, add the onion and cook, stirring, for 2 minutes. Add the garlic and cook until aromatic, about 1 minute. Add the shrimp and toss to coat with the onion and garlic. Let the shrimp cook for about 1 minute, then add the tomatoes. Add ¼ cup water, cover, and cook until the shrimp are bright pink and in the shape of a "C" and the tomatoes are tender and starting to wrinkle, 4 to 6 minutes.

TRANSFER the contents of the pan to a serving dish, and toss with the pesto.

dry-rubbed grilled steak

SERVES 4

PREP TIME: 5 minutes

MARINATE TIME: 15 to 30 minutes

COOK TIME: 15 to 25 minutes

TOTAL TIME: 20 to 30 minutes, plus marinating

---

3 tablespoons salt

2 tablespoons paprika

2 teaspoons dried oregano

2 teaspoons ground mustard

2 teaspoons onion powder

2 teaspoons black pepper

1 teaspoon ground turmeric

1 teaspoon garlic powder

¼ teaspoon cayenne pepper

4 steaks (5 to 8 ounces each) for grilling
(sirloin, strip, rib eye, tenderloin)

TO make the dry rub, mix all the seasonings together in a small bowl. Reserve 2 tablespoons and store the rest in an airtight container. Good news—you can make this weeks ahead of time. Feel free to double the recipe and save more of the rub for the next time you grill.

SEASON each steak evenly on both sides using 1½ teaspoons of the dry rub. Let the steaks marinate at room temperature for 15 to 30 minutes.

WHILE the steaks are marinating, preheat the grill to high heat (500°F) and the oven to 350°F.

LAY the steaks on the hot grill at a 45-degree angle to the grates. Let the steaks sear for 2 to 3 minutes—you'll know a steak is ready to move when it pulls off the grates easily. When ready, use grill tongs to turn the steaks 90 degrees, and sear for 2 more minutes. This creates a nice pattern of grill marks on the steaks. Flip the steaks and repeat the two-step searing process on the other side.

TRANSFER the steaks to a baking sheet or cast-iron skillet. Place the baking sheet or skillet in the oven and bake for 8 to 12 minutes, depending on the thickness of the steak and the desired temperature (see page 154 for guidelines). Use a meat thermometer until you learn how to judge this by the look and feel of the steak. Remember to pull the steak out of the oven when it's 5°F below the desired temperature, as it will continue to cook as it rests.

LET the steaks rest at room temperature for 5 minutes before serving.

grilled vegetables with balsamic glaze

SERVES 4

PREP TIME: 20 minutes

COOK TIME: 35 minutes

TOTAL TIME: 55 minutes

---

1 cup balsamic vinegar

1 bunch asparagus, ends trimmed, cut into 1-inch pieces

1 zucchini, cut into large dice

1 yellow squash, cut into large dice

1 sweet or yellow onion, cut into 1-inch slices

2 bell peppers, seeded, ribs removed, and cut into 1-inch slices

¼ cup extra-virgin olive oil

½ teaspoon salt

½ teaspoon black pepper

2 tablespoons finely chopped fresh parsley

TO make the balsamic glaze, bring the vinegar to a boil in a small saucepan over medium-high heat. Turn the heat down to medium low and simmer until the balsamic is reduced by about half, 20 to 30 minutes. Remove from the heat, allow to cool, and reserve. (You can do this up to a week ahead of time; store in a covered container at room temperature.)

TO grill the vegetables, preheat the grill to high heat (500°F).

PLACE the asparagus, zucchini, squash, onion, and peppers in a large bowl and drizzle in half the olive oil. Toss or mix the vegetables with your hands until they are well coated, place in a grill basket.

PLACE the basket on the grill and close the lid. Grill for 15 to 20 minutes, shaking the grill basket occasionally. You're done when the peppers and onions are charred on the edges and tender enough to eat.

PLACE the vegetables in a serving bowl. Drizzle evenly with ¼ cup of the balsamic glaze and the remaining olive oil. Season with the salt and pepper and garnish with the parsley. Serve warm or at room temperature.

✷ GRILL TECHNIQUES *If you've got decent grill experience (or an extra set of hands to help), you can slice the vegetables and grill them right on the slats, as described in the technique on page 164. It's a little more work, but this method will impart those pretty char marks on your vegetables (as in our photo on page 358) and lets you throw some fruit (like slices of pineapple or mango) into the mix, too.*

date night

THIS DATE NIGHT DISH is our only Fancypants Meal that serves two—just double the ingredients if you've got chaperones. We set this one up for you so that you can prepare most of it the day before or morning of, leaving you more time to entertain your date. (The last thing you want is to be distracted by searing scallops as he or she is walking in the door!)

MENU

Seared Scallops with
Ginger-Blueberry Sauce

Cabbage, Kale, and Bell
Pepper Slaw with Apple
Cider Vinaigrette

Coconut Cauliflower Rice

Lemongrass Chicken
Skewers

Here's how we'd set this one up: The morning of your date, prepare the marinade and marinate the chicken in the fridge. You'll also want to prepare the vinaigrette and the slaw, storing the dressed dish in a serving bowl or glass container in the fridge. We'd also make a pitcher of infused water—add some orange slices and mint leaves to plain old water, and let it infuse in the refrigerator or on the counter.

Plan on serving everything out of serving dishes, instead of straight from the stove. It's extra clean up, but it's classier, and avoids the awkward waiting-for-your-turn-by-the-stove scenario.

A half-hour before your date is due to arrive, start soaking your wooden skewers (if necessary), do your mise-en-place (page 187) for the cauliflower rice by pulsing the florets, chopping the onion, and measuring out the coconut milk and shredded coconut. Set these items in individual bowls by the stove, clean your food processor so it's ready for the blueberry sauce, and thread the chicken onto the skewers and place on a baking sheet.

Five minutes before your date is due to arrive, preheat the oven to 350°F. The goal is to put the chicken appetizer in the oven as he or she is walking in the door, giving you time for a relaxed greeting and drink offerings while filling the kitchen with the inviting scent of lemongrass chicken.

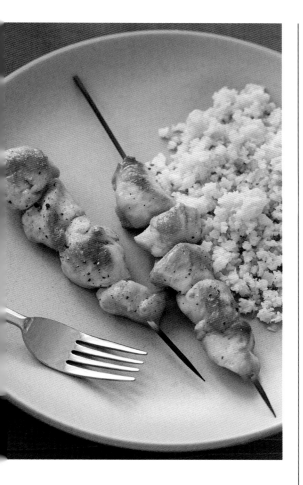

Offer your date a seat as you pull the slaw out of the fridge, and the chicken out of the oven. Have a pretty serving plate ready for the chicken, and sit and talk while you both enjoy the appetizer. Don't rush—you have all night, and you want to enjoy both the meal and the social experience.

When you're ready, it's time to impress your date with kitchen wizardry. A polite date will ask to help, so have him or her transfer the slaw to a serving bowl, and set the table. (In fact, ask for help if it isn't offered: It may feel like too much pressure if your date just sits there and watches you cook.)

Don an apron—blueberry juice is very hard to remove from clothing—and get your cauliflower rice started while you chop the ginger and prepare the blueberry sauce. While the sauce is cooking, you can season the scallops* with salt and pepper.

After you've got the blueberry sauce blended and staying warm in a small pot and the cauliflower rice simmering, it's time to cook the scallops. Have another serving dish ready, in case you have to cook them in batches. Cook the scallops and place in the serving dish when done. Add the warm blueberry sauce to a small pitcher or bowl, transfer the coconut cauliflower rice to a serving bowl, and bring everything to the table—the scallops, the sauce, the rice, and the slaw—with the appropriate serving tools.

Your table should already be set, so all that's left is to top off your waters, light some candles, and gracefully accept the compliments from your date.

*If your date is allergic to shellfish, you can substitute Perfect Oven-Baked Salmon (page 160) for the scallops. When the chicken comes out, turn the oven up to 450°F. Put the salmon in the oven when you start preparing the blueberry sauce—it should all be done around the same time.

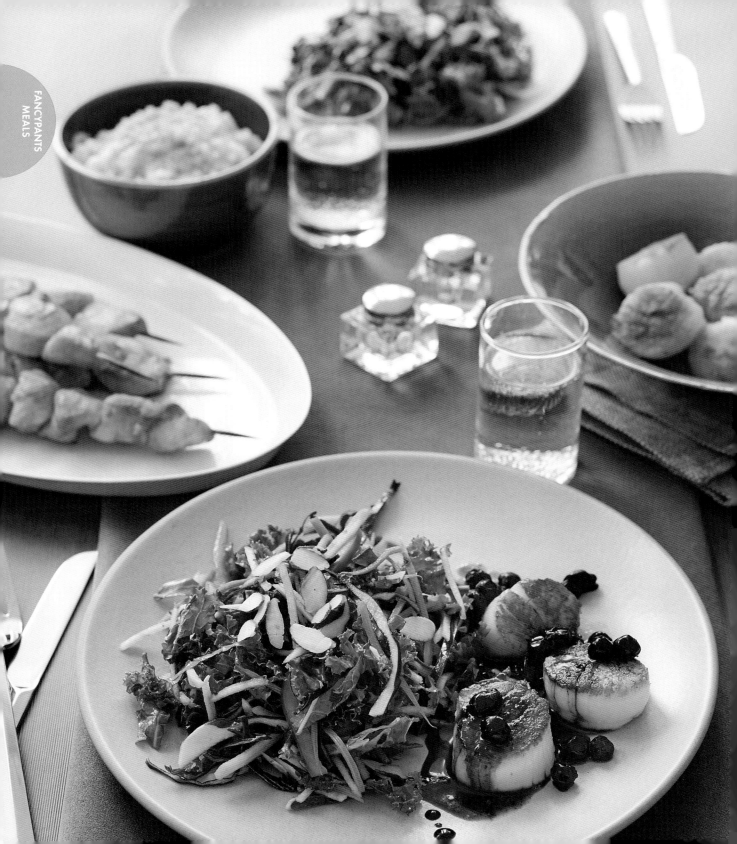

seared scallops with ginger-blueberry sauce

SERVES 2

PREP TIME: 10 minutes

COOK TIME: 10 to 15 minutes

TOTAL TIME: 25 minutes

FOR THE GINGER-BLUEBERRY SAUCE

1 cup fresh or frozen blueberries

1½ teaspoons finely chopped fresh ginger

¼ teaspoon salt

FOR THE SCALLOPS

¾ pound sea scallops, patted dry

½ teaspoon salt

½ teaspoon black pepper

3 tablespoons cooking fat

TO MAKE THE GINGER-BLUEBERRY SAUCE: Defrost your blueberries (if necessary), then combine with 1 cup of water in a small saucepan over medium-high heat. Let the mixture reach a boil, then add the ginger and salt. Reduce the heat to medium and cook for 5 minutes, letting the blueberries burst and release their juice and the ginger steep.

The sauce can be left chunky, but it looks prettier if you blend it in a food processor or with an immersion blender to a smooth consistency. Just return it to the pan after blending to keep warm.

TO MAKE THE SCALLOPS: Season both sides evenly with the salt and pepper. Heat the cooking fat in a large skillet over medium-high heat. When the fat is hot, add the scallops in a single layer (you may need to cook them in batches). Cook until the scallops begin to pull away from pan and brown, 2 to 3 minutes. Using kitchen tongs, turn the scallops and repeat the searing on the other side, for another 2 minutes.

TRANSFER the scallops to a serving dish or individual plates. Top with ¼ to ½ cup of the blueberry sauce. Serve warm or at room temperature.

cabbage, kale, and bell pepper slaw with apple cider vinaigrette

SERVES 2

PREP TIME: 20 minutes

FOR THE VINAIGRETTE

¾ cup extra-virgin olive oil

¼ cup apple cider vinegar

2 tablespoons finely chopped fresh parsley

1 clove garlic, minced

Salt and black pepper

FOR THE SLAW

½ head red cabbage, finely shredded

1 bunch kale, stems removed, ribbon chopped

½ bell pepper, seeded, ribs removed, and cut into very thin strips

½ cup shredded carrots

½ cup julienned apple

2 tablespoons slivered almonds

1 teaspoon salt

½ teaspoon black pepper

TO MAKE THE VINAIGRETTE: Combine the olive oil, vinegar, parsley, and garlic in a salad dressing bottle or bowl. Shake or mix well, until the olive oil is thoroughly incorporated. Season with salt and pepper.

TO MAKE THE SLAW: Combine the cabbage, kale, bell pepper, carrots, apple, and almonds in a medium mixing bowl. Mix well and toss with ½ cup of the vinaigrette. Season with the salt and pepper.

CHILL in the refrigerator for at least 30 minutes before serving. You can make the vinaigrette and the slaw up to one day ahead of time. Use the extra vinaigrette to refresh the flavor of leftover slaw, or store it in the refrigerator for up to 5 days.

coconut cauliflower rice

SERVES 2

PREP TIME: 10 minutes
COOK TIME: 15 minutes
TOTAL TIME: 25 minutes

---

1 head cauliflower, cut into florets

2 tablespoons coconut oil, ghee, or clarified butter

¼ onion, finely chopped

1 cup coconut milk

¼ cup shredded coconut flakes

½ teaspoon salt

¼ teaspoon black pepper

1 tablespoon finely chopped cilantro

TO "rice" the cauliflower florets, pulse in a food processor until they turn into small, ricelike pieces, 20 to 25 pulses. (You'll want to do this in two batches. Don't overcrowd the cauliflower in the food processor, and don't over-pulse or the florets will get mushy.)

IN a large skillet, melt the cooking fat over medium heat and swirl to coat the bottom of the pan. When the fat is hot, add the onion and cook, stirring, until translucent, 2 to 3 minutes. Add the riced cauliflower and coconut milk and mix thoroughly. Cover and steam until the coconut milk has been absorbed by the rice and the cauliflower is tender, about 10 minutes. (The best way to test for doneness is to eat a bite!) Scrape up any brown bits from the bottom of the pan with a wooden spoon and mix into the rice.

REMOVE the pan from the heat and mix in the shredded coconut, salt, and pepper. Gently stir in the chopped cilantro and serve warm.

lemongrass chicken skewers

SERVES 2

PREP TIME: 20 minutes

MARINATE TIME: 20 minutes to 24 hours

COOK TIME: 8 to 12 minutes

TOTAL TIME: 30 minutes, plus marinating

2 tablespoons coconut oil

1 teaspoon sesame oil

1 cup roughly chopped trimmed lemongrass

2 tablespoons chopped green onions

1½ teaspoons grated fresh ginger

1 clove garlic, minced

Juice of ½ lime

½ pound boneless, skinless chicken breast, cut into 1-inch strips

1 tablespoon cooking fat (melted, if necessary)

½ teaspoon salt

¼ teaspoon black pepper

IF using wooden skewers, soak them in water for 30 minutes to 1 hour to prevent them from burning.

TO make the marinade, heat the coconut oil and sesame oil in a large skillet over medium heat. When the oil is hot, add the lemongrass, green onions, ginger, and garlic and cook, stirring, for 1 minute to release the flavor. Remove from the heat and stir in the lime juice. Allow the pan to cool for 5 minutes.

PLACE the chicken strips in a glass storage dish or plastic bag and pour the marinade over the chicken. Seal the bag or cover the dish and marinate the chicken at room temperature for at least 20 minutes, or in the refrigerator overnight.

PREHEAT the oven to 350°F. Line a baking sheet with foil.

REMOVE the chicken from the refrigerator and discard the excess marinade.

CUT the marinated chicken into 1-inch pieces and thread onto the skewers. Arrange the skewers on the baking sheet, brush with the cooking fat, and season with salt and pepper. Bake for 8 to 12 minutes, until the chicken is cooked through and no pink remains in the center of the strips. Serve as an appetizer.

⭐ IF YOU *can't find lemongrass at your local Asian market, don't stress. Just double the ginger and add the zest from one lime.*

tapas party

WE CERTAINLY don't want you living in social isolation during your Whole30, but the idea of going to (or hosting!) a party may be intimidating. We promise, it's easier than you think, even though your days of serving corn chips alongside a jar of nacho cheese dip as "party fare" are long in the past.

MENU

Short Rib–Stuffed Peppers

Sun-Dried Tomatoes

Portabella Mushrooms

Anchovies

If not, they really should be. Allow us to help.

This dish is perfect to bring to a potluck, or as the main course for a book club meeting, baby shower, or football party. As it's just as good served cold as warm, you have a lot of flexibility in how far in advance you prepare the cooked ingredients. For now, let's assume you're having a small 7:00 p.m. get-together at your house and you'll be serving the cooked foods warm.

The ribs will take 8 hours in the slow cooker, so start preparations in the morning, and put the ribs in to cook by 10:30 a.m. After you get the ribs going, prepare the balsamic glaze. This isn't hard—once it boils, just reduce the heat to low, set a kitchen timer for 20 minutes, and go about your business. In fact, use this time to prepare the balsamic vinaigrette, too! When the glaze is done, allow it to cool, then transfer to a sealed storage container, and leave on the counter or in your pantry—no need to refrigerate.

Around 5:15 p.m., preheat the oven and start marinating the mushroom caps in the balsamic vinaigrette (the dressing, not the glaze). Coat the peppers with olive oil and put in the oven at 5:30.

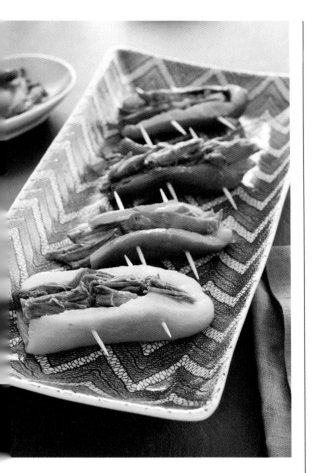

You'll pull your peppers out to cool around 6:10 p.m., give or take. The mushrooms go in the oven at the same time, on the same pan. At 6:30, the mushrooms come out and start cooling. By 6:40, you can peel the skin off the peppers and slice up the mushrooms.

And look! Your short ribs are done cooking and staying nice and warm in the slow cooker—perfect timing. Reduce the sauce, shred the rib meat, and toss them together in a bowl. Then start stuffing the peppers and securing with toothpicks.

You may have an early-bird guest or two arriving right about now—also great timing. Recruit them to help you by plating the sun-dried tomatoes, mushrooms, and anchovies as you stuff the peppers and add them to your serving dish. When the plates have been arranged, drizzle the peppers and mushrooms with the balsamic glaze, sprinkle with the capers and salt, and serve.

Oh, we forgot to mention, you've got time to get dressed and fix your hair while the peppers roast and the mushrooms marinate. Just don't forget to don an apron when you come back—do you know how hard it is to get balsamic glaze out of cotton?

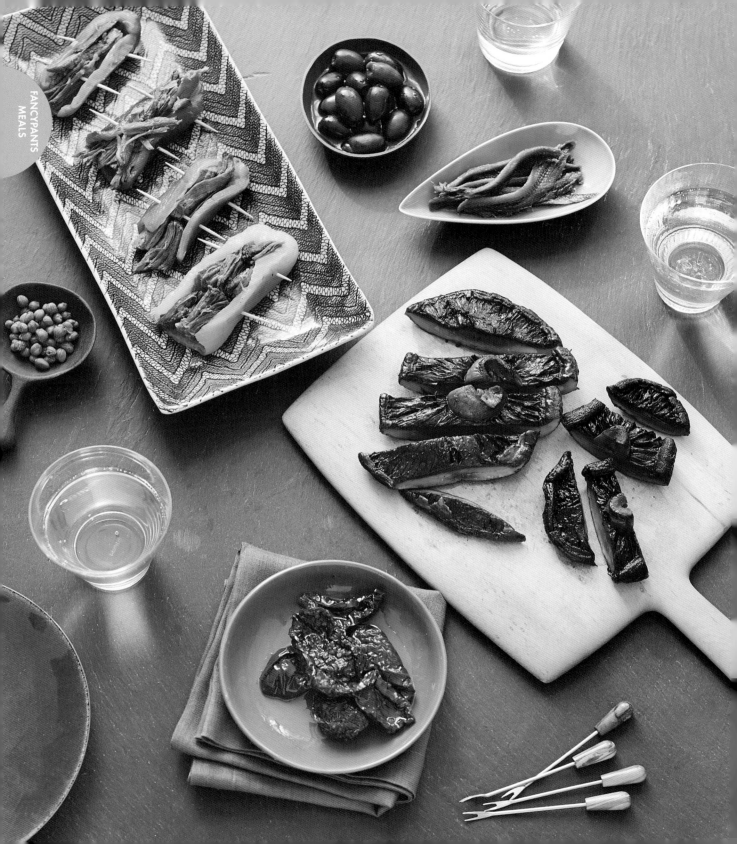

braised beef short ribs

SERVES 8

PREP TIME: 10 minutes

COOK TIME: 8 hours

TOTAL TIME: 8 hours 10 minutes

---

3 teaspoons salt

2 teaspoons black pepper

3 pounds beef short ribs, trimmed

4 to 6 tablespoons cooking fat

1 onion, quartered

6 cloves garlic, peeled

4 sprigs fresh thyme

2 cups apple cider

MIX 2 teaspoons of the salt and all the pepper in a small bowl and use to season the short ribs evenly on both sides.

IN an oven-safe heavy pot or Dutch oven, melt 4 tablespoons of the cooking fat over medium-high heat. When the fat is hot, sear the short ribs until each side is golden brown, about 1 minute on each side. (You'll likely have to do this in batches, adding another tablespoon of cooking fat to each new batch.)

TRANSFER all the ribs to a slow cooker. Add the onion, garlic, thyme, apple cider, and 8 cups of water and cook on low for 8 hours. When done, the short ribs should be fork-tender.

TRANSFER the short ribs to a bowl and shred, discarding the bones and excess fat. Ladle the cooking liquid, onion, and garlic into a food processor or blender, removing the thyme stems, and blend on low until thoroughly mixed. Transfer the blended sauce to a medium sauce-pot and bring to a simmer over medium heat. Cook until thickened, about 5 minutes. Season the sauce with the remaining 1 teaspoon salt.

TRANSFER the shredded short ribs to a serving bowl, toss with the sauce, and reserve. (You'll be using all of it to stuff the peppers for your tapas plate.)

short rib–stuffed peppers, sun-dried tomatoes, portabella mushrooms, and anchovies

SERVES 8

PREP TIME: 20 minutes

COOK TIME: 50 to 60 minutes

TOTAL TIME: 1 hour 20 minutes, plus cooking the short ribs

---

4 portabella mushroom caps, stems removed

½ cup Balsamic Vinaigrette (page 328)

1 cup balsamic vinegar

8 bell peppers (red, yellow, or orange)

¼ cup extra-virgin olive oil

Braised Beef Short Ribs (page 371)

2 cups sun-dried tomatoes in oil

2 cups Kalamata or black olives, pitted

4 ounces anchovies in oil, drained

2 tablespoons capers, drained

1 teaspoon coarse salt

PREHEAT the oven to 450°F. Line a baking sheet with parchment paper.

IN a shallow dish or plastic re-sealable bag, marinate the mushroom caps in the prepared balsamic vinaigrette for 30 minutes at room temperature.

WHILE the mushrooms are marinating, prepare the balsamic glaze: bring the balsamic vinegar to a boil in a small saucepan over medium-high heat. Turn the heat down to medium low and simmer until reduced by about half, about 20 to 30 minutes. Remove from the heat, allow to cool, and reserve. It should be thick enough to stick to your spoon, but still easy to drizzle. (You can do this step up to a week ahead of time; store in a covered container at room temperature.)

IN a large mixing bowl, coat the bell peppers with the olive oil, and place on the prepared baking sheet. Roast in the oven for 30 to 40 minutes, turning once during cooking, until the skins are wrinkled and charred. Transfer the peppers to a bowl and cover with aluminum foil. Allow the peppers to cool for 30 minutes.

WHILE the peppers are cooling, reduce the oven heat to 350°F. Remove the mushroom caps from the marinade and discard the vinaigrette. Using the same lined baking sheet, roast the mushrooms in the oven for 10 minutes, then flip them over and roast for another 10 minutes, until the center is soft. Let cool, then slice into strips.

RUB the charred skin off the peppers, leaving just the roasted flesh. Remove the stems and seeds, and cut each pepper into four equal quarters. Fill each pepper quarter with a spoonful of short ribs, wrap the pepper around the meat, and secure with a toothpick.

ARRANGE the stuffed peppers, roasted mushroom strips, sun-dried tomatoes, olives, and anchovies on one or more serving dishes. Drizzle a very thin stream of the balsamic glaze over the stuffed peppers and mushrooms. Sprinkle with the capers and coarse salt and serve warm or cold.

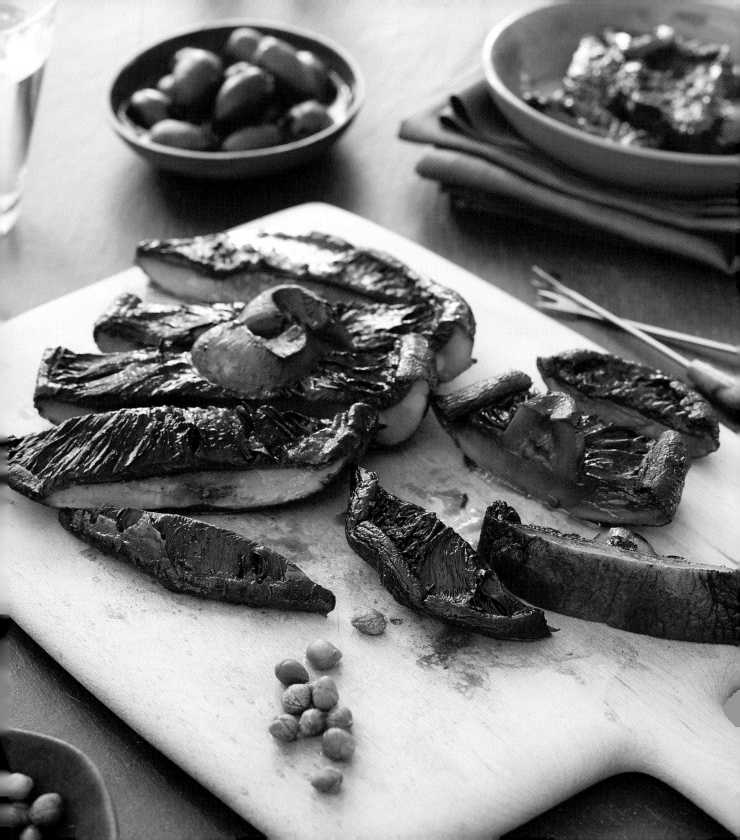

family lamb dinner

DINNER DOESN'T GET more traditional than a hunk of meat, a vegetable mash, and a side salad—but we've put some twists into these dishes to keep them tasty and Whole30-compliant. There's no way your family members will leave the table hungry after this hearty meal, and even the most skeptical will be forced to admit that this "crazy diet" you're on is actually full of familiar, nourishing, delicious foods.

MENU

Bone-in Leg of Lamb

Cauliflower-Broccoli Mash

Roasted Beet Salad with Grapefruit-Thyme Vinaigrette

Most of this meal can (and should) be done ahead of time, leaving you to navigate your leg of lamb gracefully while still having the time and mental capacity to engage with your guests. Here's our proposed timeline:

Buy the leg of lamb no more than two days before your dinner and make sure you specify a bone-in leg. The extra flavor is worth the hassle of carving around the bone, and you'll have material for the perfect bone broth (see page 177) when you're done.

The night before your dinner (or the morning of), prepare the cauliflower mash and store in the fridge. This is the time to roast your beets, too. They can take up to an hour in the oven and peeling them can be a messy process, so you want this out of the way before your guests arrive. Plus, the salad is served cold, so you could actually do this step a full day before the dinner.

Finally, prepare the vinaigrette and store in the refrigerator.

Your lamb needs to soak for about 8 hours, so prepare the marinade either the night before or the morning of your dinner and place in the fridge to marinate first thing in the morning. (An hour of marinating time either way won't

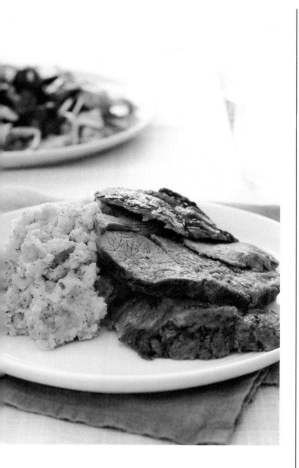

matter much.) Ideally, someone will be around to baste the lamb around the halfway mark.

Begin roasting a 6-pound leg of lamb 2 hours before dinner time; back that time up by 30 minutes or so if you have a larger leg. While it's cooking, you don't really have much to do—just set a timer for the 30-minute mark to remind yourself to reduce the oven temperature, and then again after another 90 minutes to do your first meat-thermometer check.

Ten minutes before the lamb is done, transfer the mash to a saucepan and begin to reheat on medium low, stirring once in a while. At the same time, take the vinaigrette out of the refrigerator. (This will allow some of the olive oil's cloudiness to dissipate.)

Once the lamb is out of the oven and resting, assemble the beet salad in a large serving bowl or individual side bowls.

When the lamb is fully rested, it's time to carve! Carve the lamb by first cutting thin slices parallel to the bone, until you hit the bone. Transfer those slices to a serving platter, then rest the leg on the flat surface you just created, and start cutting thin slices from the thick end of the leg, perpendicular to the bone. Continue until you hit the bone itself. Transfer those slices to the platter, continue cutting thin slices across the meat and above the bone until you reach the end. This gives you "flaps" of meat on top of the bone, which you can then carefully slice off. Slicing "against the grain" in this manner gives you more tender, flavorful meat.

Take any meat left on the bone and either clean it off for sandwiches or save it to toss into a Frittata (page 206), or take the whole thing and make lamb bone broth following our beef broth recipe on page 177.

Serve the lamb slices with a side of the warm mash and the beet salad dressed with the vinaigrette.

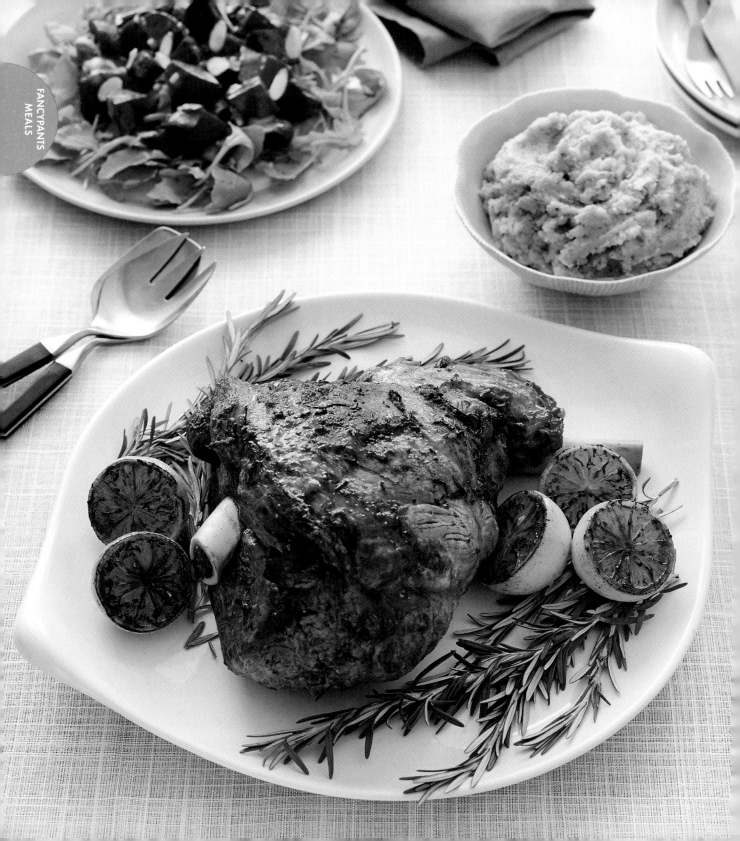

bone-in leg of lamb

SERVES 4 (WITH LEFTOVERS)

PREP TIME: 15 minutes

MARINATE TIME: 8 hours

COOK TIME: 2 to 2 ½ hours

TOTAL TIME: 2 ¼ to 2 ¾ hours, plus marinating

½ cup extra-virgin olive oil

Grated zest and juice of 1 lemon

1 tablespoon fresh rosemary

1 tablespoon fresh thyme

1 teaspoon salt

½ teaspoon black pepper

1 bone-in leg of lamb (6 to 8 pounds)

COMBINE the olive oil, lemon zest and juice, rosemary, thyme, salt, and pepper in a large non-reactive mixing bowl and whisk until blended. Pat the lamb dry with a paper towel, place in the bowl with the marinade, and turn to coat all of the meat. Cover with aluminum foil and refrigerate for 8 hours, turning the lamb and basting after 4 hours. (If you don't have a turkey baster, just use a large spoon to pour the marinade over the lamb a few times.)

PREHEAT the oven to 400°F. Place the marinated lamb in a large roasting pan and roast uncovered for 30 minutes. Reduce the oven temperature to 325°F and continue roasting for 90 minutes to 2 hours, until the internal temperature is 135°F (for medium rare) or 140°F (for medium). Cooking times will vary depending on the size of your lamb and your oven, so begin checking the temperature with a meat thermometer at the 90-minute mark, and continue to check every 10 minutes thereafter.

REMOVE the lamb from the oven and allow it to rest for 10 minutes before carving as described in the menu introduction.

cauliflower-broccoli mash

SERVES 4

PREP TIME: 20 minutes

COOK TIME: 15 minutes

TOTAL TIME: 35 minutes

---

1 ½ cups chicken or vegetable broth

1 head cauliflower, cut into florets

2 bunches broccoli, cut into florets

3 cloves garlic, minced

1 cup coconut milk

2 tablespoons clarified butter or ghee

1 teaspoon salt

¼ teaspoon black pepper

1 tablespoon minced fresh parsley

BRING the broth to a simmer in a saucepan over medium-high heat. Add the cauliflower, broccoli, garlic, and coconut milk. Cover and cook until the florets are fork tender, 12 to 15 minutes.

continued

TRANSFER the half of the florets and liquid to a food processor. (The florets are so bulky you need to puree in batches, so just estimate half the contents—it will all come back together in the end.) Blend on low speed until smooth in consistency and transfer to a bowl. Puree the remaining florets and liquid.

RETURN all the mash to the food processor and add the clarified butter, salt, and pepper, and pulse until well mixed. Add the parsley and continue blending on low until completely smooth.

YOU can make the mash up to a day before your dinner and reheat in a saucepan on the stove just before serving.

roasted beets with grapefruit-thyme vinaigrette

SERVES 4

PREP TIME: 10 minutes
COOK TIME: 50 minutes
TOTAL TIME: 1 hour

4 medium beets

¾ cup plus 2 tablespoons extra-virgin olive oil

¼ cup grapefruit juice

2 cloves garlic, minced

2 teaspoons mustard powder

2 teaspoons fresh thyme

1 teaspoon salt

½ teaspoon black pepper

1 package (about 5 ounces) arugula

¼ cup slivered or sliced almonds

PREHEAT the oven to 425°F.

RINSE the beets thoroughly and carefully stab all sides with a fork. Place in a medium bowl and add 2 tablespoons of the olive oil, tossing or mixing to thoroughly coat. Wrap each of the oiled beets separately in aluminum foil, pinching the tops closed. Place the beets in the center of a baking sheet and roast for 40 minutes. Check the beets by carefully opening the foil and sticking a thin knife into the center of a beet. If it goes in easily, the beets are done. If there's resistance, close it back up and put the beets back into the oven for 5 minutes. Repeat until they're done.

WHILE the beets are roasting, prepare the vinaigrette. Whisk the grapefruit juice, garlic, and mustard powder together in a small mixing bowl. Add the remaining ¾ cup of olive oil in a steady stream while whisking to emulsify. Add the thyme and season with the salt and pepper.

LET the beets cool until you're able to handle them. Remove the skin from each beet—you may want to wear gloves, as beet juice will stain skin. Dice the beets into 1-inch pieces and place in a glass storage container with a lid. Refrigerate for at least 30 minutes to chill before serving.

PLACE the arugula in a serving bowl, add the beets and slivered almonds, and dress with the vinaigrette.

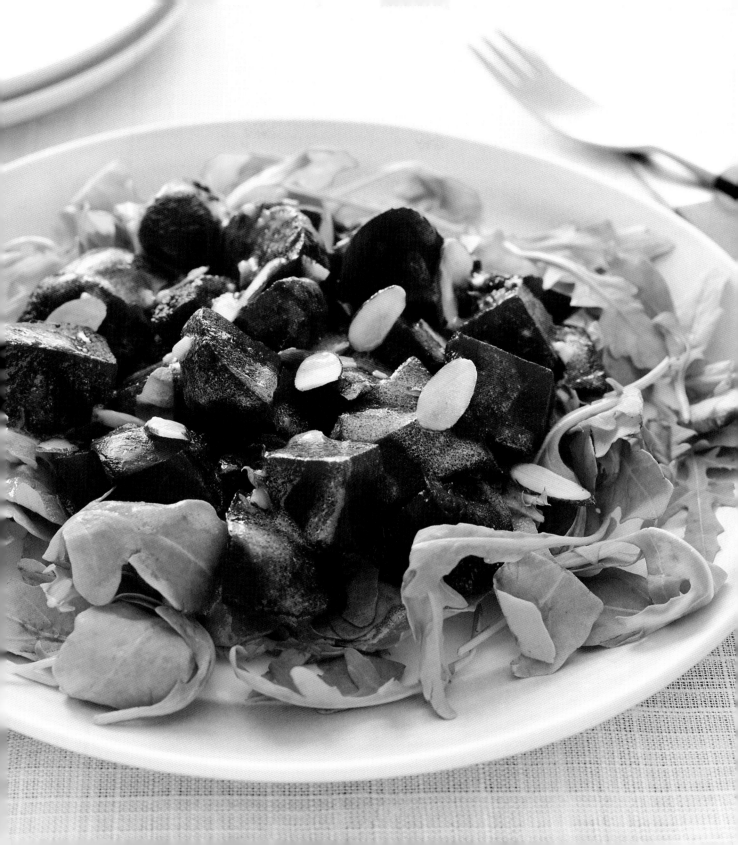

holiday dinner

THE FIRST TIME WE HOSTED a holiday dinner for family in our own home was the day we officially felt like grown-ups. People have a few misconceptions when it comes to cooking a meal like this—namely, cooking a whole turkey is really hard, and making sure everything comes out at the same time requires scheduling your day with military precision.

MENU

Green Beans with Fig Vinaigrette

Butternut Squash Puree

Sausage, Apple, and Acorn Squash Casserole

Creamed Spinach

Roasted Turkey with Gravy

Relax.

Here are three secrets: First, cooking a turkey is actually really easy. It takes a long time, but it's totally low-maintenance while it's in the oven. Second, nobody cares if things come out at different times, if not every dish is served piping hot, or if you're eating an hour after you planned. We'll do our best to help you nail your big-picture timeline below, but in the big scheme of things, it really doesn't matter.

Finally, if you're still feeling stressed, just remember that holiday dinners aren't about the food. Our family has had a few holiday kitchen disasters, but nobody cared because we were all together and that was what mattered. So don't worry about things turning out perfect, because they probably won't, and it won't matter a bit.

That having been said, we designed this Fancypants Meal to make you look like a holiday rock star. (You're welcome.) We even sent the entire menu to a few Whole30ers during the holidays to road test our hour-by-hour timeline. The recipes are simple but delicious, there's a lot you can do ahead of time, and we're going to lay out our strategy to help you prepare, cook, and serve this meal without getting so much as a spot of gravy on your apron.

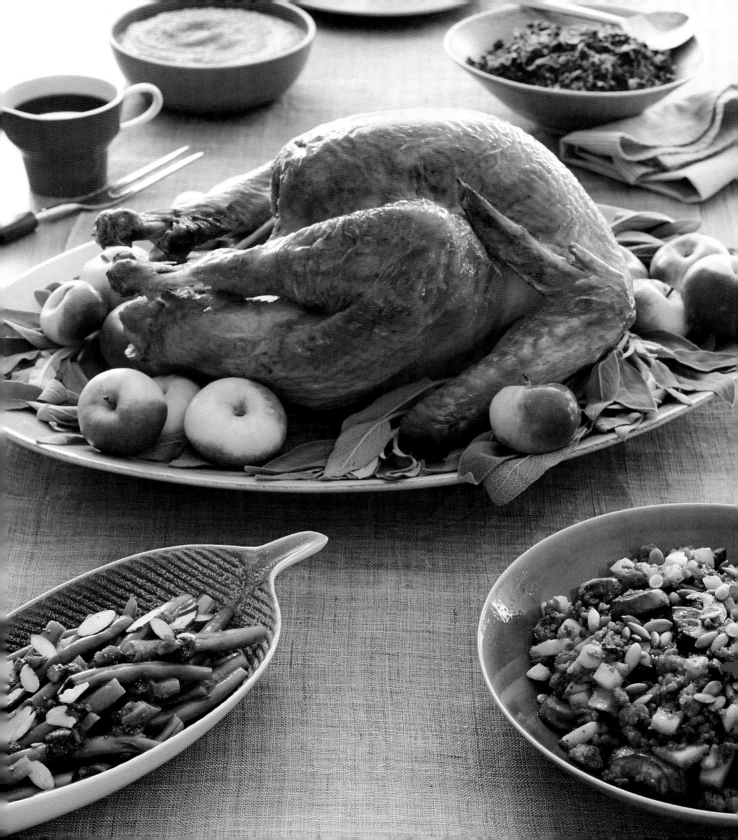

A WEEK OR TWO BEFORE

This meal requires some specialty kitchen items—things you may not use more than once a year, but you really should have for this occasion. Make sure your kitchen is stocked well before the big day.

- Large brining pan or plastic bag (big enough to hold a turkey)

- Roasting pan

- Turkey baster

- Meat thermometer (which you should already have)

- Pastry brush

- Serving dishes (a bowl for the butternut squash and sausage casserole, platters or bowls for the green beans and spinach, a large carving board and platter for the turkey, and a salad dressing bottle and gravy boat if you really want to get fancy*)

- Serving utensils (a carving knife and fork, and multiple serving spoons)

*Buy this, because grown-ups should not serve gravy out of a coffee mug.

OUR SAMPLE TIMELINE: Dinner for a family of six on Sunday at 2 p.m., which really means sometime between 2:15 and 2:30 by the time everyone sits down and the dishes are served. (Adjust our timeline accordingly if your dinner falls on another day of the week, or at a different time.)

WEDNESDAY NIGHT OR THURSDAY MORNING

First, clean out your refrigerator, because you're about to use 42 percent of your available shelf space for the next three days with a giant turkey. Next, buy a frozen turkey. You'll need to start thawing your turkey no later than Thursday morning, assuming you've bought an 8- to 10-pound frozen bird. (If buying fresh, purchase your turkey no more than two days before the big event, to ensure freshness.) Place the frozen turkey in a pan or plastic bag before placing it in the refrigerator, as it will release moisture and juices as it thaws.

SATURDAY MORNING OR AFTERNOON

Make the sausage and pop the meat mixture in the fridge (uncooked) for tomorrow, or even easier, defrost the pound of sausage you've got sitting in your freezer. Make the butternut squash puree, and once it cools, save it in a covered container in the refrigerator. Make the fig vinaigrette, and transfer it to a Mason jar, glass shaker, or container with a lid and refrigerate. Place the spinach in an uncovered container or on a plate in the refrigerator to thaw. (It will shed moisture as it thaws, so make sure you've got something to catch it.) Once your turkey is completely thawed, prepare the brine, add the turkey to the pan or bag with the brine, and put in the fridge. (These last two steps may require an extra set of hands!)

SUNDAY MORNING

Check the spinach to make sure it's fully defrosted. If it still feels hard in the center, leave it on a plate on the counter to defrost.

Prepare your kitchen for the influx of ingredients, pots and pans, and sous chefs (otherwise known as "well-meaning family members"). Pull out your serving dishes and utensils, recruit someone to set the table, and do a final

SIDE NOTE: If anyone offers to bring anything (or if you assign dishes to family members), you can have them make the butternut squash puree, which is easy to reheat on your stovetop before serving, and the fig vinaigrette—which leaves you with two fewer tasks for Saturday afternoon.

check of needed ingredients. (An hour before dinner is not the time to find out your spouse used the last can of coconut milk for a post-workout shake.)

Finally, figure out your kitchen timer strategy. You'll have a lot of dishes going at once, and it's going to be helpful to have alarms or timers set to remind you when to baste the turkey or pull the casserole out of the oven. If you use kitchen timers, make sure each one is labeled—e.g., "baste turkey" or "start spinach." Or, use your smartphone alarm to set custom timers to prompt for everything you'll be doing, making it easy to remember exactly what all that beeping is about.

SUNDAY, 9:30 A.M.

Begin preparing the turkey (stuff and rub with fat) and preheat the oven, with a goal of putting the turkey in to roast at 10:00 a.m. We are giving you lots of time with your turkey here, so you don't have to rush the cooking, resting, or carving process. If your meat thermometer is oven-safe, insert it into the meaty part of the turkey leg, and place the bird in the oven at 10 a.m. sharp.

Now would be a good time to peel and dice your acorn squash for the "stuffing," too, as peeling these suckers can take a while. Just set the diced squash in a covered dish in the fridge until you're ready to use it.

Once that's done, you have nothing more to do for a few hours, so now would be a good time to shower, get dressed, and do any last-minute cleanup.

SUNDAY, 1:00 P.M.

Pull your vinaigrette and squash out of the fridge. Drain the spinach and set it aside, still in the colander. (No need to dirty another dish.) Start your mise en place for the sausage casserole, creamed spinach, and green beans (including creating the ice bath), but don't start cooking them yet.

From here on out, pay less attention to the actual time listed, and more attention to what's actually happening with your turkey. It's been three hours since your bird went in the oven, so check the temperature now to see how far you have to go. If you're getting close to 160°F, continue checking the temperature every 10 minutes. If it's done, pull it out of the oven and let it rest. Don't worry that it's early—a longer rest

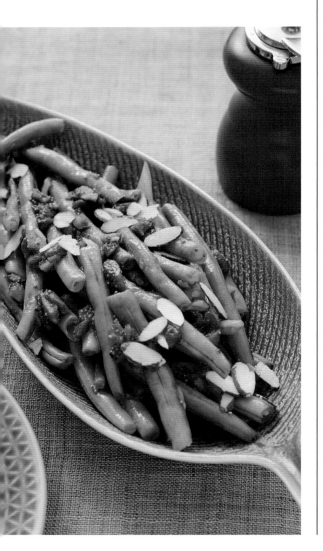

time is actually fine here, and you'll warm the turkey up with the gravy when you serve it. (Leave the oven on at 375°F, as you'll need it for the casserole in a half-hour.)

Start preparing your gravy now. You'll finish it with the turkey drippings and arrowroot powder once the turkey comes out of the oven.

SUNDAY, 1:30 P.M.

Transfer the butternut squash purée to a saucepan. Leave it on the stove, but don't turn on the burner yet. Begin cooking your sausage casserole on the stovetop.

SUNDAY, 1:45 P.M.

Place your sausage casserole in the oven. Start the water for the green beans boiling, then blanch and shock them. Place both the squash puree and gravy over medium-low heat, and add the turkey drippings to the gravy. Stir them each occasionally as they start to heat up. Cook your spinach.

Are things starting to heat up in your kitchen? All of your dishes are now in play, which is good because according to our calculations, you are officially out of stovetop burners. Now would be a good time for your designated carver to start cutting up that beautiful bird. There are a number of good video tutorials available online; try this one from Cooking.com: http://w30.co/w30carving.

SUNDAY, 1:55 P.M.

Transfer your spinach to a serving dish.

Swap the pot from the green beans for a clean pan, toast your almonds, and finish cooking the beans. Dress them with the vinaigrette, sprinkle the almonds, and transfer them to a serving dish.

Remove the gravy from the heat and add the arrowroot powder slurry. Stir well and transfer the gravy to your gravy boat.

Pull your sausage casserole out of the oven (*now* you can turn it off!) and transfer it to a serving dish.

SUNDAY, 2:00 P.M.

Hang up your apron and bring everything to your beautifully set table. Happy holidays! It's time to eat.

green beans with fig vinaigrette

SERVES 4 TO 6

PREP TIME: 20 minutes

COOK TIME: 10 minutes

TOTAL TIME: 30 minutes

FIG VINAIGRETTE

¼ cup white wine vinegar or champagne vinegar

¼ cup balsamic vinegar

½ teaspoon mustard powder

1 clove garlic, minced

¾ cup extra-virgin olive oil

¼ cup dried figs, finely chopped (5 to 6 figs)

2 teaspoons minced fresh thyme leaves

½ teaspoon salt

½ teaspoon black pepper

GREEN BEANS

2 cups ice

2 tablespoons salt

1 pound green beans, trimmed

2 tablespoons cooking fat

¼ cup slivered almonds

TO MAKE THE VINAIGRETTE: Whisk together the white wine vinegar, balsamic vinegar, mustard powder, and garlic in a medium bowl. Continue to whisk while slowly drizzling in the olive oil. Stir in the figs and thyme and season with the salt and pepper.

TO MAKE THE GREEN BEANS: Create an ice bath for "shocking" the beans by filling a large bowl halfway with cold water, then adding the ice.

COMBINE 3 cups of water and the salt in a large saucepan and bring to a boil over high heat. Add the green beans and blanch for 20 seconds. Using kitchen tongs or a slotted spoon, immediately transfer the beans to the ice bath to shock. As soon as the green beans are chilled (about 1 minute), transfer to a colander and drain.

MELT the cooking fat in a large skillet over medium-high heat, swirling to coat the bottom of the pan. When the fat is hot, add the slivered almonds and toast for 30 seconds, shaking the pan often so they don't burn. Remove the almonds from the pan and reserve. Add the green beans, tossing to coat in the cooking fat. Cook, shaking the pan often, until the beans are crisp-tender, about 2 minutes. (The easiest way to check for doneness is to taste them.)

TRANSFER the beans to a serving dish, sprinkle on the toasted almonds, and drizzle lightly with ¼ cup of the vinaigrette (add more if desired, but a little goes a long way here). Toss until evenly dressed. Serve immediately.

butternut squash puree

SERVES 4 TO 6

PREP TIME: 15 minutes

COOK TIME: 15 to 20 minutes

TOTAL TIME: 30 to 35 minutes

---

3 tablespoons clarified butter or ghee

3 pounds butternut squash, peeled, seeded, and cut into large dice (6 cups)

2 cloves garlic, minced

½ cup coconut milk

2 cups chicken broth

1 teaspoon salt

½ teaspoon black pepper

MELT the butter in a Dutch oven or large pot over medium heat. Add the squash, stirring to coat with the fat. Cook for 5 minutes, stirring once or twice, allowing the squash to begin to brown. Add the garlic and stir until aromatic, about 1 minute. Add the coconut milk and chicken broth. Increase the heat to high and bring to a boil. Reduce the heat to medium and cook until the squash is fork-tender, 10 to 15 minutes.

TRANSFER the squash to a food processor and blend on low speed until smooth. If necessary, add more chicken broth or coconut milk to reach a smooth consistency. Season with the salt and pepper.

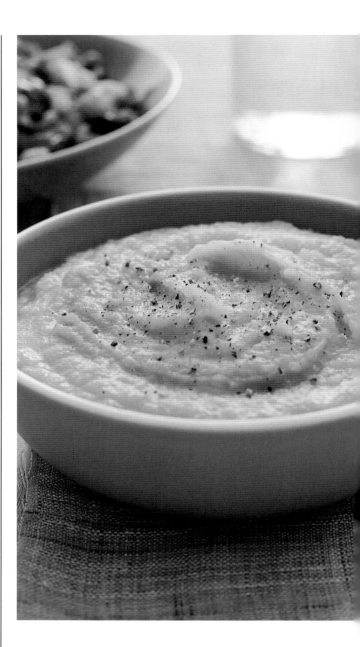

sausage, apple, and acorn squash casserole

SERVES 4 TO 6

PREP TIME: 15 minutes
COOK TIME: 20 minutes
TOTAL TIME: 35 minutes

1 pound Perfect Sausage (page 162)

1 tablespoon cooking fat

2 cups button, crimini, or portabella mushrooms, thinly sliced

1 cup diced peeled apple

2 cups peeled, seeded, and finely diced acorn squash

1 tablespoon poultry seasoning

¼ cup pumpkin seeds or chopped pecans

Salt and black pepper

PREHEAT the oven to 375°F.

HEAT the cooking fat in a medium oven-safe or cast-iron pan over medium heat. Once the fat is hot, add the sausage and cook until browned, about 2 minutes, on each side. Break the sausage into bite-size pieces with a wooden spoon, until the fat begins to release, about 2 minutes. Add the mushrooms, apple, and squash and cook until fork-tender, about 5 minutes. Add the poultry seasoning, sprinkle with the pumpkin seeds or pecans and transfer the pan to the oven. (If you don't have an oven-safe pan, transfer the mixture to a glass baking dish.) Roast for 10 to 15 minutes, until the internal temperature of the casserole is 140°F. Add salt and pepper to taste.

creamed spinach

SERVES 4 TO 6

PREP TIME: 10 minutes
COOK TIME: 10 minutes
TOTAL TIME: 20 minutes

2 packages (10 ounces each) frozen spinach, thawed

2 tablespoons clarified butter or ghee

½ onion, finely diced

3 cloves garlic, minced

1 can (13.5 ounces) full-fat coconut milk

¼ teaspoon salt

¼ teaspoon black pepper

DRAIN the thawed spinach by placing it in a colander over the sink and wringing the spinach out with your hands (like you're wringing out laundry). You can also place a clean dishtowel or paper towels over the top of the spinach and press hard, until the excess water is gone and the spinach is relatively dry.

MELT the cooking fat in a large skillet over medium heat, swirling to coat the bottom of the pan. When the fat is hot, add the onion and cook, stirring, for 2 minutes. Add the garlic and cook until aromatic, about 1 minute. Add the spinach and mix well with a wooden spoon or spatula.

ADD the coconut milk, salt, and pepper and increase the heat to medium high. Bring to a boil, cook until the coconut milk thickens, 5 to 6 minutes. Serve warm.

roasted turkey
with gravy

SERVES 4 TO 6 (WITH LEFTOVERS)

PREP TIME: 35 minutes
BRINE TIME: 12 to 24 hours
COOK TIME: about 3 hours
TOTAL TIME: about 3 ½ hours, plus brining

BRINE AND TURKEY

8- to 10-pound turkey

5 quarts hot tap water

1 cup salt

2 cups apple juice

1 tablespoon black peppercorns

2 bay leaves, torn in half

1 orange, quartered

2 lemons, quartered

3 sprigs fresh thyme

3 sprigs fresh rosemary

3 quarts ice

LEMON BROTH AND TURKEY FIXINGS

3 cups chicken broth

Juice of 2 lemons

2 teaspoons salt

1 teaspoon black pepper

1 apple, peeled and cored

2 carrots, peeled and cut into 1-inch pieces

1 white onion, peeled and quartered

Leaves of 4 sprigs fresh thyme

Leaves of 2 sprigs fresh rosemary

¾ cup clarified butter, ghee, duck fat, or coconut oil

GRAVY

2 tablespoons cooking fat

Neck and giblets from the turkey

1 large onion, diced

1 celery rib, diced

1 carrot, diced

2 cups chicken broth (page 177)

½ teaspoon salt

¼ teaspoon black pepper

2 tablespoons pan drippings (or clarified butter/ghee)

3 tablespoons arrowroot powder

IF you've bought a frozen turkey, make sure it's completely thawed before brining. (Allow approximately one day of thawing in the refrigerator for every 5 pounds of turkey.) Remove the neck and giblets (usually contained in a bag) from the turkey's cavity and save them in the refrigerator—you'll use them for the gravy.

TO MAKE THE BRINE: Pour the hot water into a very large pot. Add the salt and whisk to dissolve. Continue to whisk while adding the apple juice, peppercorns, and bay leaves. Juice the orange and lemons into the brine. Add the thyme and rosemary and mix well. Whisk in the ice, adding 1 quart at a time.

PLACE the thawed turkey in a large pot or a plastic brining bag and cover with the brine. Refrigerate the brining turkey for 12 to 24 hours.

TO MAKE THE LEMON BROTH: Mix the chicken broth and lemon juice in a large bowl and set aside.

PREHEAT the oven to 325°F.

REMOVE the turkey from the brine and pat it dry with paper towels. Season inside and out with the salt and pepper. Stuff the cavity with the apple, carrots, onion, half of the thyme, and half of the rosemary. Using your fingers, carefully work ¼ cup of the cooking fat and the remainder of the thyme and rosemary leaves evenly under the turkey skin. Brush or rub the skin with the remaining ½ cup cooking fat.

SET the turkey breast-side up in a roasting pan. Cover it loosely with foil, securing around the edges of the pan to create a tent. Roast for 2 hours.

REMOVE the turkey from the oven and discard the foil. Baste the entire turkey with 1 cup of the lemon broth, then increase the oven temperature to 375°F and place the turkey back in the oven. Roast for 20 minutes, baste with another cup of lemon broth. Roast for an additional 20 minutes, baste again with the last cup of broth. Roast for an additional 20 minute, until the turkey's internal temperature on the leg reaches 160°F. (A meat thermometer is important here.)

LET the turkey rest for 20 to 40 minutes, or until the internal temperature reaches 165°F. Transfer the turkey to a carving board. Scoop the stuffing from the middle of the turkey and discard, then begin carving.

TO MAKE THE GRAVY: Heat the cooking fat in a large pot over medium-high heat. When the fat is hot, sear the turkey neck and giblets for 5 minutes, turning to prevent burning. Add the onion, celery, and carrot. Cook, stirring occasionally for 5 minutes, until the onions are translucent. Add the chicken broth and bring to a boil. Reduce the heat to medium and simmer the ingredients for 10 minutes, until the carrots are very soft.

REMOVE the turkey neck and giblets and discard. Transfer the broth and vegetables to a food processor, add the salt and pepper, and blend to a smooth consistency. Reserve the gravy until the turkey is out of the oven.

CAREFULLY pour the turkey pan drippings into a pot with the gravy mixture (or add 2 tablespoons of clarified butter or ghee, if the drippings prove hard to transfer). Return the gravy to a pot on medium heat and bring to a simmer.

IN a small bowl, mix the arrowroot powder and ⅓ cup of cold water and mix well. It should feel like a paste at first, then blend into a milky-white consistency. (Do not mix the powder directly into the gravy, or it will clump instead of mix!)

TAKE the gravy off the heat and immediately add the arrowroot and water mixture. The heat from the gravy will activate the thickening power of the starch; stir well until the gravy thickens.

DRINKS

ONE OF THE MOST COMMON QUESTIONS we hear from those new to the Whole30 is, "How do I handle social gatherings where everyone is drinking alcohol?"

Our tough love answer: Simply say, "No thank you," and move on, because you are a grown-up and stopped succumbing to peer pressure in seventh grade. But we understand that some situations, like client dinners, weddings, or wine tastings may require a little more help to see you through.

Wait—why are you at a wine tasting during your Whole30, anyway?

The first thing to remember: you are just as fun, witty, entertaining, and charming sober as you are with a glass of wine in your hand. The second thing to remember: if you make a big deal about how you're not drinking, they will too. Conversely, if you treat it as a non-issue, no one will care. Or, likely, even notice. (If you're really uncomfortable, belly up to the bar and order a sparkling water with a slice of lime—instant vodka tonic camouflage.)

Your strategy for sober social survival on the Whole30 depends on how you're approached. If someone offers you an alcoholic beverage, start by simply saying, "No, thank you" or "Oh, I already have water, thanks." If you get any sort of follow-up, simply stick to your guns and then casually change the subject; people should take the hint and move on.

If you find someone giving you a hard time about your decision to abstain, don't make up an excuse, because excuses are just begging for a fix. Saying, "I can't, I have to meet my trainer

at 6 a.m." may prompt them to say, "I'll run with you after work, how about that margarita?"... and now you're stuck.

In this case, if you think the person will be responsive and respectful, say, "I've committed to abstain for 30 days as part of a health reset, and I'm sticking to it." If you'd prefer not to talk about your health or diet, offer a direct "no, but thank you" in a full eye-contact, slightly-more forceful manner. Or take it one step further and say, "I'm taking time off from drinking," which suggests this is a personal decision not open for discussion. At this point, most people will back off . . . unless they're intoxicated.

Which brings us to your final strategy: if absolutely necessary, opt for the public shaming. They're being incredibly disrespectful of your decision, so call them out on it. "What's up with the peer pressure? I don't want a margarita tonight, but I'm not telling you not to have one. Can we please move on?" Then, excuse yourself to another group, or step outside for a moment to give them a chance to save face (and yourself a moment to stay centered).

In summary, the Whole30 doesn't have to put a cramp in your social life, and you'll be high-fiving yourself the next morning when you wake up feeling like a champ. Plus now you've got some delicious mocktails to help you celebrate a good day at the office or keep you feeling festive during a family party. Cheers!

lemon lime zinger

SERVES 2

PREP TIME: 5 minutes

½ lemon, juiced

½ lime, juiced

1 teaspoon fresh ginger, zested

12 ounces sparkling water

Garnish your zinger with fresh raspberries or strawberries—they add a pretty pop of color.

SQUEEZE the lemon and lime into a glass and add ginger zest. Top with ice and the sparkling water. Give it a quick stir before serving.

⭐ A ZINGER *can be made with a variety of juices. Try this mix: ½ lemon juiced, ½ lime juiced, 1 orange juiced, and 2 tablespoons of pomegranate juice, top with ice and sparkling water. Using juice from a bottle? Try ¼ cup of pineapple juice and 1 teaspoon of fresh ginger, zested, top with ice and sparkling water. Looking for something less sweet? How about ¼ cup of unsweetened cranberry juice plus ½ lemon juiced, top with ice and sparkling water.*

rosemary berry smash

SERVES 2

PREP TIME: 5 minutes

¼ cup raspberries (fresh or frozen)

1 sprig fresh rosemary leaves

½ lemon, juiced

12 ounces sparkling water

To muddle means to press the ingredients against the side or bottom of the glass. Muddling helps to release the flavors of the fresh ingredients. You can buy an actual muddler for around $10, or you can use the heavy end of a butter knife or the round end of a wooden spoon.

MUDDLE raspberries and rosemary leaves in a large glass. Add the lemon juice and sparkling water, and shake or mix thoroughly. Strain the mixture into a new glass, discarding the rosemary leaves. Add ice if desired.

⭐ TO REMOVE *the rosemary leaves from the stem, hold the top of the stem between your thumb and index finger. Use the same fingers on your other hand to strip the needles from the stem in a downward motion.*

blood orange paloma

SERVES 2

PREP TIME: 5 minutes

---

1 blood orange, juiced

½ lime, juiced

12 ounces sparkling water

Serving this at a fancy gathering? Garnish with a grapefruit or lime wedge. To add another dimension to this mocktail, try adding fresh squeezed grapefruit juice; it pairs nicely with the blood orange and lime.

ADD the blood orange and lime into a glass. Top with ice and the sparkling water.

⭐ STORE YOUR BLOOD ORANGES *in the fridge— they'll last up to two weeks, compared to just a few days on the counter. Blood oranges are in season from December through May, so if you're serving this in the summertime, feel free to substitute any other variety of orange. (And if you're using orange juice from a carton, use ⅓ cup.)*

white tea-a-sangria

SERVES 2

PREP TIME: 5 minutes
TOTAL TIME: 40 minutes

---

1 white tea bag

1 ginger tea bag

1 cup boiling water

¼ cup halved white grapes

¼ cup golden delicious apple, diced

8 ounces sparkling water

Lemon slices

Peaches, apricots, and nectarines pair nicely with this drink. Slice into wedges and add to the grapes and apple, or use them as a garnish.

HEAT 1 cup of water to boiling, let it cool for 5 minutes. Add the tea bags to the hot water and steep for 7 to 10 minutes; remove and discard the tea bags. Chill in the refrigerator for 25 minutes.

PLACE the fruit into a large glass and add ice if desired. Pour tea over the fruit and top with sparkling water. Garnish with lemon slices.

⭐ ALLOWING THE FLAVORS *in the sangria to blend together will give this drink another dimension. Triple the recipe and refrigerate overnight in a glass pitcher. Serve over ice.*

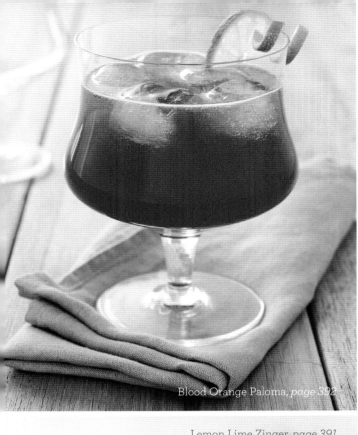

Blood Orange Paloma, *page 392*

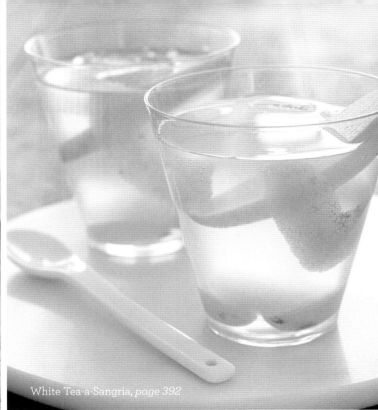

White Tea-a-Sangria, *page 392*

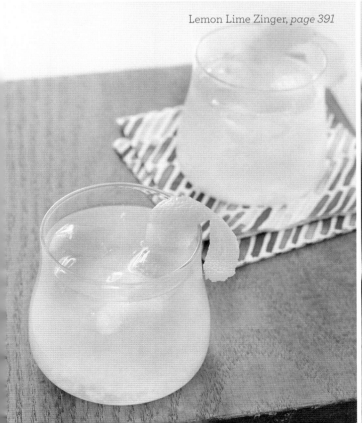

Lemon Lime Zinger, *page 391*

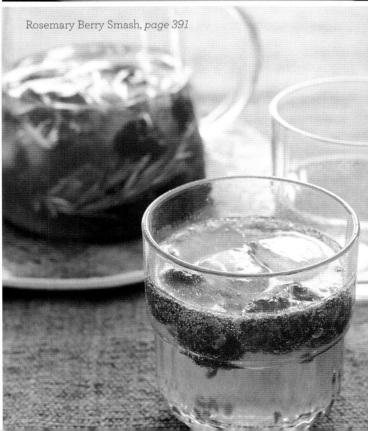

Rosemary Berry Smash, *page 391*

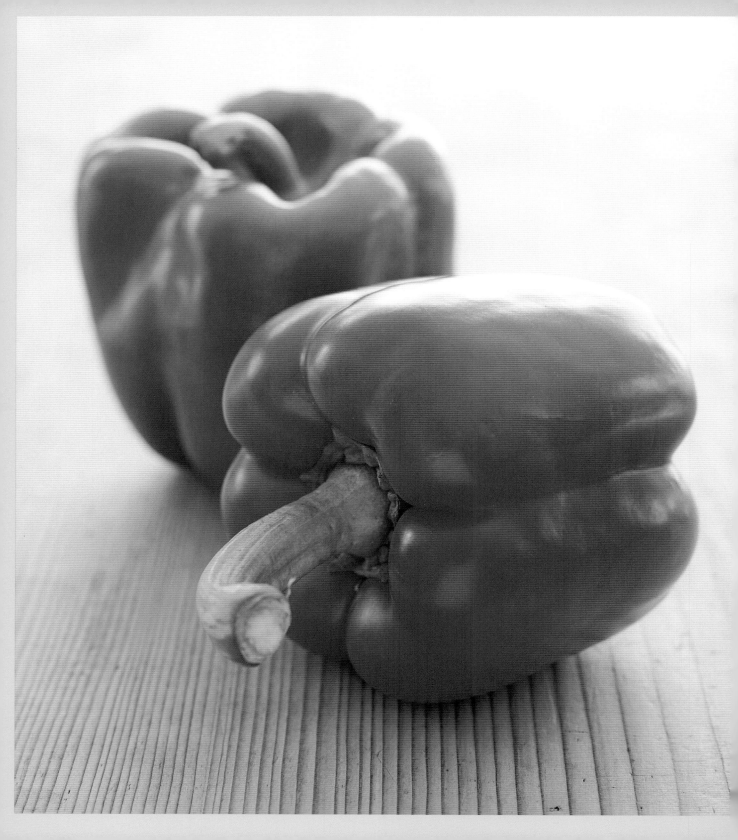

in closing

"*My mom was killed instantly in a car crash almost exactly ten months ago. Since then, my diet went from mostly Paleo to excessive alcohol, ice cream, and cookie dough, or just not eating at all. I gained 30 pounds, hated my life, and would sit for several hours a day, too depressed and exhausted to do anything. I also developed a sleeping problem, going back and forth between insomnia and extreme hibernation. I had heard about the Whole30 and decided to try it. Now, everyone around me sees a huge difference, including myself. Not just in my size (I'm starting to fit into clothes I wore before my mom's death), but in my energy and attitude, too. I no longer sit for hours at a time. I smile and sing around the house. I have a desire to see friends and connect with people. I don't cry every day. I sleep a perfect nine hours. For the first time in ten months I feel like I can enjoy life again, and I have the energy to do it. My family and friends see so much of a transformation in me that they want some of it, too—many of them are starting the Whole30! I feel like I'm getting my life back.*"

—MORGAN B., ESCALON, CA

In just over 30 days, you've committed to something really scary, overcome significant obstacles to see your commitment through, and effectively changed your life by changing the food you put on your plate.

But now, you have one last question.

Now What?

Your Whole30 is over, your reintroduction is done, you've learned how foods impact how you look, how you feel, and your quality of life. Your tastes have changed, your cravings have diminished or disappeared, and you have a newfound love of cooking. You've created new, healthy habits,

TRAINING WHEELS

The rules of the Whole30 program are very specific, and completely non-negotiable. They remove some of the stress from making your own food choices, take all the guesswork out of our expectations, and give you a clear goal. The program also gives you an easy fallback when faced with social pressures—a built-in excuse for why you don't want that piece of cake or glass of wine. (Blame us. We can handle it.) The rules of the Whole30 function much like training wheels on a bike, giving you all the support you need while allowing you to complete the program under the power of your own pedal strokes. But when your 30 days are up, the training wheels come off! Now, you'll have to figure out how to make your own Good Food choices, without the comforts of our rules, or your built-in excuses— otherwise known as riding your own bike.

broken old patterns, and discovered new ways to reward, comfort, and treat yourself.

But, now what?

Now you live your life guided by this new-found awareness and your new, healthy habits. This is what we call "riding your own bike."

At this point, you should not be surprised that we're going to ask you to create a plan for life after your Whole30. We'll provide the general template, but you have to fill in the details based on what you learned during your program, your goals and context, and what you have decided is or is not "worth it."

For those of you who followed our Slow Roll reintroduction schedule (page 49), this plan is going to look awfully familiar.

STEP 1: Eat Whole30-ish all the time.

Relax on some of the rules, reincorporating some desirable ingredients, foods, or drinks that you've determined have a negligible negative impact on how you look, feel and live. This may mean eating bacon cured with sugar, adding heavy whipping cream to your morning coffee, ordering your sushi with white rice, or enjoying the corn tortillas that come with your fish tacos.

We can't tell you specifically what this looks like, because it's entirely based on what you learned during your Whole30 and rein-troduction. Still, you get the picture, right? Your everyday foods should still be foods that make you healthy, even if they're not all strictly Whole30-compliant.

Plan on eating like this for every meal, all the time, forever and ever. This should be easy, right? It feels totally sustainable, completely sat-isfying, isn't at all stressful, and keeps you living in the Tiger Blood zone. Really, it's a piece of . . . Never mind.

STEP 2: Hit "pause" when something really special or delicious pops up.

One day—could be today, could be a month from now—something is going to cross your path that you may think is worth going significantly off-plan. Who knows what it will be: your favorite bottle of wine, your mom's chocolate chip cookies, a Cadbury Crème Egg. (We're not judging. Only you can decide what's special or delicious for you.)

When this happens, press "pause" on everything—your diet, your grabby hands, your salivating mouth. Just. Press. Pause. Buy yourself a moment to breathe, think, and use the Whole30 lessons you learned to help you make the right choice for you.

Ask yourself a series of questions, and be honest with yourself: Is this truly special, symbolic, culturally significant, or delicious? Is eating or drinking this going to seriously mess me up, psychologically or physically? Do I really think the consequences will be worth it?

Do I really, truly want it?

This last one is the most important question of them all. We often eat or drink things because they're there, or we told ourselves we could, or because we're sad/lonely/anxious/bored. But post-Whole30, you have the capacity to create enough distance between you and the food to honestly evaluate whether you *really* want it, and whether the consequences will be worth it.

Take the time to do this. If you decide it's not really that special or delicious, it would mess you up too much, it's not going to be worth it, or you don't really want it, take a pass. Why eat something you know makes you less healthy if you don't even want it? In this instance, you'll recognize that you're not actually missing out on anything, and deliver yourself exactly the kind

> **OUR GUIDE TO NUTRITIONAL OFF-ROADING**
>
> For you visually inspired people, we've actually turned this series of self-reflective questions into a fun little flow chart, called our Guide to Nutritional Off-Roading. You can download it at www.whole30.com/pdf-downloads.

of small victory that will reinforce your new, healthy habits and your sense of self-confidence.

If you decide it is special, it will be worth it, and you do really want it, proceed to Step 3.

And if you have to think too long about it, you don't want it bad enough. You're welcome.

STEP 3: Eat it, savor it, then move the heck on.

You've made a conscious, deliberate decision to consume this special, worth-it, "yes, I really want it" thing. Now, eat (or drink) it—but don't you dare spoil this moment by hoovering it down in two bites or mindlessly consuming it while watching TV. That would be a shameful waste of a delicious treat.

Say the food in question is the plate of chocolate chip cookies your mom dropped off earlier in the day. We want you to bring the same awareness and attention you learned during your Whole30 to these cookies. Here's what you do: Put one cookie on a fancy plate. Sit down in a place where you can really focus on your cookie—maybe it's with your family after dinner, maybe it's by yourself at the table, maybe it's in a bubble bath with your favorite music playing.

That would be awesome.

Now, eat the cookie.

Take small bites. Chew thoroughly. Savor the flavor, smell, and texture. Make it last. Share the experience with a friend or your family, or simply enjoy the quiet time. Since we indulge partly to provide mental satisfaction, squeeze as much satisfaction as possible out of what you are eating.

With this approach, you should have plenty of time to notice that your desire has been fulfilled, and that satisfaction has been achieved. So when it has, stop eating. Maybe that's half a cookie. Maybe it's four cookies. It doesn't matter, as long as you are mindful of the process every step of the way.

And when you're done, you're done. There is no guilt. You made a conscious, deliberate decision. You paid attention. You enjoyed the heck out of it. You decided when to stop eating.

CRAVING CAUTION

After your decision to eat the cookie, you may find you wake up the next morning with the strong desire to eat 17 more cookies. You should anticipate this, and build an extra layer of "pause" into your evaluations today. Have a plan: If I wake up craving sugar, then I'll deliberately make today a Whole30 day, and evaluate whether another cookie is worth it in a day or two. You could also legitimately go through our evaluation the next morning and decide the cookies are once again worth it. In that case, go ahead and enjoy! Just know with each indulgence, your Sugar Dragon gains some strength, so make a solid plan to get back on track when the cookies run out.

There is no guilt.

There may be consequences, but that's not the same thing. Consequences are knowing your skin might break out, your stomach might bloat, or your energy may flag. Deal with those, but then, move the heck on. Wake up the next day and go back to Step 1. Wash, rinse, repeat until the end of time.

You may go weeks before stumbling across something truly "worth it." You may consciously, deliberately choose to consume less healthy foods and drinks every day for eight days straight. (That's called "vacation in wine country.") But as long as you stick to our three-step plan, you will continue to retain your new, healthy habits; your current waistline; and the excellent quality of life you've achieved with the Whole30.

Derailed

Now, let's get real. Inevitably, at some point sooner or later, you will fall back into old habits. In truth, we'd be shocked if you didn't. Think about it—your brain has experienced years (or decades) of less healthy habits, emotional connections to foods, and powerful craving-reward cycles. Do you really expect 30 days of the Whole30 to permanently replace those habits with new, healthy behaviors?

We don't. So let's not pretend you and your waistline are going to live happily ever after effortlessly, shall we?

Do not panic. Everything will be okay, because (of course) we have a plan for this, too.

If you find your food choices have slipped more into "less healthy" territory; when your Sugar Dragon is roaring, your symptoms are flaring, your energy flagging, and you no longer feel in control of your food choices, then . . .

Come back to the Whole30.

It's so easy. You already have a plan to quash cravings, reduce symptoms, boost your energy, and bring you back to food freedom. So, come back. Do another Whole30. Return to our community. Get back to that place where everything is humming and your self-confidence is high and you're back in the driver's seat. Go through the full program again, by the book, exactly as written—including reintroduction. Learn even more about how the foods you've been eating impact you in even more subtle ways.

Then, kick off the training wheels and ride your own bike again.

Wash, rinse, repeat.

With repeated exposure to the program and dedication to the awareness and introspection the program promotes, we near guarantee that over time, the number of days and months you spend living a "more healthy" life grows, and the time and depth of your "less healthy" forays shrink.

Translation: you'll find it easier and easier to eat this way, and have less and less trouble sticking to the healthy plan you've created for yourself.

That is our wish for you—that you use the structure, the community, and the resources provided by the Whole30 to attain true, sustainable, lasting food freedom. We've done it, and hundreds of thousands of people have done it, and we know you can do it, too.

We wish you the best in health.

appendix

Resources

This first part of our resources section includes websites, cookbooks, and social-media feeds we really like, from people with whom we have developed a close personal and professional relationship. They're smart, talented people who are Whole30 experts in their own rights. They've done the program, offer specific resources for your Whole30 success, and really get the spirit and intention of the Whole30.

Not everything in their website, cookbook, or social media feed is Whole30-compliant, but you already knew that, right? They don't eat Whole30 all the time, and neither will you. This isn't a criticism—in fact, it's great to see! All of our friends featured here keep it real, and exemplify what "life after your Whole30" should look like: mostly healthy, Whole30 foods; indulgences when, where, and how often they've decided is "worth it"; with foods they've identified as "worth it" for them, thanks to their Whole30 experience.

We're just pointing this out because you have to read your website content, recipes, and social-media hashtags just as carefully as you have to read your labels.

Anyone on the internet can say a meal or ingredient is "Whole30 Approved" or "Whole30-compliant." They can, and they do, in fact—we've seen horrifically sugary, salty, fatty desserts; processed whey-based protein shakes; and even fat-burning supplements labeled "#Whole30" on Instagram. The moral of the story?

Use your own judgment as to whether something is *really* "Whole30."

Unless it's coming from us (our website, this book, or our social-media feeds), don't take any label of "Whole30-compliant" at face value. Use your critical thinking skills, read your labels/ingredients/recipes carefully, and decide for yourself whether the item in question fits into our Whole30 program.

The good news is that you can trust everyone we have listed here to tell you with 100 percent accuracy whether something on their website, in their cookbook, or on their social media feed is Whole30-compliant. (They're experts, we told you.) So use our site, this book, and the folks we have listed here as your primary resources during your program, and supplement with things you find in the blog-o-sphere on your own . . . just proceed to Pinterest with caution.

WEBSITES

Whole30
www.whole30.com
The official home of the Whole30 program. This is where you'll find our Whole30 Forum, all of our free downloads, Whole30 Approved products and affiliates, and more Whole30-related articles than you could possibly hope to read in 30 days. Spend lots of time exploring here before, during, and after your Whole30—this is the very heart of our community.
Facebook: whole30
Instagram: @whole30, @whole30recipes
Twitter: @whole30
Pinterest: whole30

Whole9

www.whole9life.com

Whole9 is the health and lifestyle community from which the Whole30 program was born. The "9" comes from the nine factors we believe come together to bring you to optimal health: nutrition, sleep, healthy movement, stress management, socialization, natural environment, personal growth, fun and play, and temperance. Use our articles and resources to help you navigate life after your Whole30, and use all that self-efficacy you built during your program to help you take on the other health initiatives we recommend.

Facebook: whole9
Instagram: @whole9life
Twitter: @whole9life
Pinterest: whole9

The Clothes Make The Girl

www.theclothesmakethegirl.com

Not only is Melissa Joulwan the author of two Whole30 Approved cookbooks (*Well Fed* and *Well Fed 2*), she's also a brilliant food, fitness, health, and lifestyle blogger with hundreds of Whole30-friendly recipes, meal plans, and resources freely available on her site.

Facebook: theclothesmakethegirl
Instagram: @meljoulwan
Twitter: @meljoulwan
Pinterest: melissa-joulwan-the-clothes-make-the-girl

Nom Nom Paleo

www.nomnompaleo.com

Nom Nom Paleo is the creation of mom, foodie, and self-described "culinary nerd" Michelle Tam. Since 2010, she has been religiously taking pictures of her Whole30 meals and sharing her Whole30 meal plans and recipes. She also penned the *New York Times* best-selling book *Nom Nom Paleo: Food For Humans*, featuring a large number of Whole30-friendly meals.

Facebook: nomnompaleo
Instagram: @nomnompaleo
Twitter: @nomnompaleo
Pinterest: nomnompaleo

Popular Paleo

www.popularpaleo.com

Ciarra Hannah is on a mission to promote wellness through whole foods centered around meat, vegetables, fruits, and healthy fats. Her site is full of everyday meals, most of which are Whole30-compliant and appropriate for those following an autoimmune or chronic pain/fatigue protocol.

Facebook: popularpaleo
Instagram: @popular_paleo
Twitter: @popularpaleo
Pinterest: popularpaleo

Rubies and Radishes

www.rubiesandradishes.com

Arsy Vartanian's experience healing her own body with a paleo-style diet led her to pursue her passions and interests: a love of cooking, shopping for fresh, organic, grass-fed ingredients, and creating delicious meals for her family and blog readers.

Facebook: rubiesandradishes
Instagram: @rubiesandradishes
Twitter: @rubies_radishes
Pinterest: arsy

Stupid Easy Paleo

www.stupideasypaleo.com

Stephanie Gaudreau is a talented chef, teacher, and athlete. Her delicious meals, sauces, dressings, and sides are simple enough for even budding chefs to re-create flawlessly, and her *Performance Paleo* books are a must-read for athletes and exercisers looking to begin a Whole30 or implement a general Paleo framework.

Facebook: stupideasypaleo
Instagram: @stupideasypaleo
Twitter: @stupideasypaleo
Pinterest: stupideasypaleo

Whole Life Eating

www.wholelifeeating.com

Whole30 team member Tom Denham is both an expert facilitator of our program and the creator of more than 300 delicious, easy, often one-pot recipes offered for free on his website. The best part? One hundred percent of his recipes are Whole30 Approved! Start here if you're new to the Whole30 and want to make absolutely sure the recipes you choose are perfect for our program.

COOKBOOKS

There is only one book where 100 percent of the recipes featured are Whole30 Approved. You're reading it right now.

However, there are dozens of cookbooks that feature delicious Whole30-compliant recipes, or recipes that could easily be adapted for our program. In fact, once you gain experience with the program, you'll be able to take just about any cookbook and make it Whole30-friendly!

As always, however, watch carefully for non-compliant ingredients, learn to swap or eliminate ingredients that don't fit the bill, and save the dessert or "treat" section for life after your Whole30.

Nom Nom Paleo: Food for Humans, by Michelle Tam and Henry Fong
www.nomnompaleo.com
Nom Nom Paleo features more than 100 recipes by award-winning food blogger Michelle Tam, and photography and illustrations by her husband, Henry Fong. We *love* their kid-friendly approach to cooking, and step-by-step photographs.

Paleo Comfort Foods and *Quick and Easy Paleo Comfort Foods,* by Julie and Charles Mayfield
www.paleocomfortfoods.com
The Mayfields are two talented chefs with an immense joy for growing, cooking, and eating fantastic food. In their Paleo Comfort Foods series, they've brought their southern roots into your Whole30 kitchen, proving that heathy food can both nourish and nurture.

Well Fed and *Well Fed 2,* by Melissa Joulwan
www.theclothesmakethegirl.com
Melissa Joulwan's best-selling cookbooks include more than 300 mouthwatering recipes and meal ideas from every corner of the world, but more importantly, her meal prep and cooking tutorials are what make this series indispensable for every Whole30er.

The Frugal Paleo Cookbook, by Ciarra Hannah
www.popularpaleo.com
This cookbook features nearly 100 recipes, and combines great taste with a practical approach. Utilizing tried-and-true cooking methods known for bringing out the best in meat and vegetables, the recipes are both Whole30-friendly and easy on your budget.

The Performance Paleo Cookbook, by Stephanie Gaudreau
www.stupideasypaleo.com
Stephanie's specialized book delivers 100 delicious, nutrient-packed recipes specifically designed to deliver a better performance in your sport or the gym, highlighting carb-dense, nutrient-boosting meals.

Paleo Breakfasts and Lunches on the Go, by Diana Rodgers
www.radiancenutrition.com
Diana Rodgers, a nutritional therapist and Paleo-community activist, created 100 delicious packable meals without bread: perfect portables that are as healthy and easy to make as they are gourmet.

The Paleo Foodie Cookbook and *The Paleo Slow Cooker,* by Arsy Vartanian
www.rubiesandradishes.com
Featuring nearly 250 healthy everyday meals, these cookbooks feature delicious, creative dishes using a wide range of ingredients, with plenty of grocery shopping ard cooking tips for the budding real-food chef.

The Autoimmune Paleo Cookbook by Mickey Trescott
www.autoimmune-paleo.com
More than 100 recipes perfect for those following and egg- and nightshade-free Whole30, or a Paleo AIP.

WHOLE30 APPROVED PRODUCTS

Our Whole30 Approved label is designed to let you know a product is 100 percent compliant with the rules of our Whole30 program. In addition, it lets you know this product, and the company who stands behind it, have been vetted personally by the Whole30 team. We have a personal relationship with every Whole30 Approved producer, and feel confident that not only their products, but their core values and mission, are in line with ours and that of our readers.

This is just a sample of our Whole30 Approved vendors—for the full list, visit www.whole30.com/whole30-approved.

EMERGENCY FOOD: Pre-Made Paleo
www.premadepaleo.com
Pre-Made Paleo was founded by Chef Richard Bradford, the Culinary Institute of America-trained chef who designed the recipes in The Whole30! Chef Richard creates, packages, and delivers delicious Whole30 Approved meals just like those featured here straight to your door, with both nutrition and convenience in mind. Order complete meals (with protein and vegetable sides), breakfast skillets, or a 5-meal "Whole30 Emergency Pack" for those nights when you come home late, hungry, and too tired to cook.

ON-THE-GO: Epic Bars
www.epicbar.com
Epic Bars are 100% grass-fed animal-based protein bars infused with nuts, seeds, fruit, herbs, and spices; perfect for on-the-go snacks, travel meal replacements, or endurance athletics like hiking and biking. Available online, in most Whole Foods Markets, and in health stores throughout the U.S.

ON-THE-GO: Primal Pacs
www.primalpacs.com
Whole30 Approved, 100 percent grass-fed, organic jerky, sourced responsibly and produced with integrity. Perfect for on-the-go meals; order the complete snack kit or just the jerky. Available online.

ON-THE-GO: Chomps Snack Sticks
www.gochomps.com
One hundred percent grass-fed beef snack sticks that are gluten, soy, hormone, and antibiotic free. The perfect on-the-go protein with a tender texture and no additives. Available online.

ON-THE-GO: SeaSnax
www.seasnax.com
Toasted nori sheets in a variety of flavors. An excellent source of micronutrients (including iodine) unique to sea vegetables. Available online and in many health food stores.

GHEE: Pure Indian Foods
www.pureindianfoods.com
One hundred percent grass-fed organic ghee made using ancient Indian traditions. Available online.

Tin Star Foods
www.tinstarfoods.com/tin-star-ghee
Seasonally produced pastured, organic ghee and cultured ghee. Available online.

OMghee
www.omghee.com
Small-batch pastured, organic ghee and cultured ghee. Available online.

DRESSINGS/SAUCES: Tessemae's All Natural
www.tessemaes.com
A family-run company featuring a line of olive-oil based dressings, sauces, marinades and condiments. Available online and in health food stores.

SAUCES: Horsetooth Hot Sauce
www.horsetoothhotsauce.com
A Colorado-based company featuring Whole30 Approved hot sauces ranging from mild to seriously spicy. Available online and in health food stores.

Red Boat Fish Sauce
www.redboatfishsauce.com
An all-natural, first press, "extra virgin" Vietnamese fish sauce with no added water, preservatives, or MSG. Available online and in health food stores.

SPICES: Spice Hound
www.spicehound.com
More than 100 high quality spices, salts, and blends sourced locally and from around the world. (All salts and spices and 20 offered spice blends are Whole30-compliant.) Available online and at various markets in San Francisco, CA.

BROTH: Bare Bones Broth
www.barebonesbroth.com
Nutritious, healing bone broth from naturally raised animals. Choose from chicken, beef, or seasonal turkey. Available online.

BEVERAGES: Choffy
www.choffy.com
Made from 100 percent premium cacao (cocoa), beans roasted and ground to create a rich drink low in caffeine.

BEVERAGES: Crio Brü
www.criobru.com
Made from 100 percent cacao (cocoa) beans, roasted to perfection, naturally low in caffeine, and brewed just like coffee.

SOURCING GOOD FOOD

US Wellness Meats
www.w30.co/grasslandbeef
Meat and seafood; Whole30 Approved sugar-free bacon; soup bones.

5280 Meat
www.5280meat.com
Beef, lamb, pork, and chicken (including organ meat); soup bones.

The Honest Bison
www.thehonestbison.com
Bison meat, soup bones.

Naked Bacon
www.nakedbaconco.com
Whole30 Approved (no sugar added) bacon.

Pre-Made Paleo
http://premadepaleo.com/products/bacon
Whole30 Approved (no sugar added) bacon.

Heritage Foods
www.heritagefoodsusa.com
Beef, pork, lamb, goat, and poultry.

Loki Fish Co.
www.lokifish.com
Alaskan salmon.

Barefoot Provisions
www.w30.co/w30barefoot
Whole30 Approved pantry items and Emergency Food Kits.

Eat Wild
www.eatwild.com/products/canada.html
Resources for the U.S. and Canada.

Eat Well Guide
www.eatwellguide.org
Resources for the U.S. and Canada. (Global resources: www.eatwellguide.org/i.php?id=international).

Local Harvest
www.localharvest.org
Community Supported Agriculture (CSA) programs.

Environmental Working Group
www.ewg.org/foodnews
Annually updated list of "clean" and "dirty" produce.

SUPPLEMENTS

Note, these featured products are brands and supplements we like based on their ingredient list, and the fact that they are all available for purchase by the general public (without going through a medical professional). However, we always recommend that you speak with your health care practitioner before taking any new supplements, or changing supplement brands or dosage. For more information on how these supplements work in conjunction with our healthy eating plan and our general dosing recommendations, please refer to Chapter 22 in *It Starts With Food*.

OMEGA-3 FATTY ACIDS: SFH SO3 Omega-3 Oils
www.sfh.com
Use the discount code "whole9" to save 10 percent off your order.

OMEGA-3 FATTY ACIDS: Green Pastures Fermented Cod Liver Oil
www.greenpasture.org

MULTI-VITAMIN: Pure Encapsulations Nutrient 950 with Vitamin K
www.pureencapsulations.com

VITAMIN D3: Pure Encapsulations Vitamin D3 Liquid
www.pureencapsulations.com

MAGNESIUM: Pure Encapsulations Magnesium Glycinate (capsules)
www.pureencapsulations.com

MAGNESIUM: Natural Calm Magnesium Citrate (powder, original flavor)
www.naturalvitality.com/natural-calm/

DIGESTIVE ENZYMES: Pure Encapsulations Digestive Enzymes Ultra with HCl
www.pureencapsulations.com

PROBIOTICS: Klaire Labs Ther-Biotic Complete
www.klaire.com

LIVER: Dr. Ron's Ultra Pure
www.drrons.com

SUPPORT ON THE WHOLE30

We spoke at length about how to find support at home in Step 2 of "Getting Started with the Whole30" (page 19). Still, it can't hurt to have some support, motivation, and accountability back-up! Here are all the links you'll need to find the help you'll need online, with our community.

The Whole30 Forum
www.w30.co/w30forum
If you have a question, we can almost guarantee it's been answered. Find those answers, solicit expert advice from our moderators, and get support from fellow Whole30ers on our free forum.

Whole30 Daily
www.w30.co/w30daily
A subscription newsletter delivering a daily dose of Whole30 wisdom, support, and tough love straight to your inbox every morning. Designed to guide you through the program step-by-step, offer you additional resources to help you succeed, and provide you with the accountability to see it through.

Wholesome
www.whole30.com/wholesome
Our free monthly newsletter filled with Whole30-related interviews, recipes, events, media, testimonials, discounts, resources, and more.

Free Whole30 PDF Downloads
www.whole30.com/pdf-downloads
Find a host of helpful PDF downloads, including our shopping list, meal template, Guide to Sneaky Sugars, Seasonal Produce Guide, and more on our website.

Free Whole30 Graphics
www.whole30.com/graphics
Announce your commitment to the Whole30, brag about completing the program, and share our mission and mantras with your friends, family, and social media followers with a variety of free downloadable graphics!

Whole30 on Facebook
www.facebook.com/whole30

Whole30 Recipes on Facebook
www.facebook.com/OfficialWhole30Recipes

Whole30 on Instagram
www.instagram.com/whole30

Whole30 Recipes on Instagram
www.instagram.com/whole30recipes

Whole30 on Twitter
www.twitter.com/whole30

Whole30 on Pinterest
www.pinterest.com/whole30

SHARING YOUR SUCCESS STORY

We love seeing readers' before-and-after photos, non-scale victories, and testimonial stories. Seriously—we live for this. There are a number of ways you can share your Whole30 story with us, and we promise if you send it to us privately, we'll secure your express permission before sharing any piece of it. (And if you want us to keep it just between us, that's okay, too! We want to hear about your experience either way.)

Via email

headquarters@whole30.com

Send us your Whole30 story (as short or as long as you'd like), along with your name, city/state, and any photographs you'd like us to see. We often turn these emails into features on our Whole30.com blog or our "A–Z" testimonial page, so feel free to be creative!

On Instagram

@whole30 and #whole30

We'll be sure to see your before-and-after photo, non-scale victory, or other expression of your Whole30 success.

On Facebook

Share your story and/or photos on our Whole30 Facebook wall, or tag us @whole30 in your post.

On Twitter

Tweet at @whole30 with a link to your Whole30 success story—or keep it short and sweet and brag to us in 140 characters or less!

FINDING A FUNCTIONAL MEDICINE PRACTITIONER

If you have a chronic health condition, are being treated for or take medication for a specific disease, or simply want to implement a comprehensive diet and lifestyle plan specific to your unique health history and goals, we highly recommend seeking the help of qualified functional medicine practitioner. But first, what the heck is "functional medicine?"

Functional medicine addresses the underlying causes of disease, using a systems-oriented approach and engaging both patient and practitioner in a therapeutic partnership. It is an evolution in the practice of medicine that better addresses the healthcare needs of the 21st century. By shifting the traditional disease-centered focus of medical practice to a more patient-centered approach, functional medicine addresses the whole person, not just an isolated set of symptoms.

Functional medicine practitioners spend time with their patients, listening to their histories, and looking at the interactions among genetic, environmental, and lifestyle factors that can influence long-term health and complex, chronic disease. In this way, functional medicine supports the unique expression of health and vitality for each individual.

Here are three websites designed to help you find a practitioner in your local community, and provide you with helpful tips for choosing and working with your new health care provider.

Institute for Functional Medicine
www.w30.co/whole30ifm

The American Board of Integrative Holistic Medicine
www.abihm.org/search-doctors

Integrative Medicine for Mental Health
www.integrativemedicineformentalhealth.com/registry.php

WHOLE30 KIDS

Here are a few websites to help you plan, prepare, and cook during your kids' Whole30 journey.

Whole30 Kids
www.w30.co/whole30kids

Nom Nom Paleo
www.nomnompaleo.com

Everyday Paleo
www.everydaypaleo.com

The Paleo Mom
www.thepaleomom.com

acknowledgments

Our list is so long, it requires its own book. We are so incredibly blessed, and owe our ability to change so many lives to the love, support, and encouragement of so many people.

First, our abundant thanks to Justin Schwartz, our fearless editor, for sharing your invaluable experience and relentless pursuit of perfection with us and this project. Please edit everything we ever do from now through forever, thanks.

To Bruce Nichols, Natalie Chapman, Cynthia Brzostowski, Rebecca Liss, Allison Renzulli, Brad Thomas Parsons, Jessica Gilo, Marina Padakis, and the entire Houghton Mifflin Harcourt team (including Brianne Halverson), we simply say thank you. Thank you for believing in us and in our mission; for supporting the program exactly as it was designed; for your tireless dedication, incredible talent, and abundant good cheer. We are happy and proud and grateful to be a part of the HMH family.

We are also grateful to Liz Gough at Yellow Kite/Hodder and Andrea Magyar at Penguin Canada. Thank you for your support for this book and our message. Your faith in us means so much; because of your hard work and dedication, we can transform even more lives.

To Christy Fletcher, Lisa Grubka, Grainne Fox, Melissa Chinchillo, Rachel Crawford, Hillary Black, and the Fletcher and Company team, this book is yours as much as it is ours. You've been our advocates, our cheerleaders, our mentors, and our friends, and we are so grateful that we're not even going to try to get fancy about it. Thank you. For everything. Partnering with you was the best decision we could have made.

To Alexandra Grablewski, Suzanne Lenzer, and Nidia Cueva, our incredibly talented, passionate, and meticulous photography, food, and prop-stylist team, you brought the joy, the flavor, and the beauty of *The Whole30* recipes to life, and we are fully in love with every single tasty photograph in this book.

We are grateful on a daily basis for our family and friends. You believed in us when we quit our 9–5 jobs to pursue our passion, and prayed for us until we once again had health insurance. To our parents, sisters, and brother, thank you for your unending support, encouragement, and advice. For the one holdout in our family (you know who you are), it's really time for you to do a Whole30. And from Melissa to Mel Joulwan, Stephanie Gaudreau, Michelle Tam, and Julie Mayfield: our little email group has saved my life and my sanity more than once. I love you all, bless your hearts.

We are fortunate to have some ridiculously smart friends and colleagues, and so thankful that they were willing to lend their brains, their names, and their passion for changing lives to this project. To Jamie Scott and Dr. Anastasia Boulais, thank you for your science, your snark, and your constant willingness to play devil's advocate. You are our partners in every sense of the word, and we are grateful. To Dr. Emily Deans, thank you for always taking the time to answer a question, read a paragraph, and contribute your own perfect perspective. You are a good friend and the smartest woman we know. To Dr. Luc Readinger, thank you for being our biggest Whole30 supporter in the mainstream medical community. We (and your patients) are blessed to know you, and we are happy to call you a friend. To Stephanie Greunke, RD, you are the perfect combination of sunshine, smarts, and common sense. Thank you for your contributions, which extend far beyond this book.

And to our incredibly talented and fiercely loyal Whole30 team: Robin Strathdee, our Whole30 O.G., journalist extraordinaire, and our social media mistress—you are why our community thrives. Thank you for putting so much of yourself into this book. To Tom Denham, our Whole30 editor, expert, and Eeyore. You *are* the Whole30. Thank you, thank you, thank you. To Erin Handley, you worked hard on this book, and we thank you. To Crystal Ellefsen and Kristen Crandall, your help, feedback, and support has been invaluable. We are so grateful to have you on the team.

To those pioneers who paved the path of paleo—Robb Wolf, Mark Sisson, Loren Cordain, and so many more, thank you for re-introducing the idea of eating real food to the masses, and laying the foundation for so many of us to spread our shared message of health, happiness, and vitality.

Finally, but most important, to our community. To you, *The Whole30* readers, program participants, and virtual friends . . . you are *everything*. You are our motivation, our support, our encouragement, our accountability. Without you, there would be no Whole30. We are eternally grateful for your presence in our life.

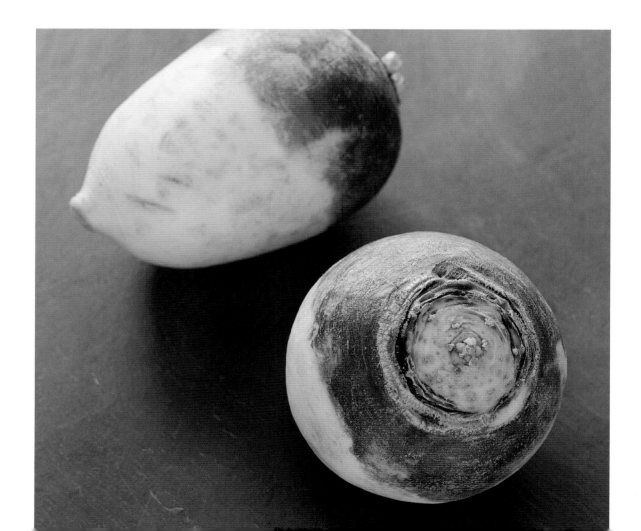

cooking conversions

Metric weights listed here have been slightly rounded to make measuring easier.

Weight

U.S.	METRIC
¼ oz	7 grams
½ oz	15 g
¾ oz	20 g
1 oz	30 g
8 oz (½ lb)	225 g
12 oz (¾ lb)	340 g
16 oz (1 lb)	455 g
2 lb	900 g
2¼ lb	1 kg

Volume

U.S.	METRIC	IMPERIAL
¼ tsp	1.2 ml	
½ tsp	2.5 ml	
1 tsp	5 ml	
½ Tbsp (1½ tsp)	7.5 ml	
1 Tbsp (3 tsp)	15 ml	
¼ cup (4 Tbsp)	60 ml	2 fl oz
⅓ cup (5 Tbsp)	75 ml	2.5 fl oz
½ cup (8 Tbsp)	125 ml	4 fl oz
⅔ cup (10 Tbsp)	150 ml	5 fl oz
¾ cup (12 Tbsp)	175 ml	6 fl oz
1 cup (16 Tbsp)	250 ml	8 fl oz
1¼ cup	300 ml	10 fl oz (½ pint)
1½ cup	350 ml	12 fl oz
2 cups (1 pint)	500 ml	16 fl oz
2½ cups	625 ml	20 fl oz (1 pint)
1 quart	1 liter	32 fl oz

Oven

FAHRENHEIT (DEGREES F)	CELSIUS (DEGREES C)	GAS NUMBER	OVEN TERMS
225	110	¼	Very Cool
250	130	½	Very Slow
275	140	1	Very Slow
300	150	2	Slow
325	165	3	Slow
350	177	4	Moderate
375	190	5	Moderate
400	200	6	Moderately Hot
425	220	7	Hot
450	230	8	Hot
475	245	9	Hot
500	260	10	Extremely Hot
550	290	10	Broiling

index

D

Dairy, 11, 14, 18
    for kids, 117
    for pescetarians/vegetarians, 121, 122
    reintroducing, 48
Dark chocolate, 62
Date night meal, 362–363
Dates, 63
Diabetes, 104
Diarrhea, 36, 125
Dice, 146–148
Digestive enzymes, 122
Digestive function, 125, 129–130
Digestive system, 5, 6, 9, 136
Dining out, 89–92
Dips, 302–303. *See also Recipe Index*
Dreaming, 37–38
Dressings, 302–303. *See also Recipe Index*
Dried fruits, 82
Drinks/beverages, 390. *See also Alcohol; Recipe Index*
    answers to questions about, 70–73
    shopping list for, 193

E

Eating disorders, 107–108
E-cigarettes, 77
Egg-free mayo, 180
Eggs, 200–201. *See also Recipe Index*
    conventionally-raised, 62
    and immune activity, 102
    number of, 82
    shopping list for, 192
Elimination diets, 56
Emergency bars, 195
Emergency dinners, 28
Emergency meal plan, 191
Entertaining, foods for. *See Fancypants meals*
Equipment, essential, 140–143
Exercise, number of meals and, 80
Exhaustion, 126

F

Facebook groups, 55
Family lamb dinner, 374–375
Family support, 23–25
Fancypants meals, 354. *See also Recipe Index*
    backyard barbeque, 356–357
    date night, 362–363
    family lamb dinner, 374–375
    holiday dinner, 380–384
    tapas party, 368–369
FAQs. *See* Frequently asked questions
Fast Track Reintroduction, 46–49
Fat(s)
    amount of, 82–83
    animal, 62
    for cooking, 190
    heating, 188
    lack of, 126
    in meal template, 194
    program-compliant, 13
    shopping list for, 193
    for vegans, 123
    when traveling, 94, 195
Fat adaptation, 35–36, 125
Fenugreek, 116
Fermented cod liver oil, 112–113
Fish, 236–237. *See also Recipe Index*
Flavored coffee, 71
Flavors, natural, 65
Flax seeds, 63
FODMAPs, 36, 129–130, 260–261
Food allergies, 90, 124, 134
Food aversions, during pregnancy, 111–112
Food fatigue, 39
Food groups, order for reintroducing, 132
Food processor, 143
Foods. *See also Recipe Index*
    amounts of, 81–83
    answers to questions about, 60–69
    clearing your house of, 23
    dressings, dips, and sauces, 302–303

eggs, 200–201
    evaluating effects of (*See* Reintroduction)
    fancypants meals, 354
    off-limit (*See* Off-limit foods)
    one pot meals, 332–333
    pork, 248
    poultry, 224–225
    red meat, 212
    relationship with, 4
    seafood, 236–237
    side dishes, 260–261
    unhealthy, 9–12
Food sensitivities, 135
French fries, 63
Frequently asked questions (FAQs), 54–137
    about amounts of foods, 81–83
    about breastfeeding, 114–116
    about dining out, 89–92
    about drinks, 70–73
    about foods, 60–69
    about grocery shopping, 84–88
    about hunger, 81
    about kids, 117–119
    about meals and snacks, 78–81
    about medical conditions, 100–108
    about off-limit foods, 95–98
    about pregnancy, 109–114
    about Reintroduction, 132–137
    about supplements, 74–77
    about the Whole30 program, 56–59
    about tracking calories/macronutrients, 99
    about travel, 93–94
    about troubleshooting Whole30, 124–132
    about vegetarians/vegans, 120–123
    about weighing yourself, 98–99
Frozen vegetables, 87, 260
Fruit(s), 260–261
    amount of, 81, 82
    canned, 61
    dried, 82

grilled, 163, 165
program-compliant, 13
seasonal, 87
shopping list for, 192–193
when traveling, 195
Fruit juice, 14, 71, 93
Fun, 191

G

Galactagogues, 116
Gallbladder, 105–106
Garlic press, 144
Ghee, 14, 183
Gluten-containing grains, 132
in alcohols, 133
reintroducing, 48, 51
Good Food Standards, 4, 5, 9, 396
Grain-like seeds, 10
Grains, 14, 18
reintroducing, 48
for vegans, 123
whole, 10
Green beans, 15, 63
Greunke, Stephanie, 109
Grill basket, 145
Grilled vegetables and fruit, 163, 165
Grilling, 356
Grocery shopping
for 7-day meal plan, 26
answers to questions about, 84–88
for omnivores, 192–193
Guar gum, 63
Guide to Nutritional Off-Roading, 397
Gum, 63

H

Habits, 19, 23, 27, 85
Hangover, 34
Hardest days, 36–37
Heating pans, 188
Hemp seeds, 64
Herbs, 86, 88, 193

High-histamine foods, 129, 130
Histamines, 129, 130
Holiday dinner, 380–384
Holidays, 59
Hot sauce, 64
House, preparing, 22–26
Hummus, 64
Hunger, 81
Hydration, 115, 129
Hyperbolic discounting, 22

I

IBD (inflammatory bowel disease), 103–105
IBS (irritable bowel syndrome), 103–105
Ice cream, Paleo, 66
If/then plans, 27–28
Immune system, 6–8, 101. *See also* Autoimmune conditions
antibodies of, 126
and food allergies/sensitivities, 136
Inflammation, 6–7, 9, 101
anti-inflammatory medications, 102
and eggs, 201
and exhaustion, 126
and legumes, 11
and unhealthy foods, 10, 11
during Whole30 program, 126
Inflammatory bowel disease (IBD), 103–105
Irritable bowel syndrome (IBS), 103–105

J

Joulwan, Melissa, 34
Julienne, 147, 148
Julienne peeler, 144
Junk food benders, 98
Junk foods, 14, 37–38

K

Ketchup, 64
Kids
answers to questions about, 117–119
meals and snacks for, 80
Kill All the Things, 34–35
Kitchen equipment and tools, 139–145
essential, 140–143
nice-to-have, 144–145
Knife cuts, 146–148
Knives, 142–143
Kombucha, 71

L

Labels, reading, 15, 190–191
Lamb dinner, family, 374–375
Larabars, 64
Leaky gut, 5, 6, 10, 102
Legumes, 10–11, 14, 18
evaluating effects of, 134
reintroducing, 47–48
Lentils, 10–11
Liver pills, 113
Lunches, 197

M

Macronutrients
and breast milk supply, 115
tracking, 99
Magnesium, 74
Marijuana, 77
Marinating, 212, 225
Mayonnaise, 64, 179
egg-free, 180
variations, 309
McClure, Michaela, 109
Meal plans, 25–26
emergency, 191
7-day, 26, 196–199
Meals, 194
answers to questions about, 78–81

recipe index

Note: Page numbers in *italic* indicate illustrations.

A

Acorn Squash Casserole, Sausage, Apple, and, *381*, 387
Aioli, Garlic, 309
Almonds, Sautéed Kale with, 298, *299*
Anchovies, Short Rib-Stuffed Peppers, Sun-Dried Tomatoes, Portobella Mushrooms, and, *369*, *370*, *372*, *373*
Apple Casserole, Sausage, Acorn Squash, and, *381*, 387
Apple Cider Vinaigrette, Cabbage, Kale, and Bell Pepper Slaw with, *364*, 366
Applesauce, Spiced, Pork Chops with, 258, *259*
Asian Vinaigrette, *329*, 330
Asparagus, Grilled, with Lemon Zest, 284, *285*
Avocado
    Grilled Steak with Garlic-Shallot Puree and, 216, 217, *217*
    Guacamole, *305*, 308
    Mayonnaise, 310, *311*
    Salad, Roasted Beet, Orange, and, 290, 291, *291*

B

Baby Back Ribs with Tangy BBQ Sauce, 256, *257*
Bacon, Perfect, 162, 163, *163*
Baked Coconut-Curry Chicken, 231
Balsamic Glaze, Grilled Vegetables with, *358*, 361
Balsamic Roasted Sweet Potatoes and Brussels Sprouts, 262, 263, *263*
Balsamic Vinaigrette, 328
Banger Sausage Patties with Sweet Potato Mash and Caramelized Onions, 249–250, *251*
Basic Mayonnaise, *179*, 179–180
Basic Vinaigrette, 184, *185–186*
BBQ Sauce, Tangy, *321*, 322
    Baby Back Ribs with, 256, *257*
Beef. *See also* Steak
    Bone Broth, *177*, 178
    Brisket, Braised, 214, *215*
    Kabobs, Chimichurri, 218, *219*
    Pot Roast, 348, *349*
    Short Ribs, Braised, 371
Beet(s)
    Roasted, Salad, Orange, Avocado, and, 290, 291, *291*
    Roasted, with Grapefruit-Thyme Vinaigrette, *376*, 378, *379*
Bell Pepper Slaw, Cabbage, Kale, and, with Apple Cider Vinaigrette, *364*, 366
Berry Rosemary Smash, 391, *393*
Blood Orange Paloma, 392, *393*
Blueberry-Ginger Sauce, Seared Scallops with, *364*, 365
Boiled Eggs, Perfect, 149, *151*
Bone Broth
    Beef, *177*, 178
    Chicken, 177, *177*
Bone-in Leg of Lamb, *375*, *376*, 377
Braised Beef
    Brisket, 214, *215*
    Short Ribs, 371
Broccoli
    -Cauliflower Mash, *375*, *376*, 377–378
    Mushrooms, Yellow Squash, and, with Red Pepper Sauce, 264, *265*

Broth
    Bone, Beef, *177*, 178
    Bone, Chicken, 177, *177*
    Vegetable, 178
Brussels Sprout(s)
    Balsamic Roasted Sweet Potatoes and, 262, 263, *263*
    Chips, 263
    Oven-Roasted Squash and, 286
Buffalo Sauce, 304, *305*
Buffalo Wings, 304
Buns
    Eggplant, 173, *175*
    Portabella Mushroom, 174, *175*
    Sweet Potato, 174, *175*
Burger, Perfect, 153, *155*
Butter
    Clarified, *182*, 183
    Compound, 181, *181*
Butternut Squash
    with Kale and Swiss Chard, 268, 269, *269*
    Puree, *381*, 386, *386*
    Roasted Pork Shoulder with Kale, Tomatoes, and, 344, *345*
    Soup, 266, *267*

C

Cabbage, Kale, and Bell Pepper Slaw with Apple Cider Vinaigrette, *364*, 366
Caramelized Onions, Banger Sausage Patties with Sweet Potato Mash and, 249–250, *251*
Carnitas, Pulled Pork, 254, *255*
Casserole, Sausage, Apple, and Acorn Squash, *381*, 387
Cauliflower
    -Broccoli Mash, *375*, *376*, 377–378
    Coconut Rice, *363*, 366–367
    Mash, 270, *271*

about the authors

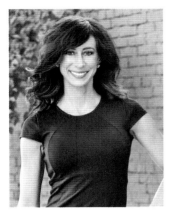

MELISSA HARTWIG, CISSN

Melissa Hartwig is a Certified Sports Nutritionist who specializes in helping people change their relationship with food and create lifelong, healthy habits. She co-created the Whole30 program in 2009, co-authored the *New York Times* best-selling book *It Starts With Food* in 2012, and has been featured in the *Wall Street Journal, Details, Redbook,* and *Woman's World.* Melissa has presented more than 150 health and nutrition seminars worldwide, and provides support to more than 1.5 million people a month through the Whole30 (whole30.com) and Whole9 (whole9life.com) websites. She lives in Salt Lake City, UT.

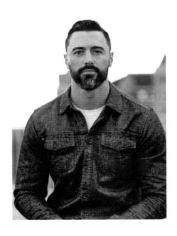

DALLAS HARTWIG, MS, PT, CISSN

Dallas is a functional medicine practitioner, Certified Sports Nutritionist, and licensed physical therapist who specializes in treating lifestyle-related hormonal, digestive, and metabolic health issues. In 2009, he co-created the original Whole30 program. In 2012, he co-authored the *New York Times* bestselling book *It Starts With Food*, and founded his functional medicine practice, mentoring under Dr. Daniel Kalish and enrolling in the Institute for Functional Medicine's certification program. Dallas has presented more than 150 health and nutrition seminars worldwide, and provides support and lifestyle recommendations to more than 1.5 million people a month through the Whole30 and Whole9 websites. He lives in Salt Lake City, UT.

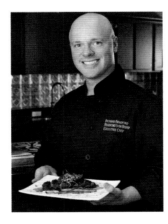

CHEF RICHARD BRADFORD

Chef Richard Bradford began his culinary career in Atlanta restaurants before studying at the prestigious Culinary Institute of America in Hyde Park, NY. Upon graduation in 2004, he returned to Atlanta to launch RSB Catering. After seven successful years, he sold the catering business and formed RSB Foods to develop Pre-Made Paleo, a nationally distributed line of gourmet prepared meals following the Whole30 program. He is now based in Dallas, TX.

CHANGE YOUR LIFE WITH
THE BEST-SELLING BOOKS FROM

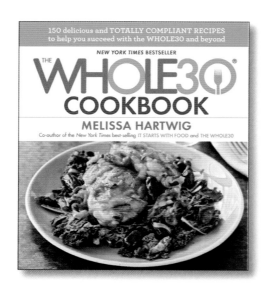

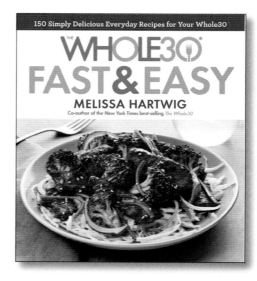

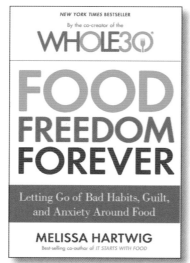

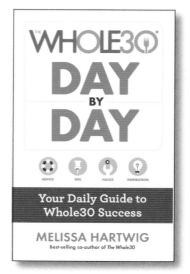

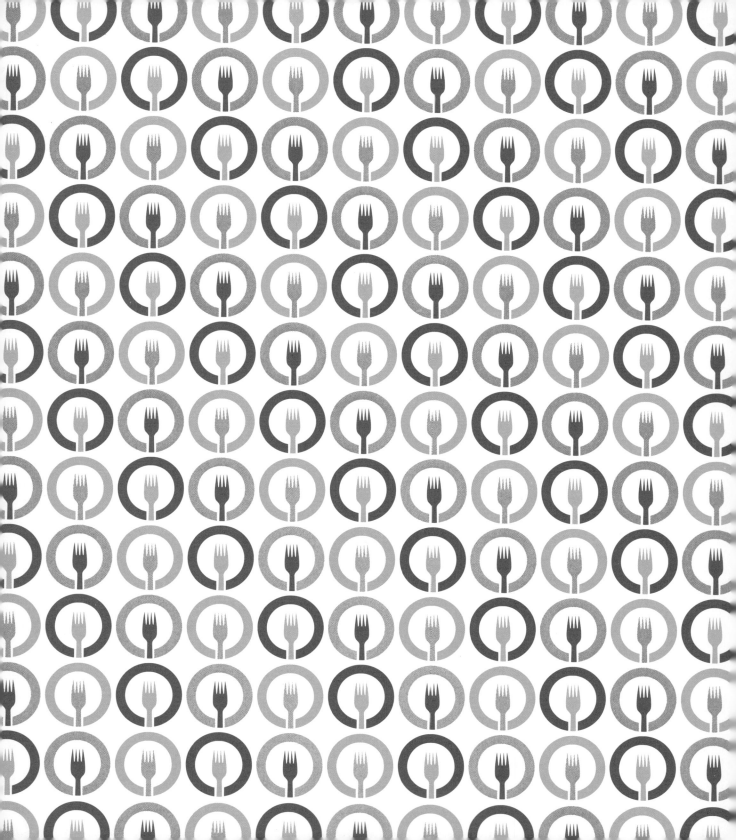